Walter J. Veith · Diet and Health

DIET AND HEALTH

SCIENTIFIC PERSPECTIVES

Walter J. Veith

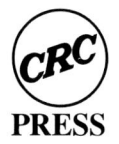

CRC PRESS

Boca Raton · Boston · London · New York · Washington D.C.

medpharm
Scientific Publishers Stuttgart 1998

Prof. Walter J. Veith
7 Hillary Close
Somerset West
7130
South Africa

Die Deutsche Bibliothek – CIP-Einheitsaufnahme

Veith, Walter:
Diet and health : scientific perspectives / Walter J. Veith. – 2nd ed. –
Stuttgart : Medpharm, 1998
  ISBN 3-88763-068-8

Library of Congress Cataloging-in-Publication Data

Catalog information is available from the Library of Congress.

This book contains information obtained from authentic and highly regarded sources. Reprinted material is quoted with permission, and sources are indicated. A wide variety of references are listed. Reasonable efforts have been made to publish reliable data and information, but the author and the publisher cannot assume responsibility for the validity of all materials or for the consequences of their use. Neither the book nor any part may be reproduced or transmitted in any form or by any means, electronic or mechanical, including photocopying, microfilming, and recording, or by any information storage or retrieval system, without prior permission in writing from the publisher.
The consent of CRC Press LLC does not extend to copying for general distribution, for promotion, for creating new works, or for resale. Specific permission must be obtained in writing from CRC Press LLC for such copying.
Direct all inquiries to CRC Press LLC, 2000 Corporate Blvd., N. W., Boca Raton, Florida 33431.

Trademark Notice: Product of corporate names may be trademarks or registered trademarks, and are used only for identification and explanation, without intent to infringe.

Sole distribution rights for North America granted to CRC Press LLC Boca Raton, Florida, USA

ISBN 3-88763-068-8 medpharm Scientific Publishers, Stuttgart
ISBN 0-8493-0289-7 CRC Press LLC, Boca Raton, Florida

The first edition of this book was published by
Southern Publishing Association, South Africa

All rights reserved. No part of this publication may be translated, reproduced, stored in a retrieval system, or transmitted, in any form or by any means, electronic, mechanical, photocopying, microfilming, recording or otherwise, without permission in writing from the publisher.

© 1998 Medpharm Scientific Publishers
Birkenwaldstraße 44, D-70191 Stuttgart
Printed in Germany

Preface to the 2nd edition

The first edition of "Diet and Health" was published at the end of 1993, and in the short time since then, some dramatic events have taken place world-wide which underline the need for a comprehensive reassessment of this often neglected field of science. Some of the concerns expressed in the first edition, regarding the impact of the animal husbandry industry on the safety of animal products in the human diet, have been found to be more than warranted. The BSE debacle, which rocked Britain and threatens the whole of Europe is but one example of the magnitude of the problem. A further example is the global increase in food poisonings, attributed to antibiotic-resistant bacteria, some of which have been heralded as national disasters in the countries where they have left their mark.

On the positive side, there seems to be an awakening among the scientific fraternity and also the community at large, in terms of alternative life-styles and their possible effects on health. Health industries with their emphasis on whole food nutrition and physical fitness have done much to raise public awareness in the field, but a sound scientific footing is needed to give credibility to these ventures, particularly since their approaches are often so conflicting. With our present state of knowledge, it is already possible to put together a substantive guideline to healthful living. Information is pouring in as is evidenced by the numerous international scientific conferences dealing with this issue. The relationship between diet and degenerative diseases such as cancer, cardiovascular disease and osteoporosis is well established, it is known what the contributing factors are, but the best alternative lifestyle is still an issue of debate. This book is an attempt at correlating the scientific data regarding the causative agents in dietary related diseases, and also to provide an insight into the field of alternative lifestyles.

I wish to thank all who contributed to this venture by providing information and advice. Special thanks go to the University of the Western Cape, my colleague Quinton Johnson for his scientific contributions and moral support, Ronald Ullmann for his editorial contributions particularly in terms of the scientific formulae used, and to my wife for her constant support and encouragement and for all the help with the recipes. I am also deeply indebted to Dr. Winfried Küsel for not only translating the manuscript into German, but also for his numerous contributions in terms of the content and layout of the book.

Introduction

The science of nutrition has only really blossomed in the last decade and there is still much to be learnt. Even so, it is becoming more and more apparent that dietary practices impact directly on health, and many diseases can be traced directly to the dinner table. In this regard it is noteworthy that degenerative diseases are particularly common in affluent societies where the consumption of refined foods and animal products is high. Eating habits have also changed drastically in these modern times and highly processed convenience foods have become an established part of the everyday diet of the majority of people living in industrialized countries. Sadly, this trend is very difficult to reverse and it will require a concerted effort to coax society back to more healthful eating practices. This book is one such attempt to provide the information necessary to encourage a change of lifestyle, and to provide an alternative dietary lifestyle, which will not only be healthier, but will also satisfy the taste buds.

Healthy eating practices are no guarantee of good health, but they can certainly sway the odds in one's favour. The foundations for disease are laid early on in life and are only manifested at a later stage, thus affecting the quality of life. It is a sad reflection on our age, that in most Western societies the senior citizens do not enjoy good health, and in the United States only 16% of persons 65 and over reported excellent health.[1] A balanced outlook on life is what is needed and in this regard it is important to note that healthy dietary practices are not the only factors that affect one's well-being. Lack of exercise, stress, insufficient leisure time and emotional trauma can do as much damage as detrimental eating practices, and due consideration must be given to these factors when planning a healthy lifestyle.

Adopting a healthy lifestyle should be an enjoyable experience for all and should not become a prison for extreme views on the subject of health. Anything that is carried to excess will eventually become a burden rather than a pleasure and the whole object will be defeated. The alternative lifestyle suggested in this book should be interpreted in this light and should be seen as an ideal, something to strive for and grow into.

1. Albrink, M.J. 1991. Age-related dietary guidance and cardiovascular risk assessment. *Nutrition Today*. July/August pp. 12–17.

Table of contents

Preface to the 2nd edition
Introduction

Part I – Diet and Health

Chapter 1 – Proteins 17

        Essential amino acids... 18
        Non-essential amino acids 18
        Protein digestion 18
        Plant and animal proteins 20
        How much protein? 21
        Amino acid requirements 23
        References... 26

Chapter 2 – Carbohydrates and fibre 29

        Carbohydrates in food....................................... 31
        Digestion of carbohydrates 31
        Diet and control of glucose levels 34
        Symptoms of hypoglycaemia 34
        NSP (fibre) and digestion resistant starch 37
        Water-insoluble fibres 38
        Water-soluble fibres and resistant starch 39
        References... 40

Chapter 3 – Fats 43

        Fats in the diet.. 44
        Triglycerides.. 44
        Saturated and unsaturated fatty acids.......................... 44
        Essential fatty acids 45
        Cholesterol 46
        Digestion and absorption of fats 47
        Fats and disease 49
        Fats and cancer... 50

Cardiovascular disease	52
Dietary lipids and immune function	53
Processed fats	55
Modern oil refining techniques	55
Margarine	57
The use of oil in the frying of food	58
References	59

Chapter 4 – Animal products — 63

Meat	66
Ammonia	67
Phenols	68
Polycyclic aromatic hydrocarbons (PAH)	69
Heterocyclic amines	69
N-Nitroso compounds	70
Biological magnification	70
Dairy products	72
Lactose intolerance	72
Milk protein intolerance	73
Calcium in dairy products	74
Dairy products and the immune system	76
Dairy products and infertility	78
Animal products and foodborne illness	81
Salmonella infections	82
Campylobacter infections	83
Listeria infections	83
Escherichia coli infections	83
Yersinia infections	83
Other organisms	84
Modern animal husbandry	84
Antibiotics	84
Additional growth promoters	88
Prion diseases	89
Mycotoxins	91
Genetic engineering	92
References	92

Chapter 5 – The vegan-vegetarian lifestyle — 97

Vegan dietary practices	98
Vegetarian dietary patterns for adults	98
Dietary patterns for pregnant and lactating mothers	100
Dietary patterns for infants and young children	100
Adolescents and young adults	104
Energy requirements	104
Health aspects of the vegetarian diet	105
Vegetarianism and obesity	106

The dangers of undernutrition.................................. 108
Diabetes mellitus.. 109
Cardiovascular disease... 110
Osteoporosis.. 111
Rheumatoid arthritis.. 113
References.. 113

Chapter 6 – Additional dietary components and hazards 117

Vitamins and minerals in vegan diets....................... 117
Vitamin A... 118
Vitamin B-6... 118
Vitamin B-12.. 119
Vitamin D... 120
Iron.. 120
Calcium... 121
Zinc.. 122
Food additives.. 122
Artificial and natural colourants............................... 125
Antioxidants.. 126
Emulsifiers and stabilizers..................................... 127
Solvents.. 127
Preservatives... 128
Flavour enhancers... 128
Sweeteners.. 129
Caffeine and alcohol.. 130
Caffeine.. 131
Alcohol and diet.. 133
References.. 134

Part II – An alternative lifestyle

Chapter 7 – The whole-food alternative 139

What is whole food?... 140
General guidelines to healthful living.......................... 141
Ensuring proper food combinations........................... 142
Combining acid- and alkaline-forming foods...................... 142
Combining fruits and vegetables................................. 146
Combining grains and legumes.................................... 147
Grains.. 149
Barley (*Hordeum vulgare* or *H. sativum*)...................... 150
Corn (maize, mealie) (*Zea mays*)............................... 151
Millet (*Panicum miliaceum*).................................... 151
Oats (*Avena sativa*)... 152
Rice (*Oryza sativa*)... 153
Rye (*Secale cereale*).. 154

Sorghum (*Sorghum vulgare*)	154
Wheat *(Triticum)*	155
Bread	156
The art of bread baking	157
Mechanical preparation	158
Other ingredients	158
Legumes	159
Carob (*Ceratonia siliqua*)	163
Chick peas (Garbanzo) (*Cicer arietinum*)	163
Kidney beans (*Phaseolus vulgaris*)	163
Lentils (*Lens esculenta*)	164
Lima and Sieva beans (*Phaseolus lunatus*)	164
Mung beans (*Vignia aureus*)	165
Soya beans (*Glycine max*)	165
Soy milk	167
Nuts and oilseeds	169
Almonds (*Prunus amygdalus* var. *dulcis*)	170
Brazil nuts (*Bertholletia excelsa*)	170
Cashew nuts (*Anacardium occidentale*)	172
Chestnuts (*Castanea sativa*)	173
Coconut (*Cocos nucifera*)	173
Hazel nuts (*Corylus avellana*)	173
Macadamia nuts (*Macadamia ternifolia*)	173
Pecan nuts (*Carya illinoensis*)	173
Pistachio nuts (*Pistacia vera*)	174
Walnuts (*Juglans regia*)	174
Seeds	174
Pumpkin seeds	174
Sesame seeds (*Sesanum indicum*)	175
Sunflower seeds (*Helianthus annuus*)	175
Fruits and vegetables	176
Fruits	176
Stone fruits	181
Apricots (*Prunus armeniaca*)	181
Cherries (*Prunus avium*)	182
Peaches and nectarines (*Prunus persica*)	182
Plums and prunes	182
Pip fruits	182
Apples (*Malus domestica*)	182
Pears (*Pyrus communis*)	183
Grapes	183
Quinces (*Cydonia oblonga*)	183
Berry fruit	183
Citrus fruits	184
Oranges (*Citrus sinensis*)	184
Lemons (*Citrus limon*)	184
Mandarins and Tangerines	184

Subtropical and tropical fruits	184
Avocado (*Persia americana*)	184
Bananas (*Musa*)	185
Dates (*Phoenix dactylifera*)	186
Figs (*Ficus carica*)	186
Guava (*Psidium guajava*)	186
Kiwifruit (*Actinidia deliciosa*)	186
Litchi (*Litchi*)	186
Loquats (*Eriobotrya japonica*)	187
Mangoes (*Mangifera indica*)	187
Melons and watermelons	187
Olives (*Olea europaea*)	187
Papayas (*Carica papaya*)	188
Passionfruit or granadilla (*Passiflora*)	188
Persimmons (*Diospyros khaki*)	188
Pineapples (*Ananas comosus*)	188
Pomegranates (*Punica granatum*)	188
Prickly pears (*Opuntia*)	189
Vegetables	189
Types of vegetables	190
Chenopodiaceae (Goosefoot family)	190
Beetroot and Swiss chard (*Beta vulgaris*)	190
Spinach (*Spinacia oleracea*)	193
Compositae (Sunflower family)	193
Chicory (*Cichorium intybus*)	193
Lettuce (*Lactuca sativa*)	193
Convolvulaceae (Morning glory family)	193
Sweet potato (*Ipomoea batatas*)	193
Cucurbitaceae (Gourd family)	194
Pumpkins and squashes (*Cucurbita*)	194
Cucumber (*Cucumis sativa*)	194
Cruciferae (Brassicaceae) (Mustard family)	194
Broccoli (*Brassica oleracea*)	195
Brussels sprouts (*Brassica oleracea*)	195
Cabbage (*Brassica oleracea*)	195
Cauliflower (*Brassica oleracea*)	195
Kale and collard (*Brassica oleracea*)	195
Kohlrabi (*Brassica oleracea*)	195
Turnip (*Brassica rapa*)	196
Radish (*Raphanus sativus*)	196
Cress (*Lepidium sativum*)	196
Leguminosae (Fabaceae) (Pea or Pulse family)	196
French beans (*Phaseolus vulgaris*)	196
Peas (*Pisum sativum*)	196
Liliaceae (Lily family)	197
Chive (*Allium schoenoprasum*)	197
Garlic (*Allium sativum*)	197
Leeks (*Allium ampeloprasum*)	197

Onions (*Allium cepa*)	197
Asparagus (*Asparagus officinalis*)	198
Malvaceae (Mallow family)	198
Okra (*Abelmoschus esculentus*)	198
Solanaceae (Nightshade family)	198
Capsicum (*Capsicum annuum*)	198
Egg plant (*Solanum melongena*)	199
Potato (*Solanum tuberosum*)	199
Tomatoes (*Lycopersicon esculentum*)	200
Umbelliferae (Apiaceae) (Parsley or carrot family)	200
Angelica (*Angelica archangelica*)	200
Aniseed (*Pimpinella anisum*)	200
Caraway (*Carum carvi*)	200
Carrots (*Daucus carota*)	200
Celery (*Apium graveolens*)	201
Chervil (*Anthriscus cerefolium*)	201
Coriander (*Coriandrum sativum*)	201
Cumin (*Cuminum cyminum*)	201
Dill (*Anethum graveolens*)	201
Fennel (*Foeniculum vulgare*)	201
Lovage (*Levisticum officinale*)	201
Parsley (*Petroselinum crispum*)	201
Parsnip (*Pastinaca sativa*)	201
References	201

Part III – Applying the concept

Chapter 8 – Guidelines and recipes 207

Introduction
Useful equipment	207
Basic shopping list	208
List of abbreviations	208
Basic recipes	211

Part 1

Diet and Health

Chapter 1
Proteins

Proteins are the most varied of all the molecules found in living organisms and play a part in virtually every aspect of that awe-inspiring phenomenon known as **life**. In fact the very processes of life are to a large extent enacted on the surfaces of proteins. Some proteins have a globular structure, and many of these function as enzymes, immunoglobulins, hormones, transport proteins as well as performing structural roles in tissues and cells. The enzymatic function of proteins is what makes life possible, and it is estimated that there are some 10 000 different enzymes in the human body, though even this figure is probably a gross underestimation. The role and structure of proteins in cells and tissues is also extremely varied, and their structure is related to their function. Besides the globular proteins which play an important part in the structure and function of cells and tissues, there are also fibrous proteins which can be hard and tough such as toe and finger nails, hair, the tough hoofs of ungulates and even the feathers of birds.

The name protein is derived from Greek and means **"primary"** or **"first"**, and indeed protein plays a vital role in nutrition. However, a clear distinction must be made between dietary significance and the quantities required to meet dietary needs. Whilst protein-poor diets are associated with developmental diseases, the metabolism of dietary protein excesses leads to the formation of a number of compounds which are potentially harmful, and too much protein in the diet is thus equally detrimental to health.

Proteins consist of molecules known as **amino acids** and these contain an alkaline amino group (NH_2) and an acid carboxyl group (COOH). The rest of the amino acid varies, and is commonly called the R-group (Figure 1.1).

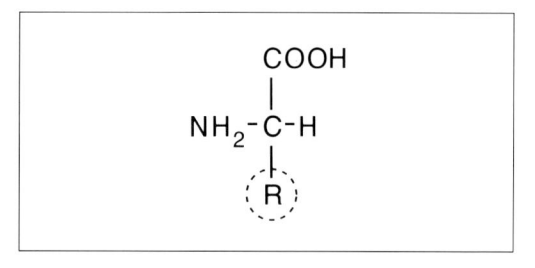

$$NH_2-\overset{\overset{\displaystyle COOH}{|}}{\underset{\underset{\displaystyle R}{|}}{C}}-H$$

Figure 1.1. The structure of a typical α-amino acid (there are 20 different R-groups in proteinaceous amino acids)

Amino acids can be strung together to form polypeptides by linking the amino group of one amino acid with the carboxyl group of another amino acid and splitting out a molecule of water (dehydration synthesis) (figure 1.2).

There are twenty common amino acids found in protein and these can be strung together in any combination, and depending on the sequence in which they are joined together, they produce the myriads of different proteins found in nature. Each organism has its own unique proteins and these are constructed from the amino acids which are either obtained from the diet, or are manufactured by the organism. Humans cannot manufacture all the different amino acids, and as

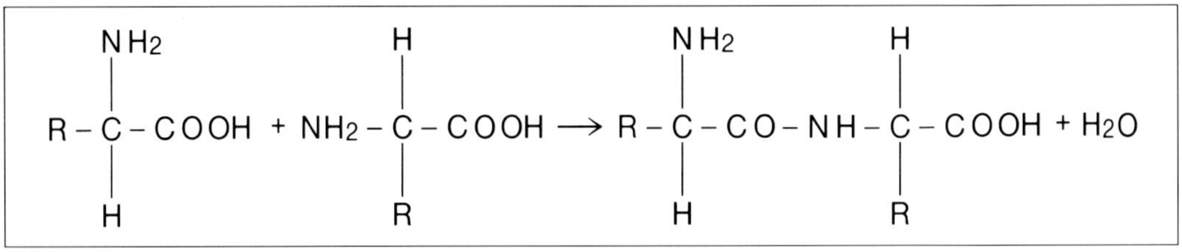

$$R-\underset{\underset{H}{|}}{\overset{\overset{NH_2}{|}}{C}}-COOH + NH_2-\underset{\underset{R}{|}}{\overset{\overset{H}{|}}{C}}-COOH \rightarrow R-\underset{\underset{H}{|}}{\overset{\overset{NH_2}{|}}{C}}-CO-NH-\underset{\underset{R}{|}}{\overset{\overset{H}{|}}{C}}-COOH + H_2O$$

Figure 1.2 Dehydration synthesis of polypeptides.

it is essential that these then be supplied in the diet, they are known as **essential amino acids**. The other amino acids are no less essential to the well-being of mankind, but because humans are able to manufacture them, it is not essential that they be obtained from the diet and they are, therefore, termed **non-essential amino acids**.

The common list of amino acids is as follows:

Essential amino acids

Isoleucine, leucine, lysine, methionine, phenylalanine, threonine, tryptophan, valine and histidine.

Histidine is not an essential amino acid for adults, but is included because infants require additional amounts of this amino acid.

Non-essential amino acids

Glycine, glutamic acid, arginine, aspartic acid, proline, alanine, serine, tyrosine, cysteine, asparagine and glutamine.

In addition to these, the amino acids hydroxyproline and citrulline are also incorporated into proteins.

The number of possible proteins that can be constructed from just these twenty amino acids is awe-inspiring. In fact, there is not enough matter in the universe to construct even one sample of each kind of polypeptide, even if the length is limited to just 60 amino acids. Indeed there are 10.240.000.000.000 different polypeptides (10^{20}) which can be constructed from the twenty amino acids if the chain is a mere ten amino acids long.[1] Human proteins, however, can contain hundreds of amino acids and some contain in excess of 1000 amino acids.

Protein digestion

The quantity and quality of proteins consumed will have a marked influence on the digestive process. Enzymes that digest proteins are divided into two groups known as **exopeptidases** and **endopeptidases**. As the names imply, the exopeptidases hydrolyse the terminal peptide bonds of the protein, and the endopeptidases, such as the enzymes **pepsin** and **trypsin**, operate on the inside of the protein by hydrolysing internal peptide bonds and cutting up the protein into smaller fragments. Pepsin is secreted by the stomach in the form of inactive **pepsinogen** which is activated by **hydrochloric acid**, which is also secreted by the stomach. Pepsinogen will only be converted to active pepsin if the pH drops to below pH 6 and protein digestion in the stomach thus takes place in an acid medium. The type of protein to be digested can influence the pH at which pepsin operates and animal proteins are usually digested at a lower pH (more acid) than plant proteins. The digestion of egg albumen, for example, requires a pH of 1,5 which is considerably lower than the pH optimum of the enzyme and much lower than the pH required for the digestion of plant proteins.

Pepsin hydrolyses proteins at peptide bonds between an aromatic amino acid (phenylalanine or tyrosine) and a dicarboxylic amino acid (glutamine or aspartic acid) and thus acts to cut up the proteins into shorter chains called **proteoses** and **peptones** (Fig. 1.3). Digestibility of a protein thus depends on the frequency and spacing of those portions of the protein where the digestive enzymes can act on the protein. As a consequence, a diet high in animal proteins will require longer periods of stomach digestion, at a lower pH, than will be required for plant proteins. The longer stomach retention time associated with a diet rich in animal products, gives a feeling of satiety, but this is not as a result of nutritional superiority. Indeed, the longer stomach retention time encourages fermentation and this, together with the higher acid levels, can contribute to sluggishness, heartburn, ulcer formation and a host of other conditions. The issue is further complicated by the high free-fat content of animal products. Fat is not digested in the stomach and the free fat thus coats the food and inhibits the water-soluble pepsin from operating optimally, thus leading to still longer stomach retention times.

A further point which needs addressing at this point, is the consumption of large quantities of liquids during a meal. Liquids should best not be consumed during a meal, as this will dilute the enzyme concentrations in the stomach and slow down the rate of protein digestion. Water should best be taken some time before or after a meal but not during a meal. All of these factors combined frequently lead to poor cleavage of the proteins and many partially cleaved molecules enter into the duodenum where the next stage in protein digestion takes place.

The enzyme **trypsin**, which is secreted by the pancreas in the inactive form **trypsinogen**, is activated in the duodenum by the enzyme **enterokinase** which is secreted by the intestinal wall. Once trypsinogen has been converted into active trypsin it too will activate trypsinogen, a process known as **auto-catalytic activation**. Unlike pepsin, trypsin requires an alkaline medium in which to operate and functions best at a pH between 7 and 9. Trypsin cleaves the proteoses and peptones in positions adjacent to the amino acids lysine

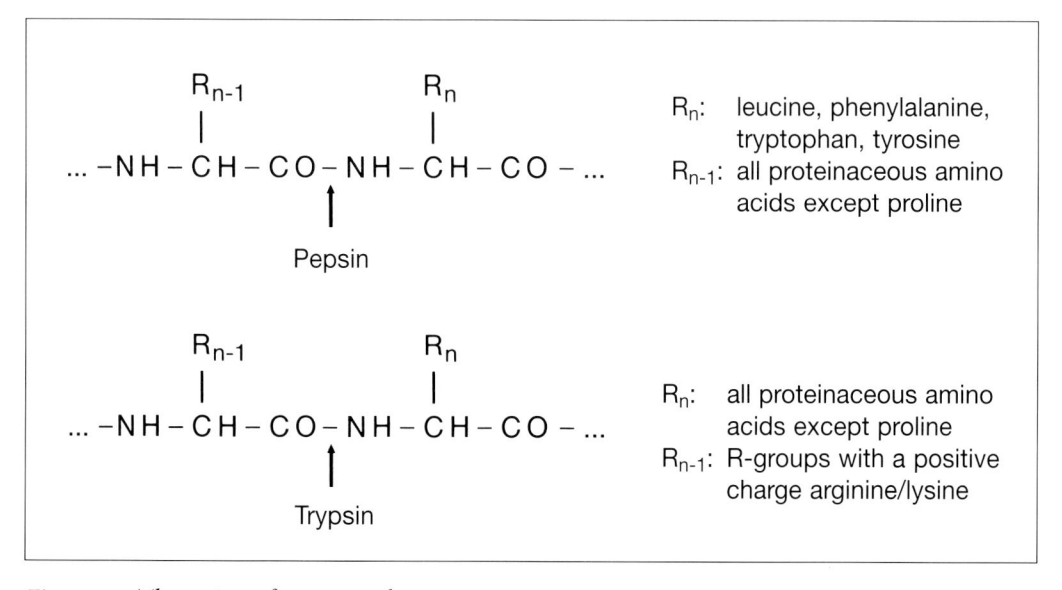

$$\ldots -NH-CH(R_{n-1})-CO-NH-CH(R_n)-CO-\ldots \quad \uparrow \text{Pepsin}$$

R_n: leucine, phenylalanine, tryptophan, tyrosine
R_{n-1}: all proteinaceous amino acids except proline

$$\ldots -NH-CH(R_{n-1})-CO-NH-CH(R_n)-CO-\ldots \quad \uparrow \text{Trypsin}$$

R_n: all proteinaceous amino acids except proline
R_{n-1}: R-groups with a positive charge arginine/lysine

Figure 1.3 The action of pepsin and trypsin on proteins.

and arginine, thus producing still smaller protein fractions. Further digestion takes place by means of exopeptidases which hydrolyse the polypeptides into **oligopeptides** which consist of residues of two or three amino acids, and finally into individual amino acids.[2,3]

Plant and animal proteins

Plants are the primary source of proteins for all heterotrophic animals, and plant proteins are thus termed **primary proteins**. When proteins are consumed, the proteins are digested, which means that they are broken down into their amino acid components, and these amino acids are then absorbed and used to construct the various proteins required by the organisms. If animal proteins are consumed as dietary protein, then the protein is obtained from a secondary source and animal proteins are thus termed **secondary proteins**. In view of human amino acid needs, proteins are also classified as complete and incomplete proteins.

A protein that contains all the essential amino acids in balanced proportions is called a **complete protein** whereas a protein that is limited in one or more essential amino acids is called an **incomplete protein**. Plant proteins are mostly incomplete proteins and animal proteins are mostly complete proteins. This has led to the general assumption that animal proteins are superior to plant proteins in terms of their nutritional value, and has led many to believe that a diet consisting solely of plants would be inferior to one which included animal products. This would certainly be true, if all plants had similar amino acid shortages, but as this is not the case, there is no sound reason for arguing that animal products supply a better protein than plants. Of course, if one were to follow a restrictive vegetarian diet, which included only a limited variety of plants, then a plant-based diet would certainly be inadequate.

A plant-based diet will supply all the essential amino acids if a variety of foods is utilized, and they will be as effective in meeting the body's needs as proteins from animal sources.[4] Plant proteins contain more branched chain amino acids than do animal proteins and they are easier to digest than animal proteins. Animal proteins, on the other hand, are rich in the sulphur-containing amino acids **cysteine** and **methionine,** and also have a greater proportion of the aromatic amino acids **phenylalanine** and **tyrosine**. Excesses of these two groups of amino acids have been associated with various degenerative diseases, in view of their degradations to **cresol** and **phenol** which are promoters of skin and colon cancer.[5]

The ratio of the various amino acids to each other may be equally as significant as the presence of essential amino acids in determining the value of a protein. Plant proteins produce higher levels of **arginine** and **glycine** in the blood than do animal proteins and the higher levels of these amino acids are associated with protection against the clogging of arteries and arteriosclerosis.[6] In our own laboratory, we have found that legumes as well as grains produce high plasma levels of arginine in all experimental animals tested thus far, which include rats, rabbits and vervet monkeys (unpublished data). The mechanism whereby high levels of arginine in particular, afford protection against degenerative diseases such as arteriosclerosis and osteoporosis is not clear at this stage, but might be related to its role in the elimination of nitrogenous waste products via the urea cycle. High protein diets will necessitate large-scale deamination of amino acids as dietary protein excesses have to be converted to carbohydrates or fats before they can be stored by the body. Deamination produces ammonia, which is toxic to the system, and high levels of arginine would aid the rapid conversion of the highly toxic ammonia to the less toxic urea, thus limiting the effects of ammonia.

Animal proteins tend to have higher proportions of essential amino acids, except for arginine, than do plant proteins. The higher values in themselves need not necessarily be regarded as a positive attribute, as some amino acids are required in higher concentrations than others. High levels of essential amino acids that are used in only small amounts, will also require the conversion of the excess, and thus lead to increased toxic loading. More important than the absolute quantity of essential and non-essential amino acids in the food we consume, is the ratio in which these amino acids occur. The more closely the ratio is attuned to our needs the fewer conversions will be required and the lower the toxic load will be. In this regard, it has been suggested that the ratio of lysine to arginine could be important in determining the ability of a protein to induce arteriosclerosis.[7,8] Early studies showed, that if animal protein is fed to rabbits, they develop arteriosclerosis and have elevated cholesterol levels even if their diet is cholesterol free. If they are fed plant proteins, such as soya, these effects are not observed. Moreover, the plant protein source was shown to decrease the degree of sclerosis even in those animals that were fed cholesterol.[7] Models of cholesterol metabolism based on experiments with rabbits have been criticised, in view of the rabbits unique hypersensitivity to dietary cholesterol, but the fact that a plant protein source could decrease sclerosis is significant.

Recent studies have shown conclusively that animal proteins increase cholesterol levels, whereas plant proteins tend to reduce the levels of cholesterol in animals and humans.[9,10] Apparently, the ratio of lysine to arginine plays a significant role in this hypocholesterolaemic effect, and the concentrations of various other amino acids are also implicated. It is therefore not surprising, that various national bodies and expert groups recommend an increase in the consumption of plant foods to improve long-term health.[11] Plant foods that are rich in proteins, also come prepacked with other macronutrients, vitamins and minerals which enhance the digestion and assimilation of these foods. The modern trend of refining plant protein sources, so as to obtain concentrated forms of protein as substitutes for animal products, thus strips them of these additional components. The use of unrefined plant protein sources, such as grains, legumes and nuts has added advantages, in that many of these foods contain phytochemicals that protect against cancer.[12]

Diets high in animal protein are normally low in carbohydrates, particularly fibre, and in typical Western diets up to 12 g of partially digested protein (approximately 2 g nitrogen) enters the colon daily in the form of protein, peptides and amino acids.[13,14] When carbohydrate levels are low the bacteria in the colon will utilize these protein residues, particularly peptides, to meet their metabolic demands and liberate ammonia, short chain fatty acids and a variety of other products including phenols and branched chain fatty acids. Urinary phenol levels increase when a high meat diet is followed and decrease when more fibre is present.[15] Phenols have been implicated as promoters of bowel cancer and ammonia increases cell proliferation and has also been linked to colon cancer.[16]

How much protein?

Estimates for daily protein requirements have undergone a considerable evolution in recent times. In the past, it was thought that a high-protein diet would impart strength and stamina, and this concept is to this day still entrenched in the minds of most people. Evidence has, however been mounting that a high-protein diet, and particularly a diet high in animal proteins, is detrimental to health. Conversely, a diet too low in proteins will lead to protein malnutrition. Low protein diets are normally associated with less affluent societies which in addition to low protein concentrations also suffer from energy deficient diets. Protein-energy malnutrition has been linked to growth abnormalities and lasting detrimental effects on mental development. Children that have experienced such malnutrition have lower IQs than their adequately nourished siblings.[17]

Hunger and malnutrition are major problems facing the world's poor. Nearly 200 million children suffer from protein-energy malnutrition and over 2 000 million experience micronutrient deficiencies.[18] In affluent societies, protein-energy malnutrition is rare, and protein-energy over-utilization which leads to obesity, cardiovascular disease, diabetes, cancer and other degenerative diseases is more prevalent. These facts have prompted many to change their lifestyles, and such changes can lead to nutrient shortages if these are not properly conducted. In this regard, minimum protein requirements become important not only to people in poorer societies, but also to those who are more affluent.

In view of the association between high protein consumption and disease, the recommended daily requirement for protein has been considerably reduced in terms of what was considered essential when the first international recommendation of 1g protein per kilogram body weight per day was made by the League of Nations in 1936. The recommended daily allowance (RDA) for protein is currently being revised, but it is generally accepted that a daily consumption of a mere 56 g for men and 44 g for women is adequate.[19] The protein requirements are, however, not the same for all age groups, and there is an age-related decline in protein needs. These age-related protein requirements were reflected in the recommended levels of protein consumption proposed by the Food and Agricultural Organization (FAO), The World Health Organization (WHO) and the United Nations University (UNU) in 1985.[20] These recommendations are presented in table 1.1 and are for an animal protein source.

Age group	male g/kg/day	female g/kg/day
3–6 months	1.85	1.85
6–9 months	1.65	1.65
9–12 months	1.50	1.50
1–2 years	1.20	1.20
2–3 years	1.15	1.15
3–5 years	1.10	1.10
5–7 years	1.00	1.00
7–10 years	1.00	1.00
10–12 years	1.00	1.00
12–14 years	1.00	0.95
14–16 years	0.94	0.90
16–18 years	0.88	0.80
Adults	0.75	0.75
During pregnancy		Add 6.0 g to total
Lactation: 0-6 months		Add 17.5 g to total
Lactation: older than 6 months		Add 13.0 g to total

Table 1.1 Safe levels of protein intake as proposed by the FAO/WHO/UNU. Values are uncorrected for the nutritional value of the protein. (Ref. 20.21)

Figures for infants are not included, but breast fed infants should have a more than adequate supply from mother's milk. There is reason to believe, that the figure of 0.75 g/kg/day of good quality protein for adults may be too low to meet the needs of adults under all circumstances. Although it is true that if people can consume enough of their traditional diets to meet their needs, then protein quantities are normally sufficient as well. However, problems can arise when illness or poverty prevents people from consuming sufficient quantities.[22] In 1994 the UNU-sponsored International Dietary Energy Consultative Group (IDECG) together with WHO and FAO representatives convened a meeting where it was concluded that the requirements for adults needed to be reassessed, but that the figures for children were probably adequate. It seems desirable at this stage to round the figure to 0.8 g/kg/day for adults, and due to the lower efficiency of protein utilization in the elderly to propose a protein intake of 1.0 g/kg/day for this group.[22]

Amino acid requirements

The quantitative need for essential amino acids also declines with age, but this need is thought to decline more rapidly than the need for total protein. Adults thus need lower concentrations of essential amino acids, per unit of protein, to maintain nutritional adequacy than do infants and young children.[21] Recent evidence, however, shows that these figures may need revision and that requirements may be somewhat higher, even for adults. In table 1.2 the amino acid requirements for children and adults are presented, and the revised estimates for adults are also included.[21]

In both infants and adults, a combination of plant protein sources will supply adequate quantities of all the essential amino acids, but variety-poor diets would be restrictive, even if a good protein source such as soy protein is used. Soy protein isolates, as sole protein source, would supply sufficient amino acids for adults but might be insufficient for children, but a restrictive diet relying solely on grains as a source of protein would be inadequate to meet the needs of even adults.[21] The combination of grains with legumes, seeds or nuts will, however, supply a high quality protein with adequate concentrations of essential amino acids to meet the needs of all age classes.

Amino acid	Children (2-5 years) mg/kg/day	Children (10-12 years) mg/kg/day	Adults (18 years and over) mg/kg/day	Adults (revised estimates) mg/kg/day
Isoleucine	31.0	28.0	10.0	23.0
Leucine	73.0	44.0	14.0	39.0
Lysine	64.0	44.0	12.0	30.0
Methionine/Cystine	27.0	22.0	13.0	15.0
Phenylalanine/Tyrosine	69.0	22.0	14.0	39.0
Threonine	37.0	28.0	7.0	15.0
Tryptophan	12.5	3.3	3.5	6.0
Valine	38.0	25.0	10.0	20.0
TOTAL	351.5	216.3	83.5	187.0

Table 1.2 Amino acid requirements for children and adults. (Ref.20,21)

The amino acid lysine seems to be one of the most important limiting amino acids, and differences between amino acid sufficiency in diets of affluent and poor societies will be greatest for lysine. Diets based largely on cereals can thus lead to shortages, and the revised estimates for lysine (30 mg/kg/day or some estimates are as high as 50 mg/kg/day) are probably closer to the actual requirements.[23,24] Comparisons between major food groups in terms of their amino acid composition per gram of protein are presented in table 1.3.

For the majority of amino acids the differences between the means are small, but levels of leucine and aromatic amino acids are low in fruits and vegetables and levels of tryptophan are high in nuts compared to the other foods. The major differences between groups are to be seen in lysine and to a lesser extent in sulphur amino acids. Lysine concentrations in cereals are only 30.5 mg/g protein compared to 84.3 mg/g protein in animal products and 67.0 mg/g protein in legumes. Vegan vegetarians with a varied diet containing grains, legumes and nuts or seeds as protein source will have no problem in meeting daily needs of essential amino acids, but restricted diets based largely on grains can be insufficient, particularly if daily intakes are low as in poorer societies.

Most people in industrialized countries consume far in excess of the recommended daily allowance for proteins, and in the United States, most adults consume 105 g to 120 g of protein per day,[25] most of which is derived from animal sources. Such high concentrations of amino acids in the intestine will stimulate the production of more amino acid receptor sites in the intestinal epithelium and will thus enhance amino acid absorption.[26] Only a fraction of these amino acids is utilized to meet the body's protein requirements, and the remainder must be converted into a form which the body can either store or utilize as an energy source. Excess proteins cannot be stored as such, as the body is geared largely for storing fat in the adipose tissues or carbohydrates, in the form of glycogen, in the liver and muscles. To meet these criteria, the amino acids must be metabolized resulting in the overproduction of potentially detrimental byproducts of amino acid metabolism. It would be wiser to limit the production of these compounds in the first place by reducing protein consumption to levels more in line with

Amino acid	Food group				
	Animal mean ± SD	Cereals mean ± SD	Legumes mean ± SD	Nuts/seeds mean ± SD	Fruit & veg mean ± SD
No samples	1726	170	153	153	572
Isoleucine	46.7 ± 4.7	39.8 ± 4.6	45.3 ± 4.2	42.8 ± 6.1	38.5 ± 10.8
Leucine	79.6 ± 6.0	86.3 ± 26.3	78.9 ± 4.2	73.5 ± 9.0	59.1 ± 19.6
Lysine	84.3 ± 7.1	30.5 ± 9.8	67.1 ± 3.8	43.5 ± 12.7	49.2 ± 13.3
Saa	37.7 ± 3.3	41.1 ± 4.8	25.3 ± 2.8	37.7 ± 11.7	23.6 ± 7.2
Aaa	74.9 ± 8.2	83.0 ± 9.2	84.9 ± 6.3	88.0 ± 16.9	64.0 ± 18.4
Threonine	43.4 ± 2.6	33.6 ± 5.4	40.0 ± 3.3	37.9 ± 5.4	35.1 ± 8.7
Tryptophan	11.4 ± 1.5	12.1 ± 3.3	12.3 ± 2.4	15.4 ± 4.6	10.8 ± 3.9
Valine	51.2 ± 5.6	51.1 ± 6.9	50.5 ± 4.0	55.6 ± 10.3	45.9 ± 12.6

Saa = sulphur amino acids, Aaa = aromatic amino acids

Table 1.3 Amino acid composition of major food groups. Data is compiled from the Massachusetts Nutrition Data Bank and is presented in mg/g protein. (From reference 24)

the daily requirements and increasing carbohydrate consumption to compensate for the concomitant energy decrease.

Many recent studies have confirmed the adverse effects of dietary excesses of proteins, particularly animal proteins. High-protein diets are not only associated with cancer, but are also associated with kidney stone formation and progressive deterioration of renal function.[27,28] Diets that are deficient in proteins can lead to the formation of bladder stones, but a strong correlation exists between the consumption of animal proteins and the formation of kidney stones. This is particularly apparent in affluent societies. In northern and western regions of India, animal protein intake is 100% higher than in the poorer southern and eastern regions and, consequently, the incidence of kidney stones is more than four times as high. Similar trends have been observed in a variety of other countries including Germany and Austria.[29,30] Diets rich in animal protein also lead to the formation of calcium oxalate crystals because the urine composition is altered in a way which inhibits its ability to prevent crystals from forming.[27] The urine levels of calcium and uric acid are increased when animal proteins are consumed whereas the levels of citrate are decreased, and it is the reduction in citrate levels which decreases the ability of the urine to inhibit crystal formation.

High-protein diets, particularly animal proteins, also have a significant calciuretic effect, that is, they cause the loss of calcium in urine,[31,32,33] and urinary calcium loss is linked to osteoporosis. Diets that are deficient in proteins have also been shown to have a negative influence on bone formation, but this is certainly not the reason for the high incidence of osteoporosis in affluent societies. Rather, it is the high consumption of proteins that gives cause for concern in these societies. Prevention of osteoporosis, through following a sensible diet, is absolutely essential, because by the time osteoporosis is generally diagnosed, 50% to 75% of the original bone material has been lost.[34]

Animal protein sources contain greater concentrations of sodium than do plant protein sources, and they also have higher concentrations of sulphur-containing amino acids both of which cause calcium loss.[29,35,36] The katabolism of dietary sulphur-containing amino acids increases the rate of acid excretion via the kidneys and this acid stress directly inhibits the renal reabsorption of calcium and leads to calcium loss. In a study done on young children, it was found that a high-protein diet increased calcium loss and the net acid excretion on the high-protein diet was nearly threefold higher than that observed with a low-protein diet.[37]

Sodium and calcium are reabsorbed at various common sites along the renal tubule, and a high sodium intake reduces the amount of calcium that can be reabsorbed from the renal filtrate, thus also leading to calcium loss. In contrast, plant protein sources such as soy protein, tend not to induce the loss of calcium,[36] and soy protein sources such as tofu and soya milk maintain calcium equilibrium. A twofold increase in protein consumption causes a 50% increase in urinary calcium, but a soy based diet maintains calcium balance at a calcium intake of 457 mg/day in spite of a 90 g protein intake. Calcium plays an important role in many physiological functions including the metabolism of proteins, and if excessive amounts of calcium are lost, because of a high-protein uptake, the body will call on the reserves in the bones, thus possibly laying the foundations for osteoporosis (for a more detailed discussion on osteoporosis see chapter 5).

Individual foods, even within food groups, vary in their protein and amino acid composition, and a comparison of these foods can thus help in the selection of food items which will ensure optimal supplies of proteins and essential amino acids, even in areas where food varieties are restricted. In table 1.4 the quantities of proteins and essential amino acids in a number of plant and animal foods are presented. Data for individual nuts and seeds is not included here as this information is dealt with later and is included in tables 7.14 and 7.15.

The total quantity of protein present, in the foods listed in table 1.4, is expressed in grams per 100 g portions (% protein), but it must be remembered that percentage protein is not the best indicator of protein availability, as not all the protein is utilizable. Nevertheless, it does give an indication of protein quantities available, and together with the information on food combinations, that will provide optimum amino acid concentrations, can still serve a useful purpose. The extent to which proteins are actually utilized is determined by a number of factors, including the concentrations of the essential amino acids present in the protein. The availability of a protein was termed its **biological value**, but the **NPU** (net protein utilization) is a better way of expressing the availability of proteins. The NPU is a combination of the **biological value** and the **coefficient of digestibility** of a protein, and is thus a more useful parameter than just the biological value. Both of these parameters, however, emphasize the importance of adequate concentrations of essential amino acids. The NPU can be improved by making the protein more digestible and by including a variety of plant protein sources in the diet to ensure a balanced supply of essential amino acids. The ways in which these objectives can be achieved, are discussed in chapter 7.

References

1. Kirk, D.L. 1980. Biology Today. Random House, Inc., New York.
2. Schmidt-Nielsen, K. 1983. Animal Physiology: Adaptation and Environment. 3rd. Edit. Cambridge Univ. Press.
3. Eckert, R. 1988. Animal Physiology. 3rd. Edit. W.H. Freeman and Company, New York.
4. ADA reports. 1980. Position paper on the vegetarian approach to eating. *J.Am.Diet.Assoc.* 77:61–69.
5. Bone, E; Tamm, A; Hill, M. 1976. The production of urinary phenols by gut bacteria. *Am.J.Clin.Nutr.* 29:148–54.
6. Sanches, A., Horning, M.C., Wingeleth, D.C. 1983. Plasma amino acids in humans fed plant proteins. *Nutrition Reports International.* 28:3.
7. Carroll, K.K. 1991. Review of the clinical studies on cholesterol-lowering response to soy protein. *J.Am.Diet.Assoc.* 91:820–827.
8. Kritchevsky, D., Tepper, S.A., Klurfeld, D.M. 1987. Dietary protein and atherosclerosis. *J.Am.Oil Chem.Soc.* 64:1167–1171.
9. Van der Meer, R. Beynen, A.C. 1987. Species-dependant responsiveness of serum cholesterol to dietary proteins. *J.Am.Oil Chem.Soc.* 64:1172–1177.
10. Sanches, A., Horning, M.C., Shavlik, G.W., Wingeleth, D.C., Hubbard, R.W. 1985. Changes in levels of cholesterol associated with plasma amino acids in humans fed plant proteins. *Nutr.Rep.Int.* 32:1047–1056.
11. Truswell, A.S. 1987. Evolution of dietary recommendations, goals and guidelines. *Am.J.Clin. Nutr.* 45:1060–1072.
12. Messina, M., Messina, V. 1991. Increasing use of soyfoods and their potential role in cancer prevention. *J.Am.Diet.Assoc.* 91:836–840.
13. Bingham, S.A. 1988. Meat, starch and non-starch polysaccharides and large bowel cancer. *Am.J.Clin.Nutr.* 48:762–7
14. Gibson, J.A.; Sladen, G.E.; Dawson, A.M. 1976. Protein absorption and ammonia production: the effect of dietary protein and removal of the colon. *Br. J. Nutr.* 35:61–5.
15. Cummings J.H., Hill, M.J., Bone, E.S., Branch, W.J., Jenkins, D.J.A. 1979. The effect of meat protein and dietary fibre on colonic function and metabolism. II Bacterial metabolites in faeces and urine. *Am.J. Clin.Nutr.* 32:2094–101.
16. Bingham, S.A. 1996. Epidemiology and mechanisms relating diet to risk of colorectal cancer. *Nutrition Research Reviews.* 9:197–239.
17. Scrimshaw, N.S. 1996. Nutrition from womb to tomb. *Nutrition Today.* 31 (2), March/April 1996. pp. 55–67.
18. FAO/WHO, 1992. International conference on nutrition: nutrition and development – a global assessment. Rome: Food and Agriculture Organization, 1992.
19. National Research Council, Food and Nutrition Board, Committee on Dietary allowances. 1980. Recommended dietary allowances. 9th rev. ed. Washington DC: National Academy of Sciences.

Proteins

Protein food	Prot. (g)	TRY (mg)	THR (mg)	ISO (mg)	LEU (mg)	LYS (mg)	MET (mg)	PHE (mg)	VAL (mg)	ARG (mg)	HIS (mg)
Animal foods:											
Milk (whole)	3.5	49	161	223	344	272	86	170	240	128	92
Cheese (cottage)	17.0	179	794	989	1826	1428	469	917	978	802	549
Cheese (cheddar)	25.0	341	929	1685	2437	1832	650	1340	1794	913	815
Eggs	12.8	211	637	850	1126	819	401	739	950	840	307
Beef (rump)	16.2	189	715	848	1327	1415	402	666	899	1045	562
Chicken	20.6	250	877	1088	1490	1810	537	811	1012	1302	593
Fish (cod)	16.5	164	715	837	1246	1447	480	612	879	929	–
Lamb (leg)	18.0	233	824	933	1394	1457	432	732	887	1172	501
Pork (ham)	15.2	197	705	781	1119	1248	379	598	790	931	525
Grains:											
Barley	12.8	160	433	545	889	433	184	661	643	659	239
Corn	10.0	61	398	462	1296	288	186	454	510	352	206
Millet (pearl)	11.4	248	456	635	1746	383	270	506	682	524	240
Oats (rolled)	14.2	183	470	733	1065	521	209	758	845	935	261
Rice (brown)	7.5	81	294	352	646	296	135	377	524	432	126
Rye	12.2	137	448	515	813	494	191	571	631	591	276
Sorghum	11.0	123	394	598	1767	299	190	547	628	417	211
Wheat	14.0	173	403	607	939	384	214	691	648	670	286
Legumes:											
Beans (Pinto)	23.0	213	997	1306	1976	1708	232	1270	1395	1384	655
Beans (Kidney)	23.1	214	1002	1312	1985	1715	233	1275	1401	1390	658
Beans (Navy)	21.4	199	928	1216	1839	1589	216	1181	1298	1287	609
Broadbeans	25.4	236	829	1593	2211	1426	106	1057	1276	1780	748
Chickpeas	20.8	170	739	1195	1538	1434	276	1012	1025	1551	559
Cowpeas	22.9	220	901	1110	1715	1491	352	1198	1293	1473	692
Lentils	25.0	216	896	1316	1760	1528	180	1104	1360	1908	548
Lima beans	20.7	195	980	1199	1722	1378	331	1222	1298	1315	669
Mung beans	24.4	180	765	1351	2202	1667	265	1167	1444	1370	543
Peanuts	26.9	340	828	1266	1872	1099	271	1557	1532	3296	749
Peas (split)	24.5	259	945	1380	2027	1795	294	1235	1372	2164	670
Soybeans	34.9	526	1504	2054	2946	2414	513	1889	2005	2763	911
Soybeans (milk)	3.4	51	176	175	305	269	54	195	186	302	121

TRY = Tryptophan, THR = Threonine, ISO = Isoleucine, LEU = Leucine, LYS = Lysine, MET = Methionine, PHE = Phenylalanine, VAL = Valine, ARG = Argenine, HIS = Histidine

Table 1.4. The protein and amino acid composition of selected protein foods. The figures are for 100g edible portions. (Ref.38)

20. Energy and protein requirements. Geneva, Switzerland: World Health Organization. 1985. Technical Report series No.724.

21. Young, V.R. 1991. Soy protein in relation to human protein and amino acid nutrition. *J.Am.Diet. Assoc.* 91:828–835.

22. Scrimshaw, N.S. 1996. Human protein requirements: A brief update. *Food and Nutrition Bulletin*, 17 (3):185–190.

23. Young, V.R. and A.E. El-Khoury. 1996. Human amino acid requirements: A re-evaluation. *Food and Nutrition Bulletin* 17 (3):191–203.

24. Pellett, P. 1996. World essential amino acid supply with special attention to South-East Asia. *Food and Nutrition Bulletin* 17 (3):204–234.

25. Blank, R.P., Diehl, H.A., Ballard, G.T., Melendez, D.D.S. 1987. Calcium metabolism and osteoporotic ridge resorption: A protein connection. *J.Prosthetic Dentistry.* 58:590–595.

26. Karasov, W.H. and J.M. Diamond. 1983 Adaptive regulation of sugar and amino acid transport by vertebrate intestine: Editorial review. The American Physiological Society.

27. Kok, D.J., Iestra, J.A., Doorenbos, C.J., Papapoulos, S.E. 1990. The effect of dietary excesses in animal protein and in sodium on the composition and the crystallization kinetics of the calcium oxalate monohydrate in the urine of healthy men. *J.Clin.Endocrinol.Metab.* 71:861–867.

28. Walser, M. 1983. Nutritional support in renal failure: Future directions. *Lancet.* 1:340–2.

29. Goldfarb, S. 1988. Dietary factors in the pathogenesis and prophylaxis of calcium nephrolithiasis. *Kidney International.* 34:544–555.

30. Goldfarb, S. 1990. The role of diet in the pathogenesis and therapy of nephrolithiasis. *Endocrinology and metabolism clinics of North America.* 19:805–820.

31. Howe, J.C. 1990. Postprandial response of calcium metabolism in postmenopausal women to meals varying in protein level/source. *Metabolism.* 39:1246–1252.

32. Einhorn, T.A., Levine, B., Michel, P. 1990. Nutrition and bone. *The Orthopaedic Clinics of North America* 21:43–50.

33. Kitano, T., Esashi, T., Azami, S. 1988. Effect of protein intake on mineral (calcium, Magnesium, and phosphorus) balance in Japanese males. *J.Nutr.Sci.Vitaminol.* 34:387–389.

34. Lukert, B.P. 1982. Osteoporosis: a review and update. *Arch.Phys.Med.Rehabil.* 63:480–7.

35. Zemel, M.B. 1988. Calcium utilization, effects of varying level and source of dietary proteins. *Am.J.Clin. Nutr.* 48:880–3.

36. Kaneko, K., Masaki, U., Aikyo, M., Yabuki, K., Haga, A., Matoba, C., Sasaki, H., Koike, G. 1990. Urinary calcium and calcium balance in young women affected by high protein diet of soy protein isolate and adding sulfur-containing amino acids and/or potassium. *J.Nutr.Sci.Vitaminol.* 36:105–116.

37. Nakano, M., Alon, U., Jennings, S.S., Chan, J.C.M. 1989. Protein intake and renal function in children. *AJDC.* 143:160–163.

38. Williams, S.R. 1989. Nutrition and diet therapy. 6th. ed. Times/ Mirror Mosby College Publishing. St. Louis.

Chapter 2
Carbohydrates and fibre

Carbohydrates are essential nutrients, that not only serve as an important fuel to meet the body's metabolic demands, but also play an important part in the digestive process. The fibre present in plant foods consists of carbohydrates known as NSP (non starch polysaccharides) which play an important part in the movement and absorption of nutrients in the intestines. For centuries it was thought that protein-rich foods supplied the body with the optimum fuel to maintain strength and stamina, and this concept is still entrenched to some extent to this day. Increasingly, however, carbohydrates are coming into their own as the fuel which keeps us functioning optimally, and it is now common knowledge that carbohydrates are the preferred energy source utilized by the body.

It has been known for some time that communities that subsist largely on high-carbohydrate diets are notable for their stamina and excellent health. One such group is the Tarahumara Indians of Mexico, whose chiefly vegetarian diet consists of 75-80% carbohydrates. Moreover, degenerative conditions such as hypertension, obesity and age-related cholesterol level increases are virtually absent from the tribe.[1,2] The stamina of the Tarahumara Indians is well demonstrated in their most popular sport which is raripuri, where participants race for 150-300 km kicking a wooden ball.[3] Achievements like these have challenged the **"proteins for energy"** concept and have encouraged an entire new investigation into the role of primary nutrients in human nutrition.

Scientific endeavours to enhance athletic and other performances have done much to explode the proteins for energy myth. In ancient times the Greek athletes consumed large amounts of meat before athletic events,[4] but today it is acknowledged that vegetarian, high-carbohydrate diets are superior to high-protein diets when it comes to enhancing stamina and endurance. Indeed, **"carboloading"** (increased carbohydrate intake) is extensively practised when preparing for sporting events. Improving the carbohydrate intake in athletes increases the quantity of glycogen which is stored in the muscles and this in turn improves the athlete's performance by delaying fatigue.[5] Training depletes the glycogen reserves in the muscles, but a high-carbohydrate intake rapidly replenishes these reserves, whereas this is not the case if a low-carbohydrate diet is followed (Fig. 2.1).

To enhance glycogen turnover, especially in athletes, a diet consisting of 65–70% carbohydrates has been suggested (550–650 g/day),[7] but few athletes consume such diets simply because modern eating habits do not cater for such high-carbohydrate intakes. It has in fact been found that carbohydrate intakes for most male endurance athletes range from 40% to 55% of total calories consumed, whereas other athletes engaged in other sports consume even lower levels of carbohydrates. To assist athletes in improving their carbohydrate intake, extensive guidelines have been developed, which list the foods with a high-carbohydrate content.[5] Many of the high-carbohydrate foods in these

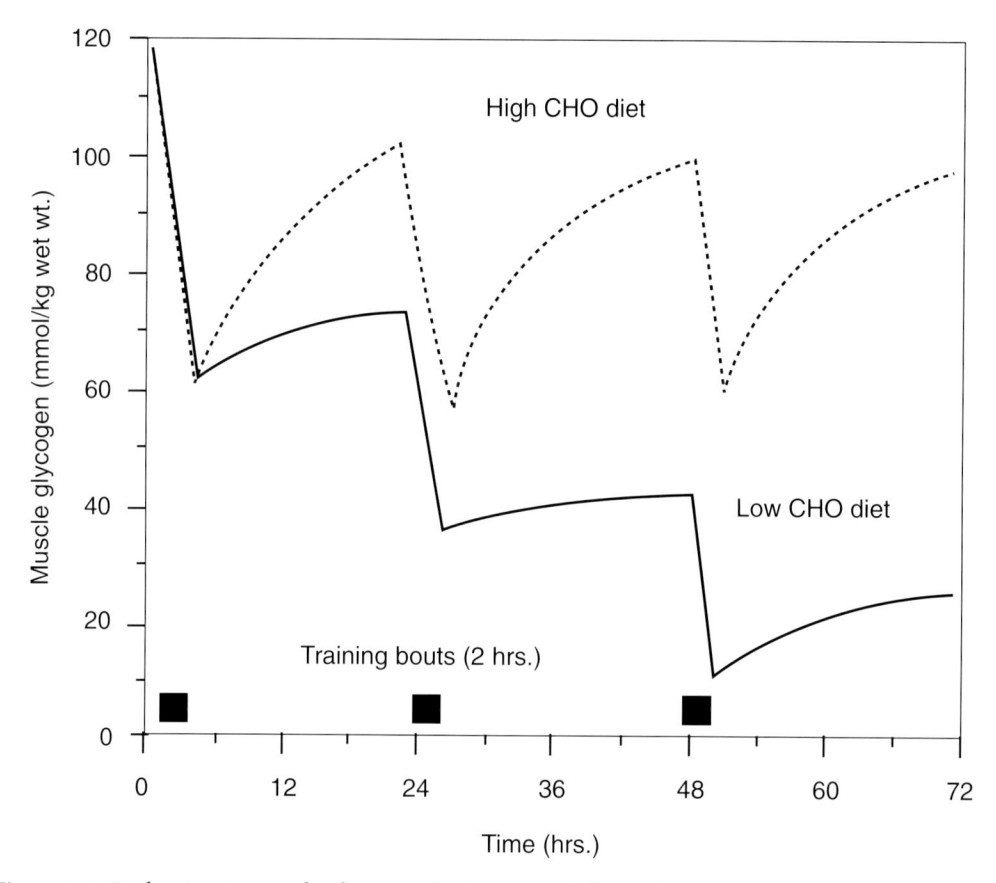

Figure 2.1. Reduction in muscle glycogen during several days of intense training. (From ref. 6)

lists are, however, refined foods and sweets, which cannot be considered as healthy.

The value of NSP (fibre) together with certain starches that are resistant to digestion in the small intestine, is now being discovered, and highly refined foods cannot meet the criteria required for healthful living. A new concept of nutrition is necessary which takes us away from modern highly refined foods and at the same time supplies primary nutrients in proper ratios. Only whole foods can supply this optimum relationship between nutrients, and will not only be of benefit to the athlete, but to every human being. Whole foods will also be of benefit to overweight individuals without being unduly restrictive in terms of the quantities of food which may be consumed. Athletes burn up more energy than non-athletes, but the ratio of nutrients required by both should remain roughly the same. For the general public, a minimum energy intake of 1200 kcal is advised, and for athletes 1600 kcal[8] (for a more detailed discussion of caloric needs see chapter 5), and a whole-food programme can certainly supply this. Fear is often expressed that a high-carbohydrate diet would be restrictive in terms of the amount of protein that is then available, but this fear is unfounded if a varied diet is followed which makes allowances for essential amino acid variations in foods, as was discussed in chapter 1. Moreover, recent evidence indicates that high-carbohydrate intakes can, without increasing protein intake, improve protein retention and synthesis.[9]

Carbohydrates in food

Carbohydrates are manufactured in plants by the process of photosynthesis using carbon dioxide and sunlight. As animal products contain virtually no carbohydrates, fruits, vegetables, grains and legumes are the main carbohydrate foods. Moreover, each of these plant foods supplies a different variety of carbohydrates, and it is therefore advisable that we know something about the structure and assimilation of carbohydrates in order to utilize these foods to our advantage. The carbohydrates in plants are largely constructed of various combinations of five simple sugars known as **monosaccharides** of which **glucose** forms the principle fuel of our bodies. The glucose molecule can have more than one configuration (Fig. 2.2), and when strung together to form polysaccharides, the properties of these macromolecules will be influenced by the type of glucose molecule incorporated.

Although α- and β-D-glucose appear very similar in structure, they are different in their biochemical properties. Whereas β-D-glucose occurs in cellulose which is a non-soluble fibre, α-D-glucose occurs in starch which is the most common storage material of plants. Starches are **polysaccharides** made up by numerous glucose molecules linked together in chains and stored as granules in various plant tissues. Not all starches are equally digestible in view of differences in stereochemistry and, whilst readily digestible starches form the main energy supply for the body (or they should form the main energy supply), starches that are resistant to digestion play an important role in the maintenance of colonic bacteria. Humans cannot digest cellulose as we lack the enzyme cellulase, but these fibres also play an important part in digestion, as they add bulk and improve gut motility. The structure of starch and cellulose is presented in figure 2.3.

Starch is broken down to glucose by digestive enzymes, and besides glucose, there are other important monosaccharides which play a significant role in human nutrition. **Fructose** is the monosaccharide found mainly in fruits and some other plant foods, and **galactose** is a component of **lactose**, the **disaccharide** found in milk. Galactose is also found in some of the storage carbohydrates of legumes and other seeds. A disaccharide consists of two simple sugars bound together. Another disaccharide that plays a significant role in human nutrition is **sucrose** (common table sugar), which is a combination of fructose and glucose. The structures of these molecules are presented in figures 2.4 and 2.5.

Digestion of carbohydrates

In natural foods the primary nutrients come prepacked with a variety of vitamins

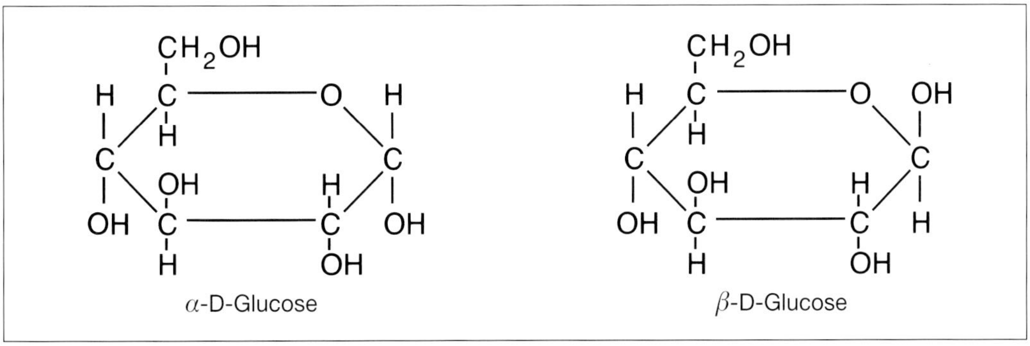

Figure 2.2 The structure of α- and β-D-Glucose.

and minerals, which enhance the maximal utilization of these foods. Whole foods contain fibres which influence the rate at which food passes through the intestine, and also control the rate at which the digestive products are absorbed. Moreover, the vitamins and minerals found in whole foods play an essential role in metabolizing the nutrients we eat. Unfortunately today's society chooses rather to eat refined foods which are poor in vitamins, and the lack must be supplied from the body's reserves, thus robbing the body of these

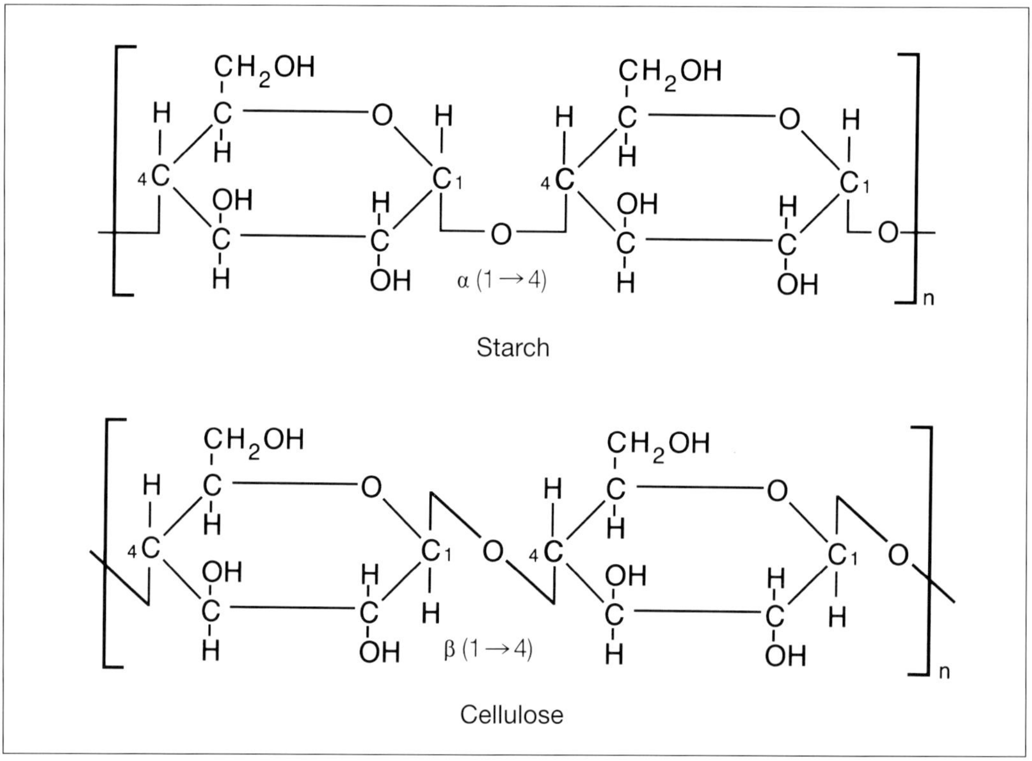

Figure 2.3. The structure of starch and cellulose.

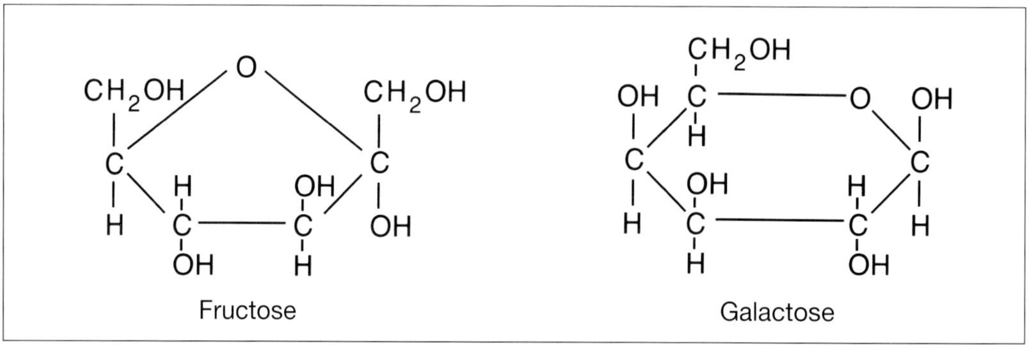

Figure 2.4. The structure of fructose and galactose.

essential components. Eating carbohydrates only in the refined state can eventually lead to numerous deficiency diseases.

The enzymes which digest carbohydrates can be divided into two categories, the **polysaccharidases** and **glycosidases**. The former hydrolyse the long chain carbohydrates such as glycogen and starch, whilst the latter act on disaccharides such as sucrose, fructose, maltose and lactose thus breaking them down into their constituent monosaccharides for absorption. The most common polysaccharidases are the **amylases (ptyalin and amylase)** which are secreted by the salivary glands and the pancreas. **Cellulase** is a polysaccharidase produced by symbiotic micro-organisms in the gut of cellulose-utilizing animals such as cattle, sheep, and termites, but humans cannot digest cellulose. Cellulose is, however, a natural fibre which supplies bulk and ensures easy passage of ingested material through the digestive tract.

Carbohydrate digestion is first initiated in the mouth, and it is, therefore, essential that food be chewed adequately to allow this process to take its course. The enzyme ptyalin occurs in saliva and it converts the starch found mainly in vegetables, grains and legumes into the disaccharide **maltose**. Ptyalin is inactivated below pH4 so that starch digestion will cease in the stomach if the pH drops below this level. The digestion of starch will continue in the stomach as long as the pH does not drop below pH4. Concentrated protein foods such as animal products will quickly induce a pH drop and consequently prevent further digestion of starch in the stomach. Proteins found in grains and legumes do not, however, require an excessive acid medium

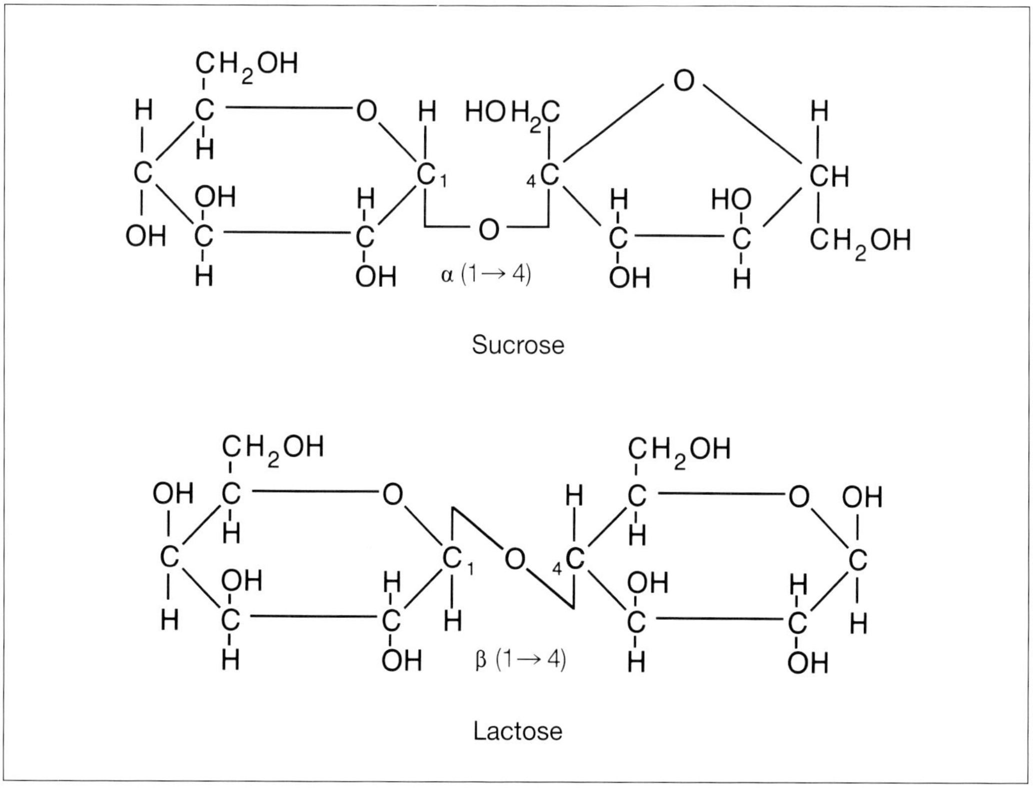

Figure 2.5. The structure of sucrose and lactose.

for digestion and are thus ideal companions for fruits or vegetables. Nuts are also an excellent source of protein but should be eaten in moderation, because excessive intake will also lower the pH in the stomach.

When food passes from the stomach into the duodenum, the environment again becomes alkaline and favours the digestion of carbohydrates. In the duodenum the enzyme amylase, which is released by the pancreas, will continue with the break-down of starch to maltose which in turn is acted upon by the intestinal glycosidase **maltase** which breaks down maltose to glucose. The glucose is then absorbed and conveyed to the liver where it is stored in the form of glycogen. Glycogen is also stored in the muscles and thus acts as an energy reservoir, and when required it will be converted to glucose again. Resistant starches and soluble and insoluble fibres reach the large bowel undigested, and some of these components are then broken down by colonic bacteria.

Diet and control of glucose levels

The body needs a constant supply of glucose, not only because it is an important energy source, but because certain tissues such as the brain and nerves cannot function without it. For this reason glucose levels are precisely controlled by the two hormones **glucagon** and **insulin**. Insulin is produced by the **islets of Langerhans** of the pancreas, and its function is to lower blood glucose levels by stimulating the conversion of glucose to a storable form of energy such as fat. The hormone glucagon has the opposite effect and increases the glucose levels. The ailment **diabetes mellitus** results from a lack of insulin production, whereas excessive insulin production results in **hypoglycaemia** or low blood sugar. Rapid uptake of glucose can be brought about by a refined food diet and can lead to hypoglycaemia or, in the case of the diabetic, it can be brought about as a result of an insulin injection.

Monosaccharides such as glucose, fructose and galactose require no digestion and are absorbed as is. The disaccharides, such as sucrose, are rapidly converted by the glycosidases in the intestine and it is easy to flood the system with glucose if refined foods are consumed. The subsequent **glucose surge** will lead to extensive insulin production, and because the glucose will then be converted to fat and glycogen, the blood sugar levels will be lowered more than normal, thus leading to hypoglycaemia. Hypoglycaemia initiates a series of bodily responses and the reduced glucose levels are recognized by the brain, which in turn triggers a response by the sympathetic nervous system. Adrenalin and other hormones are then released to counteract the fall in glucose levels, and this manifests itself in numerous symptoms of which only a few will be discussed here.

Symptoms of hypoglycaemia

These symptoms can be divided into two categories, namely: **autonomic activation**

SYMPTOMS OF HYPOGLYCAEMIA	
Autonomic activation	Neuroglycopenic
sweating (even heavy sweating), shaking, warmness, pounding heart and increased heart rate, anxiety and shivering.	confusion, drowsiness, weakness, difficulty in speaking, loss of concentration, visual disturbances such as double vision and dizziness.

Table 2.1. Symptoms associated with hypoglycaemia. (From reference 10)

and **neuroglycopenic symptoms** as summarised in table 2.1.

Many of these symptoms can manifest themselves at night or early in the morning, in view of the abstinence from food during this time, and therefore insomnia, fear and even hallucinations can be additional symptoms. The normal range of blood glucose levels should be between 80-120 mg/100ml in the morning before a good meal. After a meal, the blood sugar level will rise but should drop to this range within a few hours. Unfortunately, modern lifestyles can have a detrimental effect on the maintenance of normal blood sugar levels, and refined foods and certain stimulants are some of the main culprits.

Refined foods are used extensively in the food industry, and many processed foods as well as the myriads of sweets, cookies and soft drinks on the market contain large amounts of hidden sugars, mostly in the form of sucrose. When these foods are consumed, most of the sucrose will rapidly be converted to glucose and fructose, thus causing a glucose surge. Some of the sucrose will even enter the bloodstream unaltered and will be treated as a foreign substance as there are no enzymes to break it down outside the intestinal tract. Moreover, **caffeine**, which is found in tea, coffee and many soft drinks, as well as **theobromine** that is found in cocoa and cocoa products such as chocolates, also induce hypoglycaemia as they stimulate the conversion of stored glycogen to glucose which in turn leads to insulin release and subsequent hypoglycaemia.

The modern trend to drink large amounts of soft drinks, can prove particularly hazardous, as these contain very high levels of sugars. Although soft drink firms add only sucrose to their drinks, these beverages also contain large amounts of glucose and fructose. This anomaly is brought about by the high acidity of these drinks, which encourages acid hydrolysis of sucrose. As both glucose and fructose are less sweet than sucrose, the companies compensate for this by adding more sucrose, and an average carbonated beverage can contain as much as 136 g/l of sugar[11] which is more than ten teaspoons of sugar per 340 ml can.

Avoidance of high sugar drinks, caffeine and theobromine together with the consumption of whole foods such as unrefined grains, legumes, fruits and vegetables will prevent hypoglycaemia. The presence of soluble fibre in these foods ensures a slow release of simple sugars over a period of time, thus preventing the glucose surge associated with refined foods. Surge releases of insulin will also be avoided and in addition the whole foods come prepacked with the essential vitamins (particularly the B-group) and minerals required for their effective metabolism. People suffering from hypoglycaemia should also include more of the high energy whole foods, such as unrefined grains and legumes in their diet, because oats and bean products contain high levels of soluble fibres which offer protection against hypoglycaemia. It is not necessary to give up one's sweet tooth, but one should encourage the use of naturally sweet foods, such as dates and raisins as sweeteners, and avoid large amounts of refined sweeteners which consist largely of empty calories. In table 2.2. the chemical composition of some of the most common sweeteners, as well as foods with added sugar, is presented.

It is noteworthy that none of these sweet foods contain any appreciable amounts of fibre, and they are also vitamin poor. If these items are to be used, they should be used sparingly and preferably in conjunction with foods rich in soluble fibres such as fruits, grains and legumes. It should also be noted that brown sugar, molasses, honey and jams do at least contain some vitamins and minerals, whereas the refined products do not. In most countries in the Western world the consumption of sugar is somewhat above 100 g/person/day or more than 15% of the daily caloric intake.[13] Obviously, this is far too high, and in view of the problems associated with such a high sugar intake there has been a move away from sucrose in certain health circles, and consumption of fructose is recommended in the place of sucrose. Fructose is often considered to be the perfect substitute for sucrose as it is natural fruit sugar. Pure fructose is, however, also a refined sugar and can cause similar conditions as sucrose.

Fructose consumption does not lead to as high postprandial glucose surges as does the consumption of sucrose, and so it does seem to have some advantages over the consumption of sucrose. It does, however, lead to increases in LDL cholesterol levels, and some researchers have also found that it will increase the levels of triglycerides.[14,15] Fructose loads will also induce hypoglycaemia because fructose facilitates the formation of glycogen.[13] These facts once again underline the principle that refined foods, in whatever form, are not the most wholesome of foods and should be

Sweet food	Energy (cal)	Sugar (g)	Carb. (g)	Prot. (g)	Fat (g)	Fibre (g)	Ca (mg)	P (mg)	Fe (mg)	K (mg)
Cold drink (carbonated)	39	10.5	10.5	0.0	0.0	0.0	4	15	0.0	1
Cold drink (diluted base)	36	9.0	9.0	0.0	0.0	0.0	0	0	0.0	0
Glucose (liquid)	318	40.2	84.7	0.0	0.0	0.0	8	11	0.5	3
Honey	304	82.3	82.3	0.3	0.0	0.0	5	6	0.5	51
Jam (all kinds)	272	45.9	68.9	0.6	0.1	1.1	20	9	1.0	88
Jelly (dessert)	59	14.2	14.2	1.4	0.0	0.0	7	2	0.4	6
Molasses (light)	250	–	13.0	–	–	–	33	9	0.9	183
Mollasses (Blackstrap)	271	0.0	70.0	–	–	–	245	50	–	–
Sugar (brown)	373	96.4	96.4	0.0	0.0	0.0	85	19	3.4	344
Sugar (white)	385	99.5	99.5	0.0	0.0	0.0	0	0	0.1	3
Syrup	298	79.0	79.0	0.3	0.0	0.0	26	20	1.5	240

Sweet food	Mg (mg)	Zn (mg)	Vit.A (IU)	Vit.B1 (mg)	Vit.B2 (mg)	Vit.B3 (mg)	Vit.B5 (mg)	Vit.B6 (mg)	Fol. (µg)	Vit.C (mg)
Cold drink (carbonated)	1	0	0	0.00	0.00	0.00	0.00	0.00	0	00.0
Cold drink (diluted base)	0	0	0	0.00	0.00	0.00	0.00	0.00	0	0.00
Glucose (liquid)	2	–	0	0.00	0.00	0.00	0.00	0.00	0	0.00
Honey	2	–	0	0.00	0.04	0.30	0.04	0.04	–	1.00
Jam (all kinds)	8	–	10	0.01	0.03	0.20	0.00	0.00	0	2.00
Jelly (dessert)	1	–	0	0.00	0.00	0.00	0.00	0.00	0	0.00
Molasses (light)	–	–	–	0.01	0.01	–	–	–	–	–
Mollasses (Blackstrap)	258	–	–	0.06	0.20	–	–	–	–	–
Sugar (brown)	15	–	0	0.01	0.03	0.20	0.00	0.00	0	0.00
Sugar (white)	0	–	0	0.00	0.00	0.00	0.00	0.00	0	0.00
Syrup	10	–	0	0.00	0.00	0.00	0.00	0.00	0	0.00

Table 2.2 The composition of selected sweet foods, drinks and sweeteners. The figures are for 100 g portions. (Adapted from reference 12)

used in moderation. It is therefore advisable to cultivate the habit of substituting whole-food sweeteners for refined sweeteners wherever possible.

NSP (fibre) and digestion resistant starch

The importance of fibre in the diet is being recognized more and more. The concept that fibre could play a preventive role in colon cancer was first proposed in 1971 when Burkitt put forth the proposal that fibre could prevent colon cancer by regulating the speed and bulk of the food that passes through the intestines.[16] Since that time many studies have shown this hypothesis to be true.[17] Whole grain consumption in particular, was found to be inversely correlated to the prevalence of colon cancer.[18] Vegetable fibre was also shown to offer protection, and the NCI (National Cancer Institute of the US) has therefore recommended that a variety of foods such as whole grains, vegetables and fruits be eaten rather than fibre supplements, and that dietary fibre levels should at least be doubled over current consumption levels of 10–15g fibre/day.[19] Fibre consumption is so low in industrialized countries, because of the excessive consumption of refined foods. Modern grain mills, for example, separate the natural fibres and wheatgerm from the wheat, thus stripping the wheat of its natural fibre. The bran of wheat is rich in NSP (non starch polysaccharides or fibre) which provides bulk and aids intestinal motility. Furthermore, these outer layers of wheat include the aleurone layers which contain the B-complex vitamins, phosphorus, iron, and proteins in balanced proportions. The wheatgerm is rich in thiamin (vitamin B1) which is essential for carbohydrate metabolism and the natural antioxidant vitamin E. Vitamin E comes prepacked with the polyunsaturated oils in the wheat germ and thus offers a natural protection against the formation of free radicals when these essential oils are ingested. Whole grains or unrefined grain products such as stone-ground flour, are thus vastly superior to refined products in terms of their overall composition.

The addition of unground wheat berries or broken pieces of grain to the flour is also a poor way of adding fibre to grain products. These hard pieces pass through the intestines largely undigested, add little bulk and can even damage the delicate epithelia on their way. They do not aid in water retention in the stools and do not provide a large enough surface area for the elimination of wastes. Flour used for bread-making should be thoroughly ground and if whole grains are used for the preparation of porridges, then they must be well soaked or/and thoroughly cooked, as raw grains contain enzyme suppressants which interfere with the digestive process. Cooking or sprouting destroys these suppressants and thus allows for maximal utilization of the nutrients in the grains.

As fibre content in the diet increases, bowel transit time decreases and faeces weight and the number of defecations increase.[20,21] Furthermore, the consistency of the stool is far softer on a natural high-fibre diet than on a low-fibre diet thus eliminating constipation and its secondary effects such as **colitis, appendicitis, diverticulosis,** and **hiatus hernia**. Oats and bean products contain large quantities of water-soluble fibre and are particularly efficient in reducing blood cholesterol levels, particularly LDL-cholesterol, which is the variety which tends to clog blood vessels.[22,23,24,25,26] It was found that the inclusion of oat-bran and beans in the diet decreased LDL-cholesterol concentrations by 23% and 24% respectively in a study done on 20 hypercholesterolaemic adult males.[22] Added bran is not nearly as efficient in eliminating cholesterol as is the fibre in whole cereals,[27] thus emphasizing the importance of the consumption of whole, unrefined foods as means of controlling cholesterol levels. Some studies suggest that oat bran acts as a placebo,[28,29] but other studies have shown that this conclusion is probably unfounded.[30] By binding cholesterol and bile acids, fibre not only reduces cholesterol levels but also protects against colon cancer, as secondary bile acids, which are formed by bacterial conversion of bile acids, are carcinogenic.[31] The relationship between the incidence of colon cancer and fibre intake is presented in Figure 2.6.

Wheat-bran was also found to lower the concentrations of oestrogens in women, particularly serum oestrogen and oestradiol.[33] The presence of free and albumen-bound oestradiol has been associated with an increased risk of breast cancer,[34] and the bran can thus offer protection against this form of cancer. Precisely how fibre affords protection against this form of cancer is uncertain. When dealing with fibre, it is important to note that there are two categories of fibre, and these two differ in their function.

Water-insoluble fibres

Water-insoluble fibres include such fibres as **cellulose, lignin** and certain **hemicelluloses**. These fibres have a considerable effect on stool size and the time that the ingested food stays in the digestive tract, but they have little or no effect on intermediary metabolism,[35,36] or the growth of the bacterial population in the colon.[37] The bulking effect of water-insoluble fibre on the intestinal contents, however, dilutes the concentration of substances that can cause cancer and this type of fibre also ensures rapid elimination of harmful cancer promoters in the colon. Most studies confirm that water insoluble fibre has a protective effect against chemical carcinogenesis, and both bran and cellulose were effective in reducing the number of tumors formed under chemically induced carcinogenesis.[38]

Refined food leads to constipation, but on a high natural fibre diet stools will not only be softer, but will be passed more frequently. Two to three stools a day are consistent with

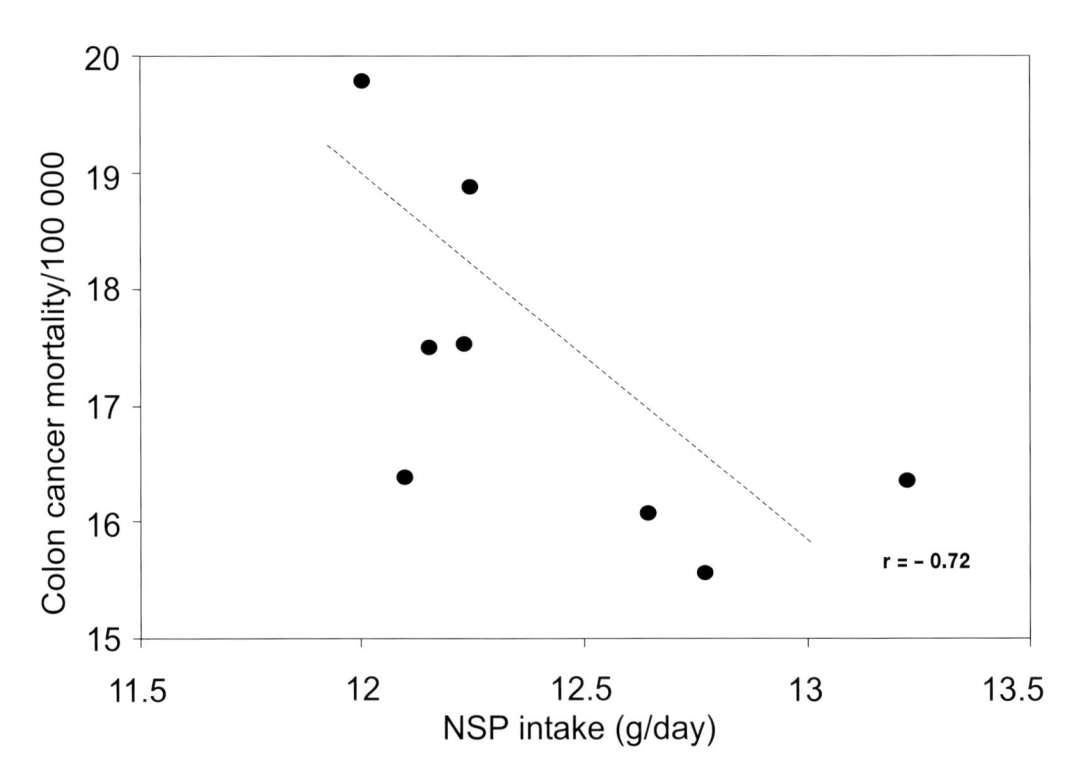

Figure 2.6 Average regional NSP intake in relation to age standardized colon cancer death rates 1969-1973 in Great Britain. (Adapted from reference 32)

healthy bowel movements, whereas one stool or even fewer per day may be categorized as constipation. This might seem excessive to those who pass stools only once a day or even less frequently. If we, however, consider that most people consume two to three meals per day, then it is only logical to eliminate the waste material more than once a day. Waste products that remain in the colon for lengthy periods of time will be acted upon by the colonic bacteria and converted to potential carcinogens. Furthermore, the compaction and pressure required to eliminate fibre-poor stools can produce **diverticulosis** of the intestinal tract (small pouches), and hardened portions of faeces can become trapped, thus eventually causing inflammation as in the case of **appendicitis**. Moreover, the increased abdominal pressure required to eliminate hard stools can also produce **hernias** and will force more blood from the large abdominal vessels into the femoral vessels thus causing **varicose veins**. Considering the high fibre content of whole-plant foods, it is thus not surprising that diverticulosis is less common in vegetarians than in omnivores.[39] There is a strong inverse association between high stool weight and colorectal cancer.[40] As there is a linear relationship between stool weight and NSP consumption (5 g increase in stool weight for every 1 g NSP consumed), both the WHO and the UK department of health have recommended an average daily intake of 18 g NSP.[41,38]

Water-soluble fibres and resistant starch

In contrast to the insoluble fibres, water-soluble fibres have little effect on stool size, transit time and mineral absorption, but they do have an important effect on secondary metabolism. As noted previously, resistant starch is starch that resists digestion in the small intestine because of the different stereochemistry of these starches. All starchy foods such as grains, legumes and starchy vegetables such as potatoes contain resistant starch. Even fruits, such as bananas that are still slightly green, contain resistant starch. When soluble fibre and resistant starch enter the colon, they are fermented anaerobically to produce **short chain fatty acids (SCFA), acetate, propionate,** and **butyrate** as well as gas. Moreover, bacterial growth is enhanced which, together with water binding to residual unfermented NSP, leads to increased stool weight, dilution of colonic contents and faster transit time through the large gut.[38] This in turn reduces the time that potentially harmful substances can come into contact with mucosal cells.

The SCFA which are produced in the colon during the fermentation process, are absorbed by the intestinal mucosa thus enhancing the functional capacity of the epithelium. Butyrate is also used by the cells in the colon, and because butyrate is formed most efficiently from resistant starch, this type of starch must be considered the prime source of this compound. Butyrate has been suggested as a protective agent against colon cancer,[38] and consumption of whole foods rich in complex carbohydrates thus offers protection against cancer in more ways than one. Diets rich in grains, legumes, fruits and vegetables are thus optimal for maintaining a healthy digestive system.

The water-soluble fibres include such fibres as **pectin, hemicelluloses,** and **storage polysaccharides** that are found mainly in fruits and vegetables, and **gums** which are found mainly in cereals. As the bacteria in the colon break down a large proportion of these water-soluble fibres, they do not contribute to faecal bulk as do non-soluble fibres. Besides contributing fermentation products, for use by the mucosal cell of the colon, soluble fibres are known to lower cholesterol levels and to prevent the postprandial (after meal) glucose surge and subsequent hypoglycaemia associated with a refined food diet. Once again, it is the fruits, vegetables, legumes and grains which contain soluble fibres which can retard the rate of glucose absorption. In the case of fruits, the soluble fibre which retards the rate of glucose absorption is pectin, and it prevents the glucose surge and subsequent hypoglycaemia associated with a refined food diet devoid of natural fibre.[42] The same effect is achieved by soluble fibres found in oat bran, and has been attributed to the presence of the oat gum **β-glucan**. This polysaccharide occurs in commercial rolled oats and is highly viscous. It has been found that the inclusion of oat gum in a meal containing glucose, significantly reduced the postprandial glucose and insulin surge that occurs in glucose meals that do not contain the oat gum (Figure 2.7).[43]

In figure 2.7 it can be seen that the glucose meal by itself produces a large increase in plasma glucose levels which is accompanied by a surge release of insulin. The result is that glucose levels rapidly drop and even drop below the fasting level (indicated by the zero in fig. 2.7), thus producing a hypoglycaemic condition. Soluble fibres probably prevent the glucose and insulin surge by slowing the rate of glucose absorption[44] and by slowing the rate at which the enzyme amylase digests the foods containing the viscous fibres.[45] This allows for a longer period of time over which glucose is absorbed, particularly as soluble fibres also slow down the rate at which glucose is absorbed across the wall of the intestine.[46] It is through the combination of these mechanisms, that soluble fibre affords protection against hypoglycaemia.

An argument which is often levelled against a fibre-rich diet, is that it will inhibit the uptake of minerals and other essential nutrients. In a recent study it was, however, found that the higher fibre intake of vegetarians did not affect mineral utilization adversely, and depending on the variety in the diet, the uptake of magnesium, iron, copper and manganese could actually be enhanced.[47] A varied whole food diet rich in carbohydrates will therefore afford the highest protection against degenerate diseases, as well as supplying all the body's energy, mineral and vitamin needs.

References

1. Conner, W.E., Cerqueira, M.T. Connor, R.W., Wallace, R.B., Malinow, M.R., Casdorph, H.R. 1978. The plasma lipids, lipoproteins, and diet of the Tarahumara Indians of Mexico. *Am.J.Clin.Nutr.* 31:1131–42
2. Balke, B., Snow, C. 1965. Anthropological and physiological observation on Tarahumara endurance runners. *A.J.Phys.Anthropol.* 23: 293–301.
3. Nieman, D.C. 1988. Vegetarian dietary practices and endurance performance. *Am.J.Clin.Nutr.* 48: 754–61.
4. Ryan, A.J. 1981. Anabolic steroids are fool's gold. *Fed.Proc.* 40:2682.
5. Moses, K., Manore, M.M. 1991. Development and testing of a carbohydrate monitoring tool for athletes. *J.Am.Diet.Assoc.* 91:962–965.
6. Costill, D.L., Miller, J.M. 1980. Nutrition for endurance sports: carbohydrate and fluid balance. *Int.J.Sports.Med.* 1:2–14.
7. Costill, D.L. 1988. Carbohydrates for exercise: dietary demands for optimum performance. *Int.J.Sports Med.* 9:1–18.
8. Hoffman, C.J. and Coleman, E. 1991. An eating plan and update on recommended dietary practices for the endurance athlete. *J.Am.Diet. Assoc.* 91:325–330.
9. Welle, S., Mathews, D.E., Campbell, R.G., Sreekumaran, N. 1989. Stimulation of protein turnover by carbohydrate overfeeding in men. *Am.J.Physiol.* 257:E413–E417.
10. Patrick, A.W., Bodger, C.W., Tieszen, K.L., White, M.C., Williams, G. 1991. Human insulin awareness of acute hypoglycaemic symptoms in insulin-dependent diabetes. *Lancet* 338:528–532.
11. Van der Horst, G., Wesso, I., Burger, A.P., Dietrich, D.L.L. Grobler, S.R. 1984. Chemical analysis of cooldrinks and pure fruit juices – some clinical implications. *S.Afr.Med.J.* 66:755–758.
12. NRIND. 1986. Food composition tables. 2nd ed. South African Medical Research Council.
13. Sestoft, L. 1983. Fructose and health. *Nutrition Update* 1:39–54.
14. Hallfrish, J., Reiser, S. Prather, E.S. 1983. Blood lipid distribution of hyperinsulinemic men consuming three levels of fructose. *Am.J.Clin.Nutr.* 37:740–8.
15. Swanson, J.E. Laine, D. Thomas, W., Bantle, J.P. 1992. Metabolic effects of dietary fructose in healthy subjects. *Am.J.Clin.Nutr.* 55:851–6.
16. Burkitt, D.P. 1971. The Epidemiology of cancer of the colon and rectum. Cancer. 28: 3–13.
17. Greenwald, P., Lanza, E., Eddy, G. 1978. Dietary fibre in the reduction of colon cancer risk. *J. Am. Diet. Assoc.* 87:1178–88.

Carbohydrates and fibre

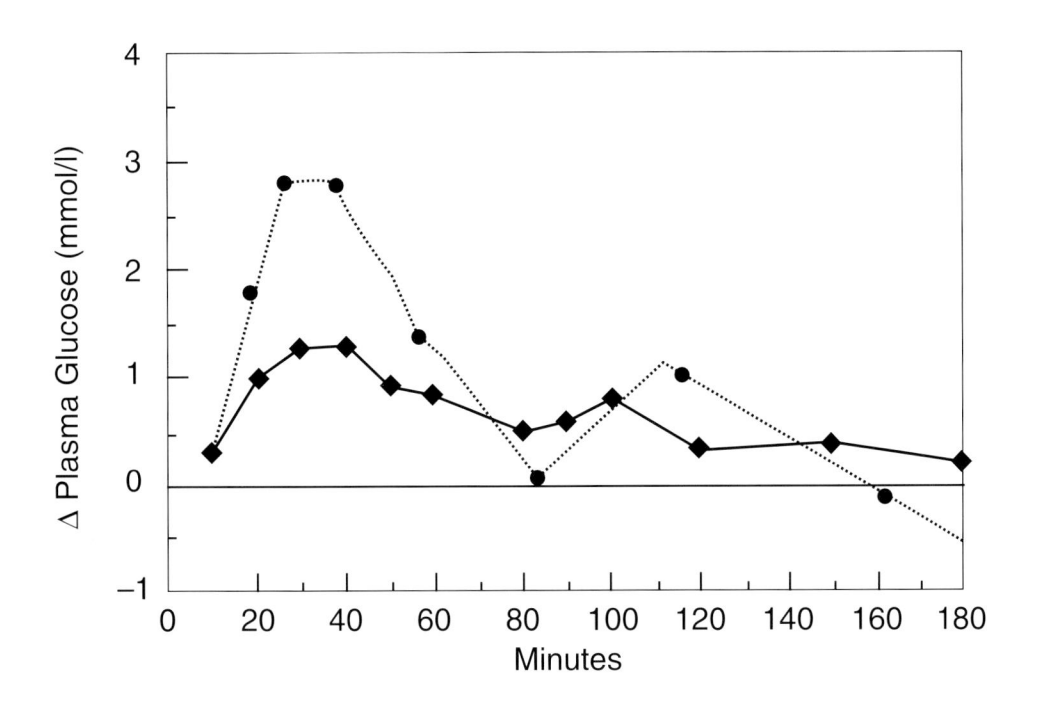

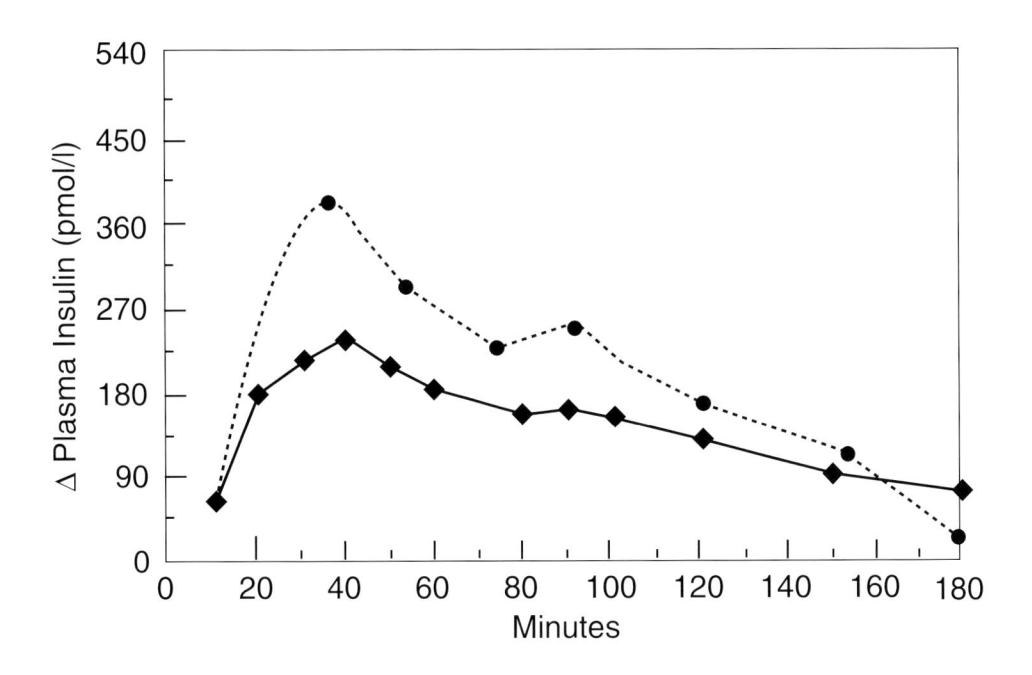

Figure 2.7. Postprandial changes in plasma glucose and insulin levels after a 50 g glucose drink (dots) and a glucose plus oat gum drink (squares). Adapted from reference 43.

18. Reddy, B.S. 1982. Dietary fibre and colon carcinogenesis: A critical review. In Vahoung,G.V.; Kritchesky, D., eds. Dietary fibre in health and disease. New York: Plenum Press. 265–85.

19. Butrum, R.R., Clifford, C.K., Lanza, E. 1988. NCI dietary guidelines: Rationale. *Am.J.Clin.Nutr.* 48:888–95.

20. Beyer, P.L., Flynn, M.A. 1978. Effects of high- and low-fibre diets on human faeces. *J.Am.Diet.Assoc.* 72 : 271-7.

21. Eastwood, M.A., Elton, R.A., Smith, J.H. 1986. Long-term effects of white meal bread on stool weight, transit time, faecal bile acids, fats and neutral sterols. *Am.J.Clin.Nutr.* 43:343–9.

22. Anderson, J.W., Gustafson, N.J. 1988. Hypocholestrolemic effects of oat and bean products. *Am.J.Clin.Nutr.* 48:749–53.

23. Anderson, J.W., Chen, W.J.L. 1986. Plant fibre: diabetes and obesity. *Am.J.Gastroenterol.* 81:898–906.

24. Gold, K.V., Davidson, D.M. 1988. Oat bran as a cholesterol reducing dietary adjunct in a young healthy population. *Western.J.Med.* 148:299-302.

25. Keenan, J.M., Wenz, J.B., Huang, Z., Myers, S.R. 1990. A randomized controlled trial of oat bran cereal for hypercholesterolemia. *Arteriosclerosis* 10:873a.

26. Anderson, J.W., Spencer, D.B., Hamilton, C.C. et al. 1990. Oat bran cereal lowers serum total and LDL cholesterol in hypercholesterolemic men. *Am.J.Clin.Nutr.* 52:495–499.

27. Burkitt, D.P 1975 Refined Carbohydrate foods and disease. Academic Press P 341.

28. Demark-Wahnefried, W., Bowering, J., Cohen, P.S. 1990. Reduced serum cholesterol with dietary change using fat-modified and oat bran supplemented diets. *J.Am.Diet.Assoc.* 90:223–229.

29. Swain, J.F., Rouse, I.L. 1990. Comparison of the effect of oat bran and low-fibre wheat on serum lipoprotein levels and blood pressure. *N.Engl.J.Med.* 332:147–152.

30. Grant, K.I. 1991. Oat bran-panacea or placebo? *S.Afr.Med.J.*(in press)

31. Nair. P.P. 1988. Role of bile acids and neutral sterols in carcinogenesis. *Am.J.Clin.Nutr.* 48: 768–74.

32. Bingham, S.; Williams, D.R.R.; Cummings, J.H. 1985. Dietary fibre consumption in Britain: New estimates and their relation to large bowel cancer mortality. *Br. J. cancer.* 52: 399–402.

33. Rose, D.P., Golman, M., Conolly, J.M. and Strong, L.E. 1991. High-fibre diet reduces serum estrogen concentrations in premenopausal women. *Am.J.Clin.Nutr.* 54(3):

34. Jones, L.A., Ota, D.M., Jackson, G.A. et al. 1987. Bioavailability of estradiol as a marker for breast cancer risk assessment. *Cancer.Res.* 47: 5224–9.

35. Munoz, J. 1984. Fibre and diabetes. *Diabetes care.* 7:297–8.

36. Crapo, P.A. 1985. Simple versus complex carbohydrate use in the diabetic diet. *Ann. Rev.Nutr.* 5:95–114.

37. Mendeloff, A.I. 1987. Dietary fibre and gastro intestinal disease. *Am.J.Clin.Nutr.* 45 (suppl):1267–70.

38. Bingham, S.A. 1996. Epidemiology and mechanisms relating diet to risk of colorectal cancer. *Nutrition Research Reviews.* 9:197–239.

39. Dwyer, J.T. 1988. Health aspects of vegetarian diets. *Am.J.Clin.Nutr.* 48:712–28.

40. Cummings, J.H., Bingham, S.A., Heaton, K.W. and Eastwood, M.A. 1992. Faecal weight, colon cancer risk, and dietary intake of nonstarch polysaccharides (dietary fibre). *Gastroentorology.* 103:1783–1789.

41. World Health Organization. 1990. *Diet, Nutrition and the Prevention of Chronic Disease (Technical Report Series* no. 797). Geneva: WHO.

42. Leeds, A.R., Ralphs, D.N.L., Ebied, F., Metz, G., Dilawari, J.B. 1981. Pectin in the dumping syndrome and plasma volume changes. *Lancet* 1:1075–8.

43. Braaten, J.T., Wood, P.J., Scott, F.W., Riedel, K.D.,Poste, L.M. and Collins, M.W. 1991. Oat gum lowers glucose and insulin after an oral glucose load. *Am.J.Clin. Nutr.*53:1425–30.

44. Meyer, J.H., Guy, G., Jehn, D. Taylor, I.L. 1988. Intragastric vs intraintestinal viscous polymers and glucose tolerance after liquid meals of glucose. *Am.J.Clin.Nutr.* 48:260–6.

45. Jenkins, D.J.A., Wolever, T.M.S., Taylor, R.H. et al. 1980. Rate of digestion of foods and post prandial glycemia in normal and diabetic subjects. *Br.Med.J.* 2:14-7.

46. Batey, I.L. 1982. Starch analysis using thermostable alpha-amylase. *Starch/Staerke.* 34:125–8.

47. Kelsay, J.L.; C.W. Frazier; E.S. Prather; J.J. Canary; W.M. Clark and A.S. Powell. 1988. Impact of variation in carbohydrate intake on mineral utilization by vegetarians. *Am.J.Clin.Nutr.* 48: 875–9.

Chapter 3
Fats

Fat is an important dietary component as it is a key energy source, and in addition is vital to proper human growth and development. Fat provides essential fatty acids necessary for the structure of cell membranes and prostaglandins and also acts as solvent for many substances including vitamins A, D, E and K. Although fat is essential in the human diet, it has been established that the free use of fats leads to numerous degenerative diseases such as cardiovascular disease and various forms of cancer. Findings such as these have prompted the US National Academy of Science to recommend a lower intake of fat, whilst encouraging the consumption of more fibre, fruits and vegetables. Moreover, they suggested an increase in the consumption of complex carbohydrates (e.g. starch), and a decrease in the consumption of pickled, salted or smoked foods.[1]

The consumption of fat in the Western world is very high and the average Western diet contains some 30–40% fat. In the United States, it has been found that both men and women consume an average of 36% to 37% fat, which is far higher than the level recommended by most health organizations.[2] Because fat is a solvent for many organic molecules it can be a powerful flavourant, and besides this attribute, fat provides a desirable mouth feel and contributes to the feeling of satiety after a meal. These attributes of fat have encouraged the use of increased quantities of fats in many traditional and commercial foods and made it extremely difficult for consumers to switch to a lower fat intake. Although the public is aware of the potential danger of high-fat diets, many are not willing to give up the tastes to which they have become accustomed, and the chemical industry has responded by developing a host of artificial foods which simulate fats. These modern fat replacement foods have similar properties to fats, but they are manufactured from carbohydrates, proteins or modified fats.[3] The modified fats differ from normal fat, in that less is required to obtain the desired effect, or in that the modified fat is not absorbed, thus enabling one to eat without concern for weight gain or other disadvantages associated with a high-fat diet.

Reduced-fat products are appearing on supermarket shelves in increasing numbers, and they contain blends of altered nutrients designed to replace fats. Protein-based fat replacements are manufactured from milk and/or egg proteins and combined with water, sugar, pectin and citric acid. Carbohydrate-based replacements include **dextrins, modified food starches, polydextrose** and **gums**, which are used as such, or combined with fats to produce the desired effects. For all the potential benefits that these replacements may provide, the long-term effects of their use must still be evaluated. It has been estimated that their use can account for 30% to 40% of the food which a person consumes instead of the 1% to 2% of other food additives.[4] The long-term effects of the fat replacement practice, particularly in young children, must surely be a matter of concern. A switch to a whole-food programme will not only solve the problem of high-fat intakes, but will also provide a solution to the taste and texture question.

Fats in the diet

Triglycerides

Most of the fat consumed by humans is in the form of neutral fats which are formed when three fatty acids combine with glycerol to form a triglyceride (Fig. 3.1).

Saturated and unsaturated fatty acids

Fatty acids consist of hydrocarbon backbones which terminate in a carboxyl group (-COOH). Carbon has a valency of four, which means that it can combine with four other atoms, and in a saturated fatty acid all the additional bonds of the carbon chain are occupied by hydrogen atoms. There are thus no double bonds in the carbon chain of a saturated fatty acid. Animal fats are rich in saturated fatty acids and they contain mainly **palmitic acid** which contains sixteen carbon atoms, and **stearic acid**, which contains eighteen carbon atoms (figure 3.2).

Unsaturated fatty acids have one or more double bonds between carbon atoms, and the carbon molecules are therefore **"unsaturated"** with hydrogen atoms. Unsaturated fatty acids are commonly found in plant foods, and can be either **monounsaturated fatty acids** or **polyunsaturated fatty acids**, depending on the number of carbon atoms which contain double bonds. The unsaturated fatty acids are classified according to the

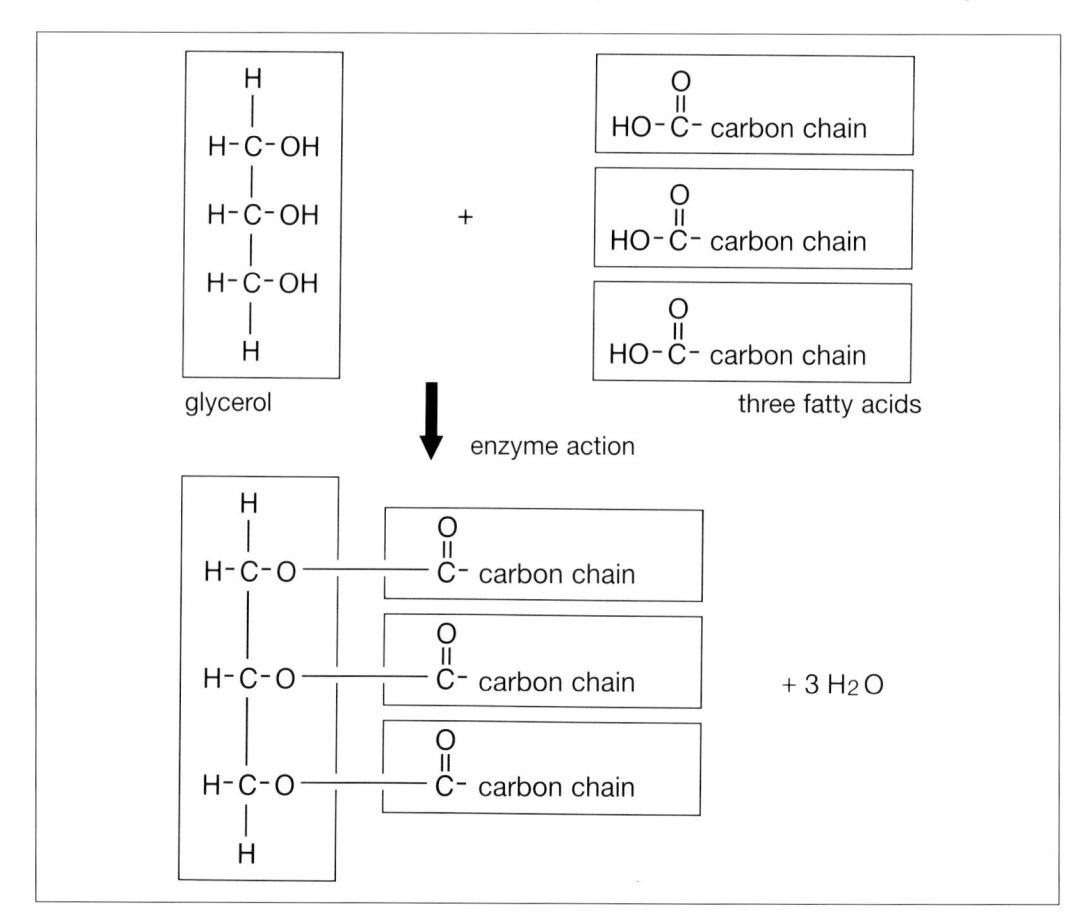

Figure 3.1. Formation of a triglyceride (a neutral fat)

position of the double bond which they contain ie, omega-9 (n-9), omega-6 (n-6), or omega-3 (n-3), then they can also have different isometric configurations, namely *cis* or *trans*. The principle fatty acid found in olive oil, for example, is oleic acid, and because oleic acid contains only one double bond in its carbon chain, it is a monounsaturated fatty acid (fig. 3.3).

Polyunsaturated fatty acids contain more than one double bond in the carbon chain and they are more common in plant foods than in animal foods. The most important polyunsaturates are **linoleic acid, linolenic acid** and **arachidonic acid**, of which linoleic acid is the most abundant. A further fatty acid in this group is **eicosopentanoic acid** which is a long-chain fatty acid found in fish oil. The double bonds between the carbon atoms of polyunsaturated fatty acids make the fat more fluid and lower the melting point, which is the reason why plant oils are normally liquid and animal fats are solid.

Essential fatty acids

Essential fatty acids are fatty acids which we cannot manufacture ourselves and which must therefore be obtained from the diet. Animals and humans are capable of elongating fatty acid chains and they can also desaturate fatty acid chains but they cannot desaturate the fatty acid carbon chain at positions six and three. Because linoleic acid and α-linolenic acid are unsaturated at these positions, they cannot be manufactured from other fatty acids and must therefore be obtained from the diet. These two fatty acids are essential components of cell membranes and act as precursors to a group of molecules known as **prostaglandins**. They are not required in large quantities, and it has been found that if they comprise 1% of total calories, then this is sufficient to prevent deficiency manifestations. Arachidonic acid is similar in structure to linoleic acid and α-linolenic acid, and originally it was also considered to be an essential fatty acid, but since it can be manufactured from linoleic acid, it is no longer considered an essential fatty acid. The structures of linoleic and linolenic acid are given in figure 3.4 and in figure 3.5 the distribution of fatty acids in plant foods is presented. In table 3.1 the major fatty acids in Western diets are presented.

$CH_3 - (CH_2)_{14} - COOH$ $CH_3 - (CH_2)_{16} - COOH$

Palmitic acid   Stearic acid

Figure 3.2. The structure of palmitic and stearic acid.

$CH_3 - (CH_2)_7 - CH = CH - (CH_2)_7 - COOH$

Oleic acid

Figure 3.3. The structure of oleic acid.

$$CH_3-(CH_2)_4-CH=CH-CH_2-CH=CH-(CH_2)_7-COOH$$

linoleic acid

$$CH_3-CH_2-CH=CH-CH_2-CH=CH-CH_2-CH=CH-(CH_2)_7-COOH$$

linolenic acid

Figure 3.4. The structure of linoleic and linolenic acid.

Cholesterol

Cholesterol belongs to a group of fats known as steroids. Cholesterol has been blamed for the coronary havoc wreaked in the world today, but cholesterol is an essential compound in all animals, and it forms an important substrate for several biosynthetic pathways. Cholesterol occurs in almost all samples of animal fats as well as in blood and bile and is thus mainly derived from the consumption of animal foods. Another source of cholesterol is endogenous cholesterol, which

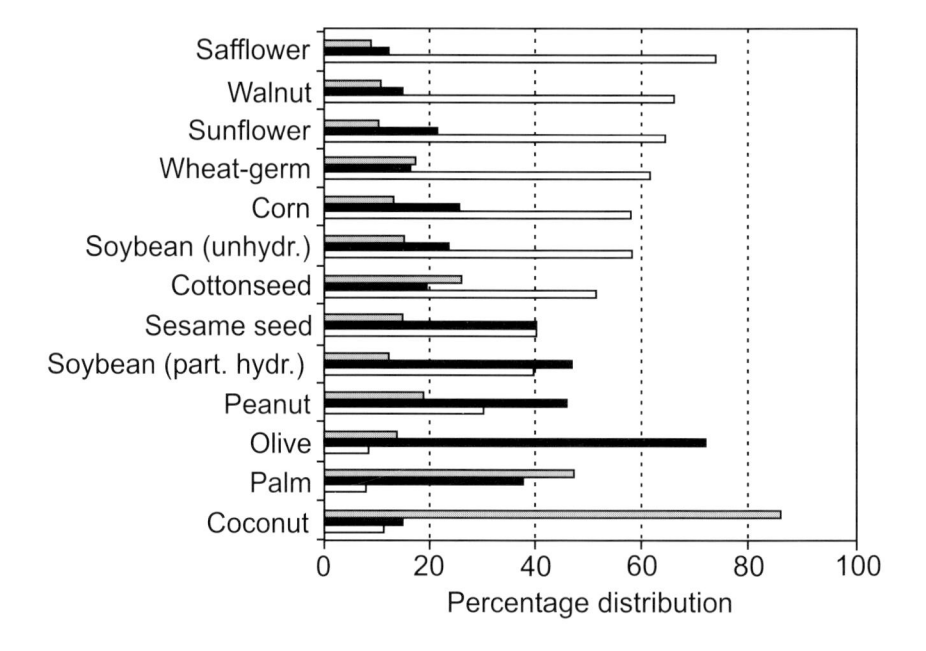

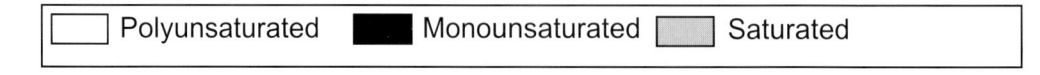

Figure 3.5. Fatty acid distribution in vegetable oils. (Adapted from reference 5)

is synthesized in the liver and intestine. Contrary to popular belief, plants do not produce cholesterol although they do produce phytosteroids. The consumption of plant foods per se, can therefore not increase cholesterol levels. In the absence of dietary cholesterol, the liver will synthesize enough cholesterol to meet all the needs of the body and a vegetarian diet will thus not lead to shortages in cholesterol.

Cholesterol is usually bound to two kinds of protein carriers which are called **high-density lipoprotein (HDL)** and **low-density lipoprotein (LDL)**. High levels of LDL are associated with vascular disease as these molecules tend to infiltrate arterial walls, whereas HDL seems to attract cholesterol out of the walls and transports it to the liver where it is metabolized. The consumption of animal fats will lead to increased levels of the harmful LDL-cholesterol, whereas plant foods tend to lower cholesterol levels. In table 3.2 the concentration of cholesterol in various foods is presented.

Fatty Acid	Common Abbreviation
Saturated	
Lauric acid	C12:0
Myristic acid	C14:0
Palmitic acid	C16:0
Stearic acid	C18:0
Monounsaturated	
n-9	
Oleic acid	cis C18:1 n-9
Elaidic acid	trans C18:1 n-9
Polyunsaturated	
n-6	
Linoleic acid	C18:2 n-6
Arachidonic acid	C20:4 n-6
n-3	
Linolenic acid	C18:3 n-3
Eicosopentaenoic acid	C20:5 n-3
Docosahexaenoic acid	C22:6 n-3

Table 3.1. The major fatty acids in the US diet. Besides these long-chain fatty acids the diets also include small quantities of short- and medium-chain fatty acids as well as other long-chain fatty acids. (From reference 6)

Digestion and absorption of fats

The digestive system breaks down food into simple components that can be readily absorbed, and these are then reconstituted into the various components of the body. Because fats are water-insoluble, their digestion and absorption is different from that of the other nutrients we eat. Fats must first be **emulsified**, which means that they must be dispersed in the aqueous medium of the intestinal contents before they can be broken down by enzymes. Emulsification is achieved by the addition of **bile salts** and **lecithin** to the gut contents which, together with the churning of the ingested material, breaks the fat up into droplets. These tiny droplets are then acted upon by enzymes known as **lipases** which are released by the pancreas. Lipases break the fat down into **fatty acids, monoglycerides** and **diglycerides**. By the further action of bile, still tinier droplets called **micelles** are formed which are polar and consist of bile and bile salts, monoglycerides, fatty acids and glycerol. Once these products have been absorbed by the absorptive cells of the intestines, they are again converted to triglycerides which together with phospholipids form protein-coated droplets known as **chylomicrons**.

About 80% of chylomicrons find their way into the lymphatic system via the lymph ducts of the gut villi, whilst the other products of digestion, such as the sugars and amino acids enter the bloodstream via the capillaries. The lymphatic system acts as a filter to remove harmful residues and bacteria before returning the fatty acids to the bloodstream. Excessive fat intake thus places severe demands on the lymphatic system and can lead to increased susceptibility to disease and common ailments such as fatigue, headaches, colds and flu.

Food item	Cholesterol (mg)	Food item	Cholesterol (mg)
Dairy products		Meat products (continued)	
Buttermilk	4	Frankfurter (chicken)	101
Camembert cheese	72	Goose (roasted)	91
Cheddar cheese	105	Ham (cooked, lean)	47
Cheese spread	55	Ham (cooked, regular)	57
Cottage cheese	26	Heart (beef)	230
Cottage cheese (low fat)	15	Heart (lamb)	260
Cottage cheese (fat free)	7	Kidney (ox)	690
Cream cheese	110	Liver (beef)	240
Fetta cheese	89	Liver (chicken)	631
Gouda cheese	114	Liver (pate)	120
Low fat hard cheese	108	Mutton (leg, roasted)	110
Milk (cow's, condensed)	34	Offal	331
Milk (cow's, powder)	97	Pork (Grilled, fat trimmed)	95
Milk (cow's, skim)	2	Pork (with fat)	94
Milk (cow's, whole)	14	Turkey (roasted)	82
Milk (goats)	11	Veal (roasted)	82
Milk (human)	14	Venison	80
*Milk (Soy)	0	Sea foods	
Parmesan cheese	79	Calamari (fried)	27
Processed cheese	94	Crab (cooked)	100
Yogurt	13	Haddock (smoked, boiled)	75
Egg products		Harder (steamed)	80
Boiled egg	548	Herring (grilled)	80
Dried whole egg	1918	Herring (pickeled)	70
Raw egg white	0	Kipper (baked)	80
Raw egg yolk	1602	Mackerel (steamed)	80
Meat products		Mussels (boiled)	100
Bacon (fried)	85	Oysters (raw)	54
Beef (braised, lean)	82	Prawns (boiled)	200
Beef (minced, lean)	82	Rock lobster (cooked)	104
Beef (rump steak)	82	Roe (caviar)	300
Brains (lamb)	2200	Salmon (red, canned)	100
Brawn	52	Sardines (canned)	100
Chicken (boiled)	83	Shrimps (boiled)	200
Chicken (giblets)	393	Trout (steamed)	80
Frankfurter (beef, pork)	50	White fish (steamed)	68

* Value for soy milk given for comparison.

Table 3.2. The cholesterol content of selected foods. The amounts are for 100 g edible portions. (Adapted from reference 7)

As there are no lipases nor emulsifiers secreted in the saliva or stomach, lipid digestion does not commence until the ingested food has left the stomach. Excess fat in the diet will also retard the digestive processes in the stomach, and protein digestion thus takes considerably longer if free fat is present. Moreover, the fat coats the ingested food making it difficult for the water-soluble enzymes in the stomach to penetrate and commence the process of digestion. This is particularly true if the protein is of animal origin, as animal proteins take longer to digest than plant proteins and also require a lower stomach pH than do plant proteins. Meat, for example, takes some 3-6 hours preparation time in the stomach, but the presence of free fat will lengthen the digestion time well beyond this point. A further consequence of this delay is that the products of carbohydrate digestion will start to ferment under these circumstances and lead to a build up of acid fermentation products. Protein foods prepared by frying or grilling will give a satisfied after-dinner feeling, but this is because of the longer time that the food remains in the stomach, and not because of the better nutrient quality of the food consumed. The presence of fats in the food retards the digestive process in the stomach because fat induces the release of a hormone known as **gastric inhibitory peptide (GIP)** which slows down the gastric activity.

Once the food has left the stomach and entered the duodenum, fatty acids in the duodenum will cause the release of another hormone known as **cholecystokinin-pancreozymin**, which induces the gall-bladder to contract and to release bile into the small intestine. This same hormone will also induce the pancreas to release sodium bicarbonate into the duodenum to neutralize the acid in the chyme so that the alkaline phases of digestion can commence. The phospholipid **lecithin**, which is produced in the liver and assists in the emulsification of fats, is also released into the duodenum. The presence of these emulsifiers makes it possible for the water-soluble enzymes in the duodenum to operate optimally, even in the presence of fat. In whole foods the fats are not in a free form (they are still surrounded by the phospholipid bilayer), and thus remain water-soluble until acted upon by the lipases in the duodenum. Even whole foods that are rich in fats, such as oil-seeds, nuts and oil rich fruits such as avocado pears and olives will thus not interfere with the digestive process in the stomach. Only once the fat has been extracted in its free form will it retard the digestive processes.

Lecithin plays a significant role in the metabolism of fats in general, and it protects against the accumulation of fatty deposits in the arteries. Lecithin is a phospholipid consisting of fatty acids, phosphoric acid, glycerol and the B-group vitamin choline. The pancreatic enzyme **phospholipase-A** liberates **lysolecithin** from lecithin and lysolecithin then acts as a detergent and assists in the emulsification process. As the liver can only produce a limited amount of lecithin per day, the regular consumption of fatty foods, particularly animal products, will lead to a reduction of lecithin reserves and lay the foundation for the development of arteriosclerosis. A regular supply of whole foods such as fruits, vegetables, grains, seeds, nuts and legumes will ensure that the body's lecithin needs are met. Legumes in particular are an excellent source of lecithin, but all whole foods will help the body to produce natural lecithin and aid in the emulsification of dietary lipids.

Fats and disease

Fats have been positively linked to numerous degenerative diseases such as cancer and cardiovascular disease, but a number of common ailments can also be attributed to a high-fat consumption. It is, however, not only the quantity of fat that is implicated in disease, but also the type of fat. In countries where fat consumption is low, the incidence of degenerative diseases is far lower than in Western countries with their high-fat consumption. The Japanese have a fat intake of only 10%–20%

of their food intake and they do not seem to suffer from the diseases prevalent in Western society, and also seem to enjoy greater longevity of life. This phenomenon is definitely linked to their lifestyle, because Japanese communities that have adopted Western lifestyles suffer from the same diseases that are prevalent in these societies.

Different fatty acids exert different effects, and though research into the role of fatty acids in disease causation is still in its infancy, some information is available. Precisely how fatty acid imbalances cause disease, is unknown, but because they are incorporated into cell membranes, changes in dietary intake of fatty acids can cause changes in membrane fluidity, responses to outside signals such as hormones, binding of ligands (ie, lipoproteins) to their membranes, lipid mediators of the intracellular signalling cascade (ie, inositol triphosphate, prostaglandin, and leukotrine production). Moreover, the oxidation products of fatty acids can cause damage and even cell death.[6]

Fats and cancer

The role of fats in cancer promotion has received much attention of late, as there is a strong correlation between various forms of cancer and total fat intake. Carcinogenic processes have two distinct stages: **Initiation** and **Promotion**. Initiation involves an irreversible interaction between a carcinogen and the genetic material of its target tissue. Not much is known about initiators, but **asbestos** (lung cancer), **viruses** (lymphatic cancers and cervical cancer) as well as **tobacco smoke** (lung cancer) are known to initiate cancer. Initiation does not generally lead to observable tumours unless promoters are present. These promoters can cause the transformed cells to form tumours. As the consumption of excess fats and certain types of fat can promote cancer, it is important to plan dietary strategies accordingly. In table 3.3 the association between fat and certain other parameters is presented. Clearly, fat is strong promoter of colon and prostate cancer, and fruits and vegetables act as anti-promoters.

Cancer of the breast, colon and prostate is common in countries with Western lifestyles such as Switzerland, the US and South Africa, but is rare in Japan. Japanese migrating to the US soon develop the same incidence of US prevalent cancers in view of a change in diet. In developing countries as much as 80% of total calories come from cereals and grains, but in industrialized countries there is a calo-

Site of cancer	Fat	Body weight	Fruits and vegetables	Alcohol	Smoked, salted and pickled foods
Lung			−		
Breast	+	+		±	
Colon	++		−		
Prostate	++				
Bladder					
Rectum	+		−	+	
Endometrium		++			
Oral cavity			−	+	
Stomach			−		++
Cervix			−		
Oesophagus			−	++	+

Table 3.3. The association between selected dietary components and cancer. (From Ref. 8)

rie intake shift towards animal fat, vegetable oil and refined sugar. This latter diet reduces the incidence of gastric cancer but increases the incidence of colon, ovarian, prostate and breast cancer. The drop in gastric cancer has been attributed to refrigeration, which has replaced salting, pickling and smoking as a means of food preservation. Countries such as Austria where smoked foods are used extensively, also have high incidences of gastric cancer.[9]

International correlation studies have shown that a high-fat intake increases the incidence of prostatic, breast and colon cancer. Prostate cancer has been correlated with diets high in animal fats such as fatty meats, cheeses, cream and eggs. The US, Britain, the Netherlands, Denmark and South Africa have some of the world's richest diets, and also have the highest incidence of breast cancer.[9] Diabetes and pancreas cancer are also positively correlated with a high-fat diet.[10] **Saturated fatty acids** in particular are associated with breast cancer, particularly in postmenopausal women,[11] colorectal adenomas,[12] and ovarian cancer, where a 20% increase in risk was observed for every 10 g of saturated fatty acids consumed.[13] The association between **polyunsaturated fats** and cancer is even more profound. Animal studies have shown that high linoleic acid consumption in particular promotes mammary tumours to a greater extent than saturated fatty acids. Safflower oil and corn oil, both rich sources of linoleic acid, where more likely to induce tumours than were olive oil or even coconut oil because these oils are poor in linoleic acid.[6]

Fibre, vitamin A, C and E, the trace element selenium, and some phytochemicals in certain vegetables, beans, seeds and herbs have been identified as **anti-promoters** which offer protection against cancer. The food types that offer this protection, as well as the distribution of phytochemicals, are discussed in chapter 7 and summarized in figure 7.3 and figure 7.4. These foods contain **sulfides, phytates, flavonoids, glucerates, carotenoids, coumarins, mono- and triterpenes, lignans, phenolic acids, indoles, isothiocyanates, phthalides**, and **polyacetylenes** which interfere with the processes of cancer initiation or promotion, and in this way block the formation of tumours (fig. 3.6).[14]

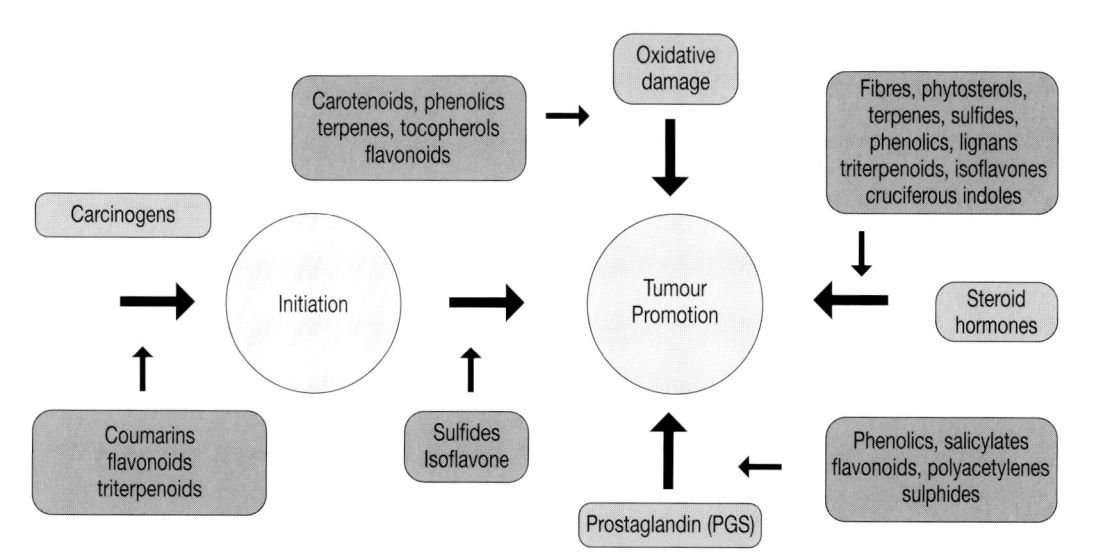

Figure 3.6. The effect of dietary phytochemicals on the processes of cancer initiation and promotion. (From reference 14)

Vitamin A probably acts as an anti-promoter for lung, colon, stomach, bladder, oesophagus and oral cavity cancers. Vitamin C and E are associated with reduced incidence of gastric cancer and selenium with a reduced incidence of breast and colon cancer.[9] Fibre on the other hand protects against cancer by decreasing the length of time that faecal matter stays in the digestive tract, thus limiting the build up of potential carcinogens.[15] Finns for example have a high consumption of whole grains and the associated high faecal mass has been cited as a contributing factor to the low incidence of colon cancer in this nation. The vegetarian lifestyle thus offers considerable protection against cancer, and a vegan diet seems to be more effective than other vegetarian diets. In studies conducted on vegetarians it was found that ovo-lacto vegetarians (vegetarians that include dairy products and eggs in their diet) have a higher incidence of prostate and ovarian cancer than do their vegan (vegetarians that do not use any animal products) counterparts.[16]

Cardiovascular disease

Coronary heart disease has become one of the biggest killers in modern societies, and the consumption of animal fats has been positively associated with this phenomenon. Arteriosclerosis does not only lead to heart disease, but can also be responsible for strokes and kidney diseases. Arteriosclerosis is a slow insidious disease which progresses slowly as a result of the deposition of fat and cholesterol in the walls of the arteries. These fatty deposits become hardened, making the blood vessels less elastic, and eventually clogging them with plaque (a mass of fat and cholesterol). It sometimes happens that blood platelets become caught on the rough edges of plaque, thus initiating clot formation. In this way blood flow to the tissues can be further diminished or stopped. If a clot stays in place it is called a **thrombus** but if it becomes dislodged and travels around it is called an **embolus**. Clogged blood vessels in turn lead to a host of secondary effects such as **ischaemia** (lack of blood supply and oxygen in the area supplied by the blood vessel) or coronary or cerebral **infarct** where the supply of oxygen is completely cut off as in the case of a heart attack or stroke. **Angina** attacks are an indication that the coronary arteries are clogged to the extent that only a quarter of the normal blood supply is being sent to the heart muscle.

It has been clearly established that high cholesterol levels can pose a serious risk of contracting cardiovascular diseases. Besides cholesterol, there are other compounding factors which increase the risk of getting a heart attack, such as high blood pressure and smoking. What is more, the risk is more than additive, as being exposed to more than one of these factors will more than double the risk of having a heart attack. Cholesterol levels per se are however not necessarily a good indicator of the overall risk, but it seems as if the relationship between HDL- and LDL-cholesterol is a better criterion to use when determining the risk factor. HDL-cholesterol has been firmly established as a predictor of protection from atherosclerotic disease. People with low HDL cholesterol levels have the highest heart attack rates, even if their cholesterol levels are in the supposedly safe range of 116 to 192 mg/dl for men and 124 to 211 mg/dl for women. LDL-cholesterol, on the other hand, appears to remain a risk factor throughout life.[17]

An elevated serum triglyceride level is also a risk factor for arteriosclerosis. This could be because high triglyceride levels are associated with low HDL-cholesterol levels. When triglyceride metabolism is efficient, the triglyceride concentration is low and the HDL concentration is high. When triglyceride metabolism is sluggish, the triglyceride concentration is high and the HDL concentration is low.[18] Elevated triglyceride levels will also lead to obesity which has also been established as a leading cause of disease. The incidence of obesity also increases with age, as do the risks of contracting cardiovascular disease.

The ratio of saturated to unsaturated fats

in the diet is also of significance when determining the risk of contracting cardiovascular disease. Saturated fat is highly correlated with the incidence of coronary heart disease.[6] A high intake of total fat, cholesterol and saturated fatty acids can also lead to thrombosis, as such diets increase the levels of fibrinogen and factor VII which could cause an increase in thrombosis tendency. Clinical studies have shown, that stearic acid is the most thrombogenic fatty acid,[6] and diets high in animal products will thus increase the risk of thrombosis. Research has focused for many years on the benefits of polyunsaturated fatty acids in the diet, and these fats have become the desirable replacement for saturated fats to lower cholesterol levels. However, this practice has raised some concern, as studies showed that polyunsaturated fats lowered the levels of the desirable HDL-cholesterol, which was not the case if foods rich in monounsaturated fatty acids were consumed.[19,20] Moreover, it was found that diets high in polyunsaturated fats increased the cancer risk[21] and had a negative influence on the immune system.[22] **Trans fatty acids** in the diet have been positively associated with cardiovascular disease. In the Nurses' Health Study,[23] a 50% increase in risk of heart disease in the highest versus the lowest levels of *trans* fatty acid consumption was reported, although there were no differences at the intermediate level of consumption. Clinical studies have also shown, that hydrogenated vegetable fats (corn, soy, cottonseed, peanut, or safflower) consistently increased blood cholesterol levels compared to the natural unhydrogenated oils.[6] Mediterranean diets rich in monounsaturated fats, on the other hand, seem to afford protection against heart disease and cancer.

Mediterranean diets include mainly olive oil as the main fat, and they contain lower levels of polyunsaturated and saturated fats. Mediterranean diets are also rich in grain products such as all kinds of breads, baked goods and pastas. They also include many legumes, seeds, nuts, fruits and vegetables. Populations on this type of diet have low cholesterol levels and a low incidence of coronary heart disease compared to counterparts in other regions of the same country.[21] Olives, canola oil, monounsaturated safflower and sunflower oils, and almonds are rich in oleic acid which is a monounsaturated fatty acid. In figure 3.7 the relationship between the various fatty acids in foods commonly used in Mediterranean countries is presented.

Vegan vegetarians consume very similar foods to those prevalent in Mediterranean diets. It has also been established that a vegan vegetarian diet can afford protection against cardiovascular diseases. Vegan vegetarians have lower LDL-cholesterol and triglyceride levels than are prevalent in the general population, but HDL-cholesterol levels are not depressed.[25] Thus the ideal relationship between these components can be maintained by a vegan diet and this lifestyle can help both adults and children to maintain or achieve desirable blood lipid levels. In view of the increase in the prevalence of cardiovascular diseases with age, a vegan vegetarian diet can contribute substantially to the quality of life during old age. There is also quite a body of evidence, that coronary lesions can even be reversed by extremely stringent diets combined with other lifestyle changes.[26] Having said this, it is essential to note, that stringent lifestyle changes may be acceptable for adults who want to reduce fat intake to prevent cardiovascular disease, but care should be taken not to enforce similar changes on children, who require higher fat intakes than adults.[27] For a more detailed discussion of these criteria see chapter 5.

Dietary lipids and immune function

The influence of fat on the immune function has only recently come under serious study. It is known that polyunsaturated fatty acids, particularly linoleic acid, are required for optimal functioning of the immune system, but there is an optimum level which should not be exceeded. In recent years there has been a tremendous increase in the consumption of polyunsaturated fats to combat heart disease, but this has brought to the fore a host of problems not previously envisaged. High levels of fats, particularly polyunsaturated fats, impact negatively on the immune system and decrease its ability to cope with cancer tumours, allergies, infections by microbial organisms and both thymic-dependent and thymic-independent antigens.[28]

Immune responses can thus be enhanced or depressed, depending on the concentration and extent of unsaturation of dietary lipids. It has been found that high-fat diets consistently depress resistance to malaria and tuberculosis in rats, and respiratory infections in chickens, but the same seems to be true for humans. Lower respiratory tract infections in infants, for example, are significantly more common in obese infants than in non-obese infants, and in one third of obese infants, adolescents and adults studied there was impairment of cell-mediated immune responses.[29]

The mechanism whereby fats interfere with the body's ability to combat the growth of cancerous tumours has also been investigated. A subpopulation of **T-lymphocytes**, known as **natural killer cells**, specifically react to destroy tumour cells before they can proliferate. Recently it has been found that diets high in polyunsaturates, particularly those rich in n-6 fatty acids (e.g. linolenic acid), impact negatively on the ability of these killer cells to seek out and destroy cancer cells.[30] The three types of blood cells associated with the immune response are the **granulocytes**, **monocytes** and **lymphocytes**. The **neutrophils** are the most abundant granulocytes and they destroy antigens by simply engulfing them. **Macrophages** of monocytic origin, are also phagocytes but they carry out other functions as well. They secrete substances known as **lymphokines** and **prostaglandins** that affect B- and T-cell activity in many ways. Examples of lymphokines are **interferon** and **interleukon 1**, of which interferon stimulates T-cell proliferation and interleukon 1 stimulates a broad range of cells, including the natural killer cells, neutrophils, and B- and T-lymphocytes. T-cells do not produce antibodies, but B-lymphocytes produce antibodies which combine with antigens, rendering them inactive and enabling phagocytes to engulf the invaders.

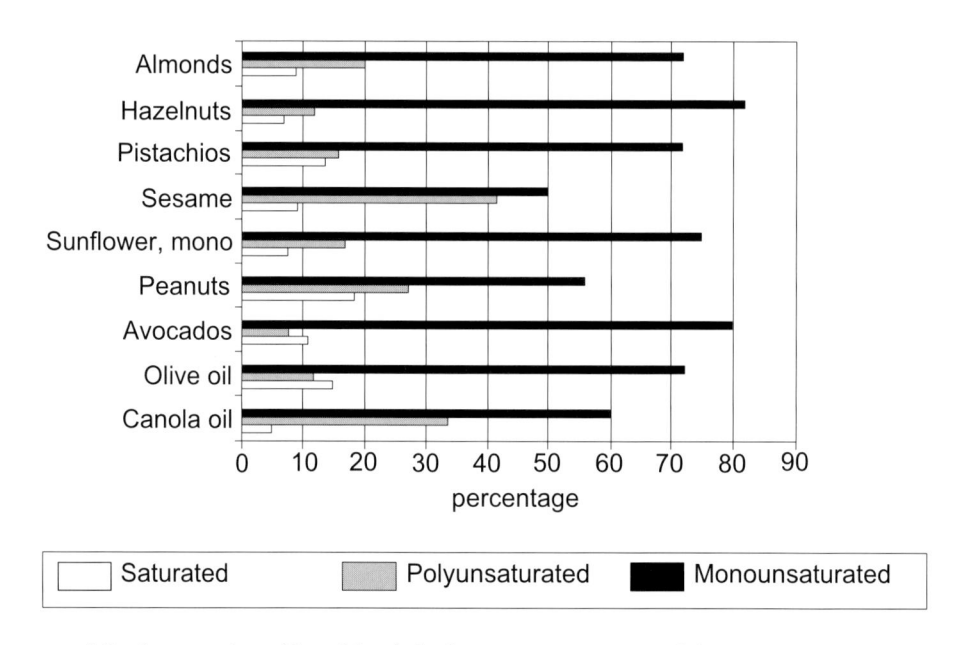

Figure 3.7. The fatty acid profiles of foods high in monounsaturated fats. (From reference 25)

Prostaglandins, thromboxanes, and **leucotrienes** are **eicosanoids** which are produced from the essential fatty acids, linolenic and linoleic acid. Generally, prostaglandins function as vasoconstrictors, thromboxanes affect platelet aggregation, and leucotrienes contract smooth muscle cells. Those prostaglandins that have a relaxing, anti-inflammatory and anti-clotting effect are generally formed from alpha-linolenic acid (**Triene prostaglandins**) whilst those with the opposite effect are manufactured from linoleic acid (**Monoene prostaglandins**) and arachidonic acid (**Diene prostaglandins**). More than one hundred different prostaglandins have been identified, and they promote or inhibit basic bodily functions such as fever, blood clotting, vasodilation and constriction, stress, allergy response, membrane permeability, eye pressure, inflammation, steroid production, appetite, fat metabolism and the functioning of the immune system.[31] When prostaglandins occur in a balanced relationship they tend to relax arteries and reduce blood pressure as well as slow down tumour formation and decrease platelet aggregation, thus lowering the risk of thrombus formation. If the balance of prostaglandins is, however, disturbed then the opposite effects are achieved. It is interesting to note that tumour cells produce large amounts of the prostaglandin PGE_2 and cancer patients can produce four times the normal amount of this prostaglandin. It has an immunorepressive effect and leucotriene B_4 is a potent chemotactic and chemokinetic agent.[6] For a summary of the effects of eicosanoids see figure 3.8.

A reduction in the amounts of polyunsaturated fats in the diet, inclusive of the essential fatty acids, can provide a substantial anticarcinogenic effect.[32,33] A whole-food diet, which includes grains, legumes, seeds and nuts will provide the ideal blend of fatty acids and total fat composition to ensure the optimal functioning of the immune system.

Processed fats

In today's world the appearance, texture and colour of food is often considered of greater importance than the nutrient value of such food. In an instant world we need instant food, and to avoid spoilage and financial loss, such food is often chemically manipulated to obtain all these desired effects. When the chemical nature of our food is changed so that it meets the requirements of the market place, then the risk is great that it no longer meets the requirements of the body. Our bodies are designed to interact with the environment in a highly specialized way, and any interference with this delicate balance may impact negatively on the system.

Modern oil refining techniques

Extracted oil undergoes a series of steps which adversely affects its nutritional value. Free fatty acids are removed by vacuum extraction and precipitation. Furthermore, the oil is filtered and heated to 220 °C to obtain a clear liquid. In order to obtain a less fluid oil, suitable for the production of margarine, the oil is further subjected to the process of hydrogenation, to which liquid oils nowadays are also partially subjected. This process was developed by W. Norman in the year 1900 and involves a catalytic reaction which changes **cis** fatty acids to **trans** fatty acids, thus rendering them less fluid by changing the shape of the molecules.

Polyunsaturated fats contain double bonds, and this gives rise to the possibility of **cis-trans** conversions. In nature, fatty acids occur mainly in the cis configuration, which means that the carbon chains on either side of the double bond are spatially arranged on the same side of the double bond, whereas in the trans configuration the chains are on opposite sides of the double bond. The cis and trans configurations of oleic acid (which has just one double bond) are presented in figure 3.9.

Trans fats do not form part of the normal diet and should not be introduced into the

```
                        Dietary Fatty Acids
                                ⇓
                        Arachodonic Acid
                        membrane phospholipids
                          ↙    ⇓    ↘
     Prostaglandins       Thromboxane        Leucotrienes

CHD, Hypertension &    CHD, Hypertension &   Cancer & Immune Response
Trombosis:             Thrombosis            – mediates immune cell
– platelet activation  – platelet aggregation   adhesion
– vasoconstriction     – vasoconstriction    – proliferation
                                             – cytokine production
Cancer & Immune                              – lymphocyte proliferation
Response:                                    – vascular permeability
– cytokine production
– lymphocyte proliferation
– antibody production
```

Figure 3.8. The effects of eicosanoid imbalances on various diseases. (From reference 6)

system as they can result in a number of biochemical changes, and together with saturated fats and cholesterol, can lead to altered membrane structure and concomitant hardening of the arteries. The essential fatty acids (linoleic and linolenic acids) also naturally have the cis configuration, and in linoleic acid the atoms are arranged in such a fashion that there is a 60° bend at each of the two double bonds, resulting in a U-shaped molecule. Trans-linoleic acid however has a Z-shape as the chains on either side of the double bond do not project into the same plane. The free use of extracted, partially hydrogenated oil, rich in linoleic acid (found in corn, safflower and sunflower oils), has been associated with

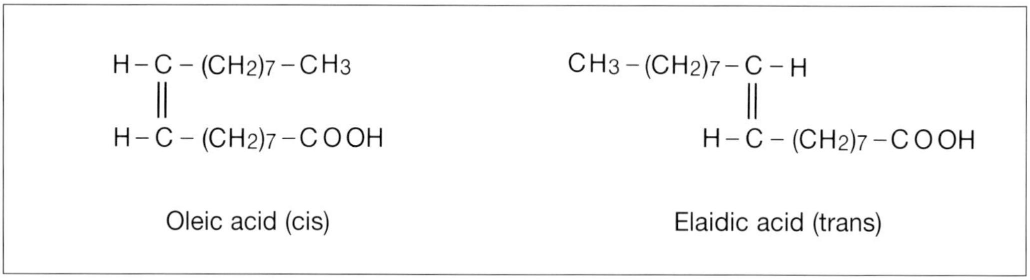

```
    H – C – (CH2)7 – CH3              CH3 – (CH2)7 – C – H
        ‖                                              ‖
    H – C – (CH2)7 – COOH             H – C – (CH2)7 – COOH

         Oleic acid (cis)                   Elaidic acid (trans)
```

Figure 3.9. The cis and trans configuration of oleic acid.

cancer promotion. Linoleic acid is the substrate from which prostaglandins are manufactured, and trans-linoleic acid can result in altered prostaglandins, thus modifying the effect of these hormones or even producing opposite effects. Because leucotrienes play an essential role in regulating the immune system in that they are involved in the production of antibodies and the destruction of viruses and cancer cells, it is essential that these molecules be produced from essential fatty acids that have the correct configuration so that the delicate balance and the function may not be jeopardized.

The molecular changes found in even partially hydrogenated oils can adversely affect the relationship between the various prostaglandins as well as changing them structurally. Trans fatty acids depress serum levels of prostaglandins, and both PGE_1 and PGE_2 were affected in a study done on rats, presumably because linoleic acid could not be converted to long chain fatty acids in the presence of a large influx of the trans-isomer.[34,35] Moreover, hydrogenated oils do not share the properties of normal unsaturated fats and will also not lower cholesterol levels as do the natural oils in whole foods.[6,36] The consumption of trans fatty acids in the Western world is quite high, and it has been estimated that in the US and in Canada, men of 20–39 years of age consume 11–12 g per person per day of these fats.[36] The British Medical Committee on Cardiovascular Diseases proposed new guidelines in 1994 on recommended consumption of fatty acids. Recognizing that trans fatty acids have an undesirable effect on HDL and LDL cholesterol and coronorary disease mortality, they suggested that no more than 2% of caloric intake come from this source, and that the amount should even be reduced.[37]

Margarine

Margarine is typically manufactured from the oil of soya beans, maize, sunflower seeds, olives, coconut and palm, with the addition of substances which enhance the flavour and act as preservatives and texturisers. The typical ingredients of margarine include a combination of oils, water, sodium chloride, vitamins A, D and E, lecithin or other emulsifier, preservatives such as sodium benzoate and/or potassium sorbate, milk solids including casein, colorants such as beta-carotene and retinyl esters, flavourants such as butter distillate or simulated butter taste chemicals. The manufacturing process of margarine involves a combination of a number of steps. The fat-insoluble gums and other substances from the crude oil are first removed and then the oil is neutralized with alkali. Subsequently it is bleached, filtered, deodorized and in most cases hydrogenated. After this the product is again subjected to further filtration, neutralization, bleaching, deodorization and blending. Finally, colorants, flavourants, vitamins, emulsifiers and preservatives are added, and proportioning (creating the desired balance between water and fat), emulsification, chilling and packaging round off the final product.

In most cases, margarines exceed the recommended maximum levels for saturated and trans-unsaturated fatty acids, but some countries (Germany) have taken cognizance of the detrimental effects of trans fatty acids and many of the margarines, shortenings and cooking fats in Germany are being produced essentially free from trans fatty acids. Nevertheless, a concentrated, chemically manipulated, unnatural food such as margarine must place excessive demands on the system, and viable alternatives should be sought. Artificial foods are however the vogue, and large quantities of spreads and non-dairy creamers are consumed annually. Non-dairy creamers also contain extracted saturated and hydrogenated plant oils of coconut and palm origin, and therefore contain no less fat than dairy cream.

There are many ways to prepare palatable meals without the use of extracted oils, and their use can thus be limited. The best way of obtaining chemically sound fats, suitable for maintaining the fine chemical balances of the body, is to eat whole food that has not been changed by modern refining techniques.

Whole grains, seeds, nuts as well as oil-rich fruits such as avocado pears and olives, together with other plant sources will supply an abundance of fats of the variety required by the body.

The use of oil in the frying of food

The frying of food in oil or lard also has detrimental effects. Studies have shown that heated oils and fats undergo autoxidation and that the rate of autoxidation is proportional to the degree of unsaturation and the presence or absence of **pro-** and **anti-oxidants**. It has been established that animal fats undergo autoxidation more readily than oils of plant origin, in spite of the fact that animal fats are saturated fats, but this has been attributed to the virtual absence of natural antioxidants in animal fats. Polyunsaturates, however, sustain the most thermo-oxidative damage when oil is heated. In this regard it is enlightening that a tri-unsaturated fatty acid will undergo autoxidation 10 000 times more readily than a monounsaturated fatty acid.[38] The rate and degree of autoxidation of unsaturated and saturated fats is presented in figure 3.10.

The products formed in fats and oils that are heated to high temperatures are **peroxides, aldehydes, ketones, hydroperoxides, polymers** and **cyclic monomers**, any one of which can have toxic effects. Subjecting saturated and polyunsaturated fats, such as butter and sunflower oil to temperatures of 170 °C for two hours will so alter the

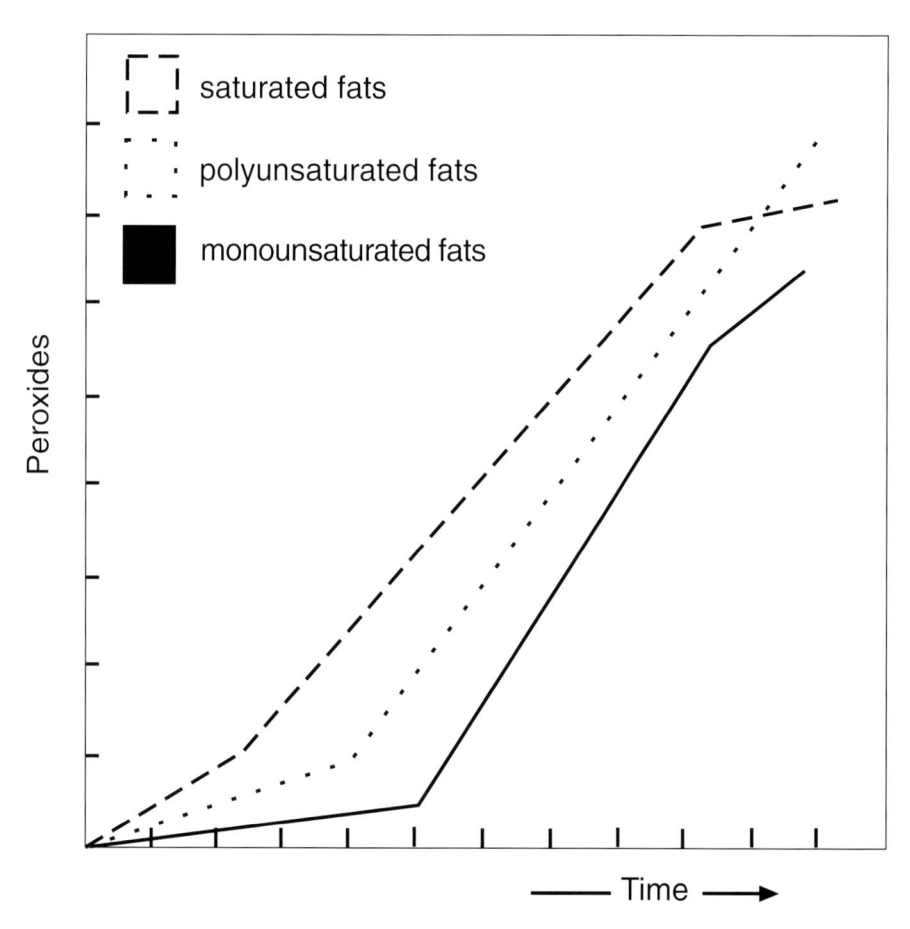

Figure 3.10. Heat damage sustained by oil. (Adapted from reference 20)

composition that if fed to experimental animals they will induce liver ailments in these animals. If animal fat, polyunsaturated oil, and even monounsaturated oil such as olive oil, is however heated to 180 °C for longer periods of time, serious liver disorders are induced in experimental animals that are fed these oils.[39] The peroxidised fatty acids in heated fats also affect the cardiovascular system, possibly even causing lesions in the cardiac muscles and arterial lining as well as enhancing clot formation.[40]

As most processed oils are heated to 220 °C during the manufacturing process, and are still further heated during the frying process, the use of free oil should for these reasons alone, not be encouraged. The frying of food should therefore be avoided if healthful living practices are introduced into the household. This does not necessarily mean that taste must be sacrificed, but it does mean that age-old habits will have to be revised and substituted with a little bit of ingenuity. If oil is used at all, it should be used in moderation and the cold-pressed variety should be used as this has been least subjected to heat during the extraction and clarifying processes. Also oils rich in monounsaturated fats, such as olive oil, should be the oils of choice as monounsaturated fats undergo the least damage during heating.

Whilst it is true that increased dietary consumption of polyunsaturated fats has led to a decrease in cholesterolaemia and associated drop in cardiovascular disease, it has been accompanied by a rise in deaths from non-vascular diseases such as cancer,[41] cholelithiasis[42,43] and a general drop in life expectancy,[44] probably resulting from the peroxidation of the polyunsaturates. Peroxidation of polyunsaturates takes place because these molecules are unstable, and the more double bonds there are in the molecules the more readily the process of peroxidation takes place. During this process **"free radicals"** are formed which are extremely reactive in view of their unpaired electron. Free radical formation is largely prevented in whole foods, as natural antioxidants, which are present in these foods, prevent their formation. A natural balance exists between antioxidants such as the fat-soluble vitamins A and E and the quantity of polyunsaturated fats that are present in whole foods. An imbalance between polyunsaturates and antioxidants will result in a rise in free radical formation with concomitant harmful results such as an increase in the rate of the aging process,[44,45,46] inflammation,[47] carcinogenesis,[48,49,50] liver disorders[51] and arteriosclerosis.[52,53]

Unfortunately modern food processing techniques often strip food of the essential fatty acids and vital prepacked antioxidants and in this way deprive the system of these essential nutrients. During the refining process grains, for example, are stripped of the germ, which contains the essential oils and fat-soluble antioxidant vitamins in a perfect biorelationship, and the lack is then substituted for with large intakes of disproportionate combinations of processed oils and fats. In this regard it is enlightening to note that the daily vitamin E requirements (which amount to about 10 mg per day) increases 200fold if polyunsaturates are added to the diet.[53] It is doubtful whether any diet will supply this additional requirement without supplementation, and it is therefore not surprising that the degenerate diseases are so prevalent in Western societies. The eating of whole foods that have not been stripped of their essential components will supply all the essential oils required in healthful combinations and should therefore be encouraged.

References

1. Bruton, R.R., Clifford, C.K. and Lanza, E. 1988. NCI dietary guidelines: rationale. *Am. J. Clin. Nutr.* 48:888–95.

2. Diet and Health Committee. 1989. Diet and health, implications for reducing chronic disease risk. Washington, DC: National Research Council, National Academy Press.

3. ADA Reports. 1991. Position of the American

Dietetic Association: Fat replacements. *J.Amer. Diet.Assoc*. 91:1285–1288.

4. Stark, C. 1988. Fake fats raise real issues. Professional Perspectives. No. 4. Ithaca, NY: Cornell University.

5. Williams, S.R. 1989. Nutrition and diet therapy. 6th. ed. Times Mirror/Mosby College Publishing. St. Louis.

6. Jonnalagagadda, S.S., Mustad, V.A., Yu, S., Etherton, T.D., Kris-Etherton, P.M. 1996. Effects of individual fatty acids on chronic diseases. *Nutrition Today*. 31 (3) May/June 1996.

7. RIND. 1986. Food composition tables. 2nd. ed. South African Medical Research Council.

8. World Health Organization. 1990. *Diet Nutrition and the Prevention of Chronic Diseases*. Technical Report Series 797, Geneva: WHO, 1990.

9. Cohen, L.A. 1987. Diet and Cancer. *Sci. Amer*. 257:42–49.

10. Dwyer, J.T. 1988. Health aspects of vegetarian diets. *Am. J. Clin. Nutr*.48:712–38.

11. Howe, G.R., Hirohata, T., Hislop, T.G., Isovich, J.M., Yuan, J.M. Hatsouyanni, K., Lubin, F. Marubini, E., Modan, B., Rohan, T., Toniolo, P., Shunzhang, Y. 1990. Dietary factors and risk of breast cancer: Combined analysis of 12 case-control studies. *J.Natl Cancer Inst*. 82:561–9.

12. Giovannucci, E., Stampfer, M.J., Colditz, G., Renim, E.B., Willett, W.C. 1992. *J.Natl Cancer Inst*. 84:91–8.

13. Rish, H.A., Jain, M., Marrett, L.D., Howe, G.R. 1994. Dietary fat intake and risk of epithelial ovarian cancer. A pooled analysis. *J.Natl Cancer Inst*. 86:1409–15.

14. Caragay, A.B. 1992. Cancer-preventive foods and ingredients. *Food Tech*. April 1992.

15. Anderson, J.W.A. and Gustafson, N.J. 1988. Hypocholesterolemic effects of oat and bean products. *Am. J. Clin. Nutr*.48:749–53.

16. Snowdon, D.A. 1988. Animal products consumption and mortality because of all causes combined, coronary heart disease, stroke, diabetes and cancer in Seventh-day Adventists. *Am. J. Clin. Nutr*.48:749–53.

17. Abbott, R.D., Wilson, P.W.F., Kannel, W.B., Castelli, W.P. 1988. High density lipoprotein cholesterol, total cholesterol screening, and myocardial infarction. The Framington study. *Arteriosclerosis*. 8:207–11.

18. Albrink, M.J. 1991. Age-related dietary guidance and cardiovascular risk assessment. *Nutrition Today*. July/August 1991.

19. Mattson, F.H., Grundy, S.M. 1985. Comparison of effects of dietary saturated, monounsaturated, and polyunsaturated fatty acids on plasma lipids and lipoproteins in man. *J.Lipid.Res*. 26:194.

20. Grundy, S.M. 1989. Monounsaturated fatty acids and cholesterol metabolism: Implications for dietary recommendations. *J.Nutr*.119:529.

21. Broitman, S.A., Vitale, J.J., Jakuba, E.V., Gottlieb, L.S. 1977. Polyunsaturated fat, cholesterol and bowel tumorigenesis. *Cancer*. 40:2455.

22. Bennet, M., Uauy, R., Grundy, S.M. 1987. Dietary fatty acid effects on T cell-mediated immunity in mice infected with mycoplasma pulmonis or injected with carcinogens. *Am.J.Pathol*. 1236:103.

23. Willett, W.C., Stampfer, M.J., Monson, J.E., Colditz, G.A., Speizer, F.E., Posner, B.A., Sampson, L.A., Hennekens, C.H. 1993. Intake of *trans* fatty acid and the risk of coronary heart disease among women. *Lancet*. 341:581–5.

24. Spiller G.A. 1991. Health effects of Mediterranean diets and monounsaturated fats. *Cereal Foods World*. 36:812–814.

25. Resnicow, K., Barone, J., Engle, A., Miller, S., Haley, N,C., Fleming, D., Wynder, E. 1991. Diet and serum lipids in vegan vegetarians: A model for risk reduction. *J.Am.Diet.Assoc*. 91:447–453.

26. Scrimshaw, N.S. 1996. Nutrition and Health from Womb to Tomb. *Nutrition Today*.31 (2), March/April 1996. pp. 55–67

27. Olson, R.E. 1995. The folly of restricting fat in the diet of children. *Nutrition Today*. 30 (6), November/December, 1995. pp. 234–244.

28. Maki, P.A., Newberne, P.M. 1992. Dietary lipids and immune function. *J.Nutr*. 122:610–614.

29. Chandra, R.K. 1981. Immune response in overnutrition. *Cancer Res*. 41:3795–3796.

30. Byham, L.D. 1991. Dietary fat and natural killer cell function. *Nutrition Today*. Jan/Feb 1991, pp. 31–36.

31. Lee, L.B. 1976. "Prostaglandins and blood pressure control" (Combined clinical and basic science seminars) *Am. J. of medicine* 61:681.

32. Barone, J., Hebert, J.R., Reddy, M.M. 1989. Dietary fat and natural killer cell activity. *Am.J.Clin. Nutr*. 50:103–106.

33. Hebert, J.R., Barone, J., Reddy, M.M., Backlund, J.Y. 1990. Natural killer cell activity in a longitudinal dietary fat intervention trial. *Clin.Immunol.Immunopathol*. 54:103–16.

34. Hwang, D.L., Kinsella, J.E. 1979. The effect of trans, trans-methyl linoleate on the concentra-

References

tion of prostaglandins and their precursors in rats. *Prostaglandins*. 17:543.

35. Kanhai, J. 1988. Hydrogenation of edible oils – Toxicological and nutritional implications: A review. *Food Chem*. 27:191–201.

36. Mensink, R.P., Katan, M.B. 1990. Effect of dietary trans fatty acids on high-density and low-density lipoprotein cholesterol levels in healthy subjects. *New Engl.J.Med*. 323:439.

37. Nutrition Today Newsbreaks. 1995. British scientists endorse new fatty acid guidelines. *Nutrition Today*. 30 (1), January/February 1995. p. 5

38. Fedeli, E. 1984. La auto-ossidazione Lipidica. In: *Simp. su „Rrilettura di un problema: I lipidi Alimentari", Rimini* (Italia)

39. Alexander, J.C. 1978. Biological effects due to changes in fats during heating. (In: Symp. on frying oils, Presented at AOCS 68th Annual meeting, New York City, New York (USA) 11.5. 1977). *J.Am.oil Chem.Soc*. 55:711.

40. Giani, E., Masi, I., Galli, I. 1985. Heated fat, vitamin E and vascular eicosanoids. *Lipids*. 20:439.

41. Oliver, M.F. 1981. Diet and Coronary Heart disease. *Brit. Med. Bull*. 37:49.

42. Stundervanti, R., Pearce, M.L., Dayton, S. 1973. Increase prevalence of cholelithiasis in men ingesting a serum cholesterol-lowering diet. *N. Engl. J. Med*. 24:288.

43. Bennion, L. J., Grundy, S. M. 1978. Risk factors for the development of cholelithiasis in men. *N. Engl. J. Med*. 29:1221.

44. Harman D. 1982. The Free-Radical Theory of Aging. In: Free radicals in Biology. Prior W.A. Ed., Vol. 5, p. 55, New York, Academic Press.

45. Timiras, P.S. 1982. Radicali liberi, malattie ed invecchiamento. *Fed.Med*. 8:890.

46. Toffano, G., Calderini, G., 1984. Nuove prospetive sperimentali dell'invecchiamento cerebrale. *Fidia Biomed. Inform., Anno* 1, n. 2, aprile maggio.

47. Babior, M.E. 1977. Oxygen dependent microbia killing of phagocytes. *N. Engl. J. Med*. 298:659.

48. Graham, S., Marshall, J., Mettlin, C., Rzepka, T.; Nemoto, T. 1982. Diet in the epidemiology of breast cancer. *Am. J. Epidem*. 116:65.

49. Vitale, J. J., Broitman, S.A. 1981. Lipids and Immune Function. *Cancer Res*. 41:3706.

50. Santamaria, L., Bianchi, A. 1984. I carotenoidi e le vitamine anti ossidantie nella prevenzione alimentare di malatti neoplastiche e dell'invecchiamento. In: *Simposio su "Rilettura di un problema, I lipidi alimentari", Rimini* (Italia) 12-13 ott.

51. Dianzani, M.U. 1978. La perossidazione lipidica nella patogenesi delle lesioni cellulari. In: *Simposio su "Il contenuto ottimale di acido linoleico nella dieta", Sestri Levante (Italia) 26–28 Maggio*, p. 143.

52. Mingrone, G., Passi, S., Gambassi, G. 1984. Lipoperossidazione e aterosclerosi: Effeto degli acidi grassi polinsaturi della dieta nella induzione dell'aterosclerosi spermentale. In: *Simp. su "aggiornamenti sull'aterosclerosi"*, Roma, 13 nov.

53. Ursini, F. 1984. Perrossidazione lipdica, invecchiamento ed aterosclerosi, possible ruolo degli acidi grassi polinsaturi. In: *Simp. su "Aaggiornamenti sull'aterosclerosi"*, Roma, 13 nov.

Chapter 4
Animal Products

It is becoming more and more evident, that many degenerative diseases can be directly linked to dietary lifestyles. Moreover, the incidence of these diseases is also higher in Western cultures than in Eastern cultures. Western lifestyles are, however, becoming popular even in the East, and with this encroachment, degenerative diseases are becoming increasingly prevalent even in societies where these diseases were virtually unknown in the past. Besides coronary heart disease, the incidence of cancer in Western societies is very high, and most of the major cancers can be linked to lifestyles thus making them potentially preventable diseases. The most common cancers occurring in Western societies are listed in table 4.1.

In table 4.1 the major cancers are listed in order of prevalence, and the rates are age standardized. However, the risk of cancer increases with age, and the **age specific** incidence of cancer can give a clearer picture of the risk for various age categories. These figures are presented in figure 4.1.

Even when age is taken into account, major discrepancies between the incidence of the various cancers occur in different countries, indicating that national lifestyle choices impact directly on the prevalence of cancer in these societies. These differences are not as a consequence of inheritable differences in resistance to cancer among the different races and nationalities, but are directly related to lifestyle choices. A well studied example of this impact, is the change in incidence of colorectal cancer in Japan with the adoption of a more Western orientated lifestyle. Whereas the rates for colorectal cancer were once low in Japan, there has been a rapid increase in age specific incidence of this cancer since

Site	Male	Site	Female
Bronchus, lung	65.4	Breast	56.1
Colorectal	30.8	Colorectal	22.4
Prostate	23.1	Bronchus, lung	20.5
Bladder	17.7	Uterus	19.9
Stomach	16.9	Ovary	11.4
Pancreas	7.4	Stomach	6.8
Oesophagus	6.5	Bladder	4.9
Kidney	5.6	Pancreas	4.9

Table 4.1. Age standardized rates for the major cancers excluding skin in men and women in England and Wales. (From reference 1,2.)

1960, and rates are approaching those recorded in Britain (fig. 4.2.)

As discussed in the previous chapters, a healthy diet is one that relies on a high complex-carbohydrate intake whilst at the same time limiting the consumption of proteins and fats. Diets rich in animal products, on the other hand, are high-fat, high-cholesterol, high-protein diets and carbohydrates, including fibre, are present in negligible amounts. By definition therefore, diets high in animal products must therefore be considered a health risk. In spite of these facts, the media encourages humanity to consume more and more animal products to prop up and maintain the vast economic empires that have been erected upon the foundations of the animal-products industry. Consumers are brought under the wrong impression by the advertising claims of manufacturers, and as a result there has been a dramatic rise in the consumption of animal products in the industrialized world over the past few decades. Moreover, some of the advertising claims have even left their mark on the medical profession, which often prescribes diets rich in animal products such as dairy products to ensure adequate supplies of essential nutrients.

Consumption of animal products has risen sharply in the United States since the US Department of Agriculture began keeping records in 1910, whereas consumption of fruits, vegetables and grains has declined drastically. Meat, fish and poultry only contributed 30% of the total protein consumption of Americans from 1909-1933, but this figure gradually rose, together with that of dairy products, so that these commodities today supply a staggering 70% of proteins consumed by that nation, and a similar trend is apparent in other industrialized nations.

The consumption of animal products has been positively associated with mortality because of disease, particularly heart disease, diabetes and cancer. In a study on the cause of mortality, carried out on vegetarians and non-vegetarians in California, it was found that the consumption of animal products could be correlated with mortality from degenerative diseases. It was found that meat consumption could be positively correlated with all causes-combined-mortality in males whereas there was a positive correlation of egg consumption and all causes-combined-mortality in females.[4] Meat consumption particularly increased the relative risk of mortality from coronary heart disease, diabetes, colon cancer and prostate cancer in males (fig. 4.3a), whereas in females, meat consumption could be positively correlated with mortality from coronary heart disease, and ovarian cancer (fig. 4.3b).

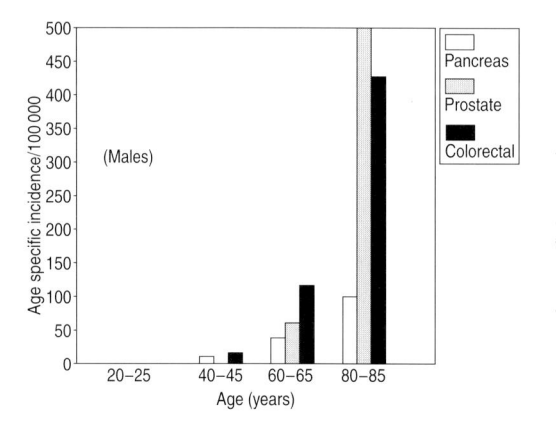

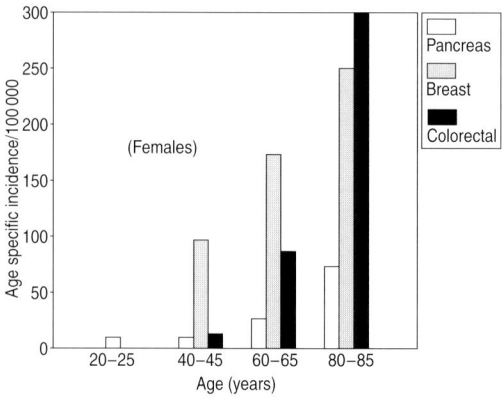

Figure 4.1. Age specific incidence rates for various cancers in males and females in England and Wales. (Adapted from references 2,3)

Animal Products

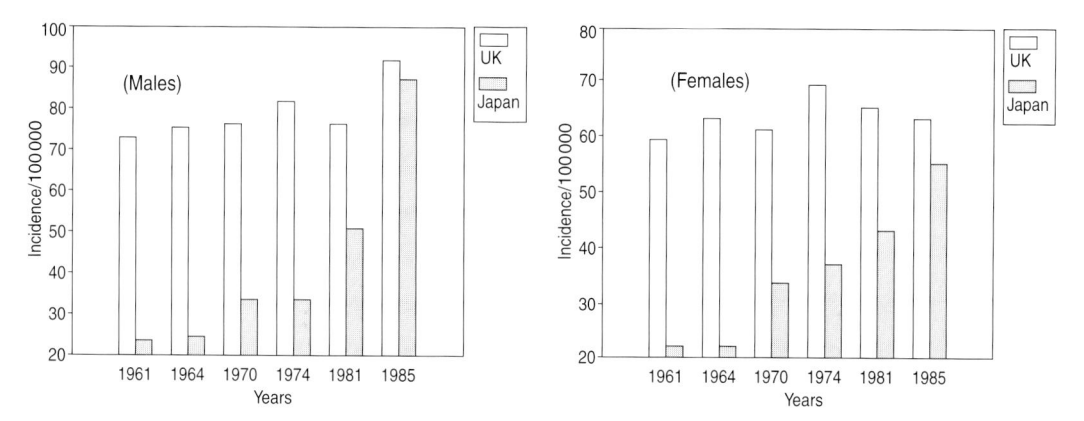

Figure 4.2. Age specific colorectal cancer incidence rates in men and women aged 55-60 in Japan and the UK. (Adapted from references 1,2,3)

Meat is not the only animal product that increases the risk of mortality. Dairy products and eggs show similar trends. In the case of eggs, there was a moderate increased risk in males from diseases such as colon cancer and prostate cancer (fig. 4.4a), and in females there was a moderate to high risk of mortality from colon and ovarian cancer (fig. 4.4b).

The consumption of dairy products could also be correlated with increased incidence of

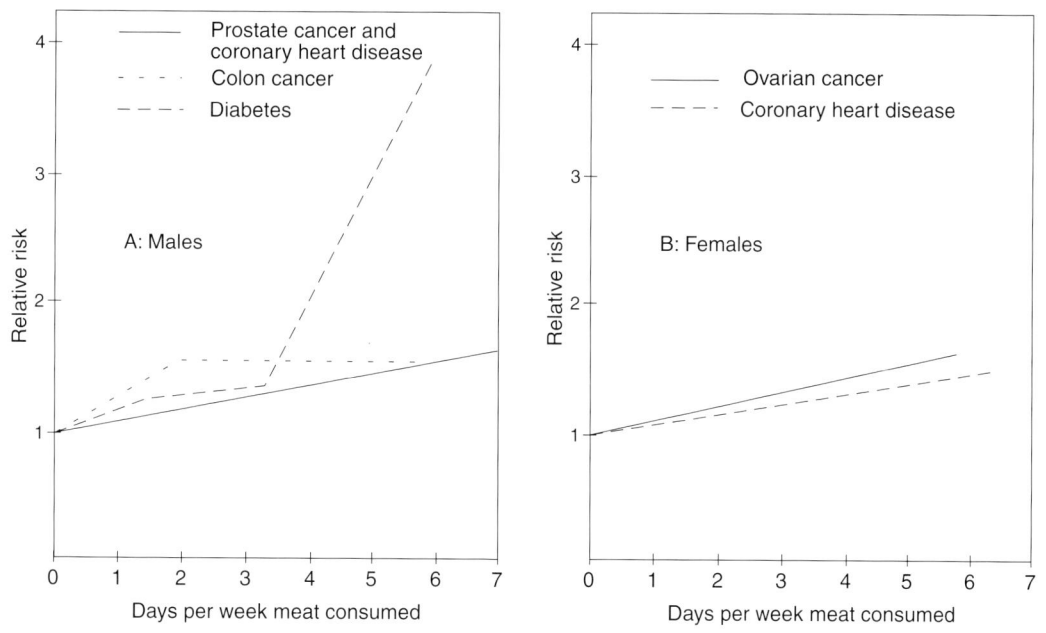

Figure 4.3. Meat consumption and age-adjusted relative risk of mortality in men (A) and women (B). The relative risk is calculated by dividing the mortality rate of meat eaters by the mortality rate of non meat eaters. A relative risk that is >1.00 (greater than one) suggests that the exposed group has a greater likelihood of dying from the disease in question than the non-exposed group. (Adapted from reference 4 and 5)

disease-related deaths, particularly as a result of prostate and colon cancer in males, and in females there was a moderate correlation with breast cancer. Milk consumption, in particular, was linked to an increased risk of prostate cancer (fig. 4.5).

It is true that opposite effects are also obtained, and that relative risk is in some cases reduced when animal products are consumed, but the bulk of the evidence strongly links their consumption to increased mortality rates from disease-related causes. The reasons for these statistics are however numerous, and vary from product to product.

Meat

Diets high in meat are usually low in carbohydrates, particularly fibre. The levels of proteins are very high, and these high protein levels can cause numerous problems. Not all the protein ingested is completely digested, and approximately 2 g of nitrogen in the form of undigested protein, peptides and amino acids (equivalent to 12 g of protein) enter the large bowel daily. The bacteria in the large bowel will preferentially utilize carbohydrate residues to meet their energy needs, but when carbohydrate levels are low and protein levels high, then amino acids will be metabolised resulting in the release of **ammonia** and **phenol**, both of which are potentially harmful. Cooked and smoked meat products, in addition, also contain other potentially harmful substances such as **polycyclic aromatic hydrocarbons, heterocyclic amines**, and **N-nitroso compounds**, which have been linked to degenerative diseases.

These potentially harmful substances should be eliminated from the system as rapidly as possible, and if sufficient fibre were present in the diet, then the time that food is retained in the intestines would be considerably reduced. In the case of a relatively high intake of cereal fibre, the partly fermented residual polysaccharides, derived from these fibres, would absorb water, and this would lead to increased faecal mass and decreased

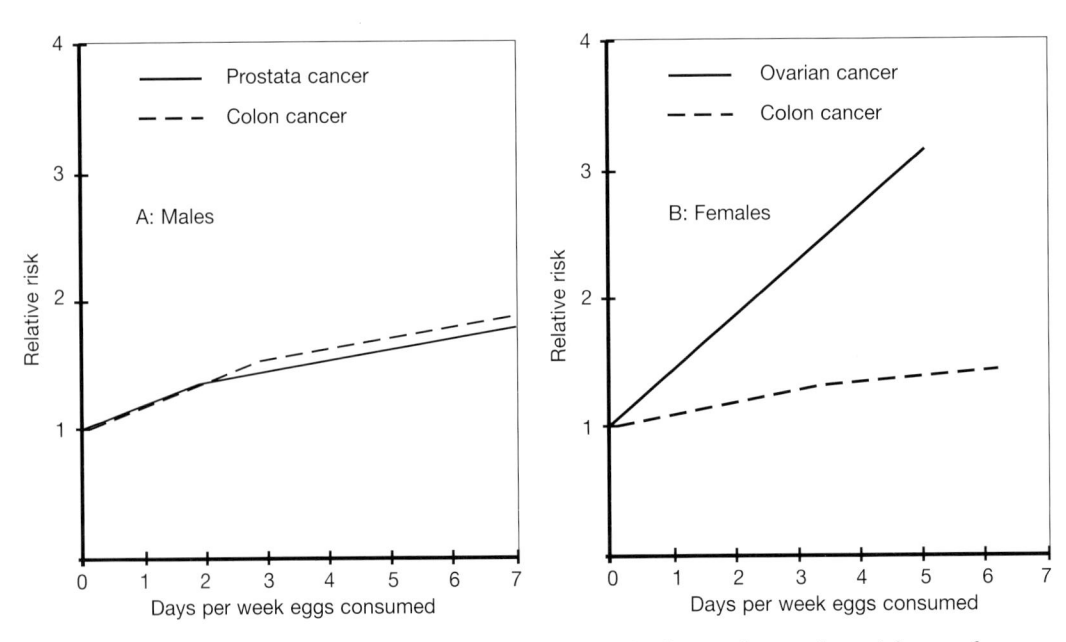

Figure 4.4. Egg consumption and age-adjusted relative risk of mortality. (Adapted from references 4 and 5)

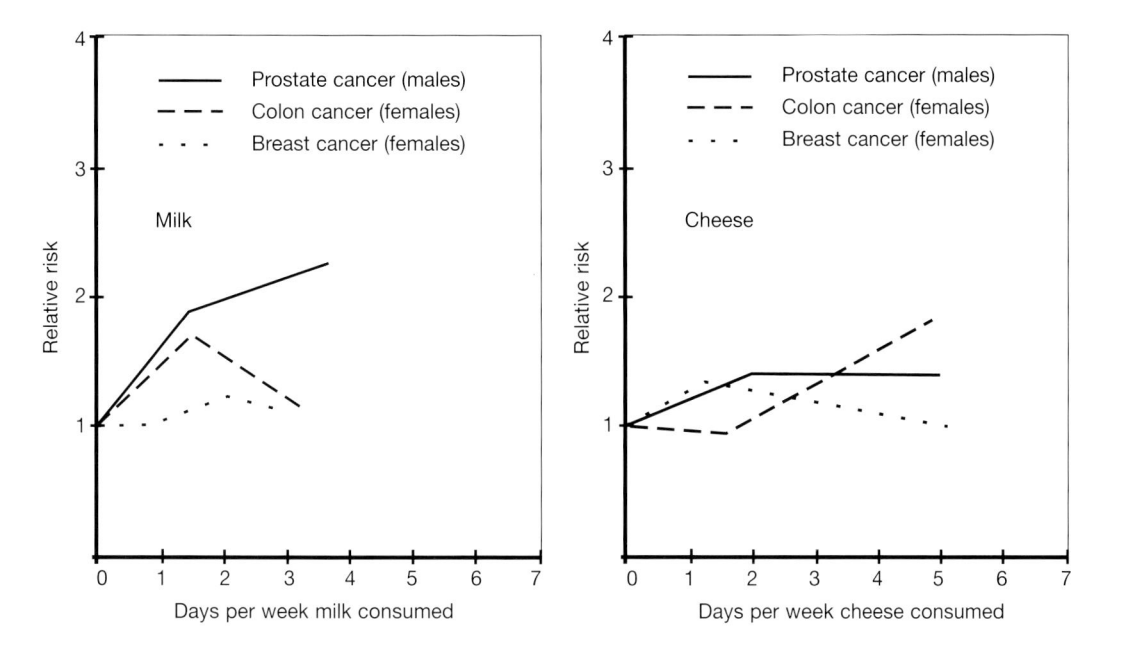

Figure 4.5. Dairy product consumption and age-adjusted relative risk of mortality. (Adapted from references 4 and 5)

transit time, thus reducing the time that potentially harmful substances such as carcinogens remain in large bowel.[4,6] With a high meat consumption, however, the harmful substances can remain in the intestines for much longer periods, and this exposure has been linked to increased cancer rates. In this regard, the relationship between colorectal cancer and meat consumption is well established and is presented in figure 4.6.

Colorectal cancer is the second most prevalent cancer in Western societies and affects up to 6% of men and women by the age of 75. Different factors seem to be responsible for colorectal cancer in the various countries, because the cancers manifest themselves differently, probably due to different induction modes. In high risk countries, the majority of colorectal cancers are located in the lower bowel, near the rectosigmoidal junction, whereas in low risk countries the majority of cancers are situated in the right side of the colon. Besides being low in fibre, the compounds in meat most commonly linked to the promotion of tumours are ammonia, phenols, polycyclic aromatic hydrocarbons, heterocyclic amines, and N-nitroso compounds.

Ammonia

Within the gut, the limited availability of carbohydrates in high-meat diets will lead to an increase in ammonia concentration in the colon because bacteria will metabolize the protein residues which enter the gut when carbohydrate levels are low. Ammonia, in turn, increases cell proliferation and alters DNA synthesis and has, therefore, been implicated in colon cancer.[4] It is known that increased cell proliferation is associated with cancer in humans.[8] Ammonia will not only be liberated from animal proteins, but from excessive intake of plant proteins as well. A high plant-protein intake is, however, usually associated with a high fibre intake and this would shorten the exposure time. This is particularly true in the case of whole foods with their high concentrations of fibre. High ammonia levels are not only a problem within the gut, but also effect the whole organism. As discussed in the chapter on proteins, the consumption of high levels of proteins will necessitate the de-amination of amino acids in order to meet the body's energy demands. This will require efficient detoxification of the produced ammonia, which in mammals is achieved via the urea cycle. As the amino acid arginine plays a principle role in this cycle, the higher level of this amino acid in plant proteins than in animal proteins offers a possible protection against ammonia toxicity.

Phenols

A high-meat, low-carbohydrate diet will also allow more aromatic amino acids, such as phenylalanine and tyrosine to enter the colon. Gut bacteria produce **cresol** and **phenol** when they metabolize these amino acids. Both cresol and phenol have been associated with the promotion of skin and colon cancer[9] and rapid elimination of these compounds seems advisable, even if their effect on the gut mucosa has not been fully resolved. A diet rich in fibre can once again assist in clearance of these compounds by decreasing the food transit time. Amino acid metabolism will also increase the concentration of these compounds in the blood, and elimination of these compounds is normally done by the kidneys. Nevertheless, consistently high levels of these compounds can be associated with diets rich in animal products, as it is known that urinary phenol levels increase when subjects are fed high-meat diets and to decrease with an increase in dietary fibre.[10] Low phenol levels could thus limit the risk of cancer, and a whole-food diet is ideal to achieve both low levels of these compounds and high levels of fibre.

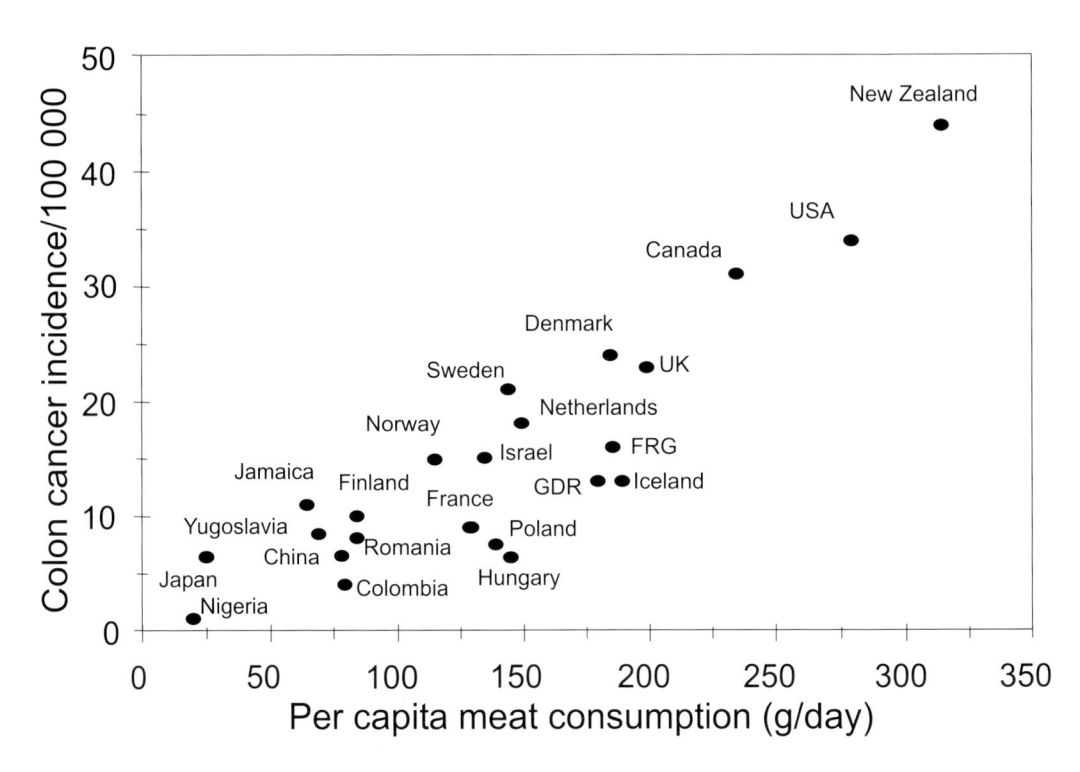

Figure 4.6. The relationship between meat consumption and colorectal cancer in various countries. (Adapted from references 2,7)

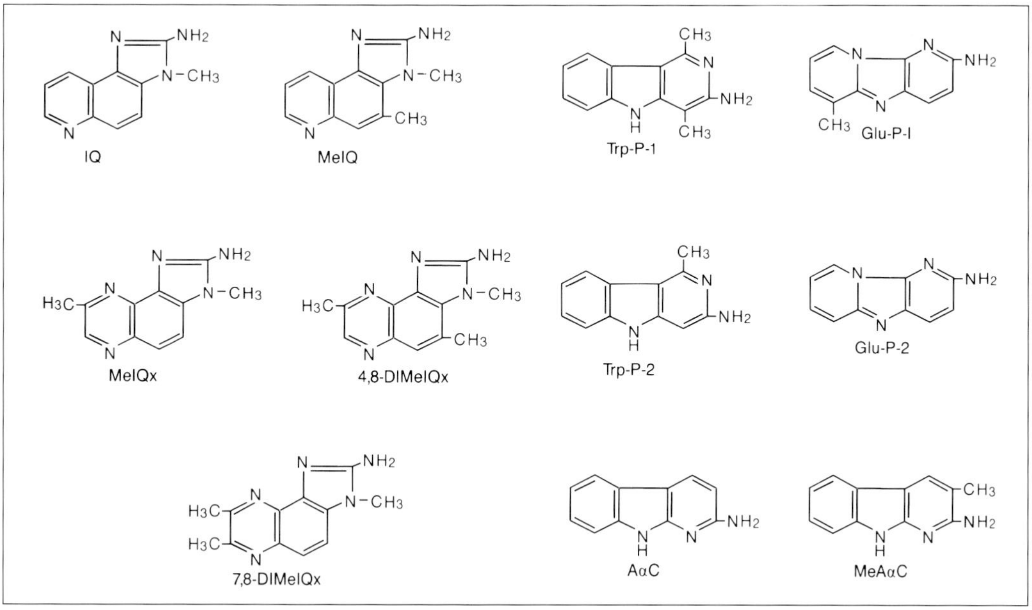

Figure 4.7. The chemical structure of heterocyclic amines. (Adapted from reference 14)

Polycyclic aromatic hydrocarbons (PAH)

Polycyclic aromatic hydrocarbons (PAH) result primarily from atmospheric deposition onto plants in smoky areas. One such hydrocarbon is **Benzo(a)pyrene**, a potent carcinogen, which is also formed in foodstuffs that are smoke-dried (such as tea) and also during the smoking and grilling of animal foods. PAH also occur in shell-fish that come from a polluted marine environment.[11] Fats are once again a prime source of PAH and smoked and grilled food in particular are subject to contamination by these carcinogens[12] Avoidance of high risk foods seems desirable if the risk from these compounds is to be curtailed.

Heterocyclic amines

Heterocyclic amines are mutagenic and carcinogenic compounds that are formed in cooked and charred foods.[12] They form particularly in meat and fish even if cooked at relatively low temperatures.[13] In fact, it is estimated that the average consumption of these compounds is as high as 100 µg per person per day,[14] but other calculations place daily consumption in the range of 0.4 to 16 µg/day.[2] Heterocyclic amines have been found to elicit carcinogenicity in the liver, lung, oral cavity, stomach and intestines of rats and mice, and have also been implicated in cancer of the lymphatic systems, blood vessels, skin and mammary glands. Over 20 mutagenic heterocyclic amines have been isolated from cooked animal products, and well done portions of meat contain higher concentrations than medium or rare portions. To obtain these compounds for experimental purposes, a standard protocol of grilling or frying for 6 min. at 200 °C is used. Generally, frying, grilling and barbecuing produce more of these compounds than does stewing, steaming, microwaving or poaching.[2]

The chemical structures of these compounds and the concentrations found in some foods are presented in figure 4.7 and table 4.2.

Heterocyclic amines are relevant carcinogens in humans, but in the case of colon cancer their relative contribution may be small

(0.25% of all colon cancers).[2] Food that will be particularly suspect in terms of heterocyclic amines will be cured and baked or fried meats. Even beer, soybeans, protein isolates and fried mushrooms were found to contribute significantly to the daily intake of these compounds. A study of heterocyclic amine formation in swine meat heated to 200 °C showed that the main reactants of the mutagen-forming reactions are amino acids and creatine.[15]

N-Nitroso compounds

These compounds have been linked to human cancer of the oesophagus, stomach, bladder and possibly lung.[16] Beer as well as nitrite-cured meat products, especially bacon after frying, and salt-dried or smoked fish, are major sources of these compounds. Incidentally, the mainstream smoke from one cigarette contains up to 65 µg volatile nitroso amines and the side stream contains up to 1000 µg,[13] a healthy lifestyle thus constitutes more than just eating correctly. It is difficult to estimate what the level of exposure to these compounds is, particularly since it is known that nitroso amines are efficiently metabolized in the liver. Nevertheless, these compounds have induced liver and oesophagus cancer in experimental animals.[12,13] Intestinal bacteria can also catalyse the formation of nitroso amines and this has been linked to gastric cancer. Nitrosated amides are direct acting carcinogens, and cause tumours near to the site they are produced, whereas nitrosated amines require hydroxylation and can initiate tumours at distal sites.[2] In one study, increased consumption of red meat caused a 3-fold increase (from 40 to 113 µg/day) in N-Nitroso compounds in the faeces of eight volunteer males who were subjected to low and high meat diets, but white meats did not seem to induce similar effects. The increase is high, when one considers that smoking 40 cigarettes a day produces an exposure to approximately 30 µg/day of tobacco-specific carcinogenic N-Nitroso compounds.[17]

Biological magnification

In addition to the aforementioned compounds, animals are also known to concentrate environmental pollutants such as heavy metals, pesticides, herbicides and industrial toxins. These toxins become concentrated in the tissues of organisms as they pass through the food chain. The concentrating process is called biological magnification and is responsible for widespread decimation of animal life on earth. Moreover, if species are harvested for human consumption from the top of the food chain (largely marine species), then these concentrated toxins are transferred to the human consumer. The extent of biological magnification of toxins such as DDT is well

Animal product	AαC	MeAαC	Glu-P-2	IQ	Me IQ	Me IQX	TRP-1
Broiled/fried beef	651	63.5	–	< 20.1	1–24	1.5	53.0
Beef extract	–	–	–	< 0.2	< 0.2	<69.0	–
Broiled chicken	180	15.1	–	–	2.1	–	–
Broiled/sun–dried sardine	–	–	–	158.0	72.0	–	13.3
Broiled/sun–dried cuttlefish	–	–	280	–	–	–	–

Table 4.2. The occurrence of heterocyclic amines in animal products. Concentrations are in µg/kg. (Adapted from reference 14)

documented, and it has been shown that the concentrating potential can induce several million fold increases in the concentration of these substances in the tissues of animals. Concentrations of DDT in the water as low as 0.000005 parts per million can be concentrated to over 26 parts per million in top carnivores.

Animals accumulate toxins particularly in their fatty tissues, and when called upon to utilize their fat reserves, the release of these toxins into the bloodstream can lead to various diseases and death. In this regard, it has been established that the deaths of hundreds of thousands of marine mammals can largely be attributed to lowered immune capacity owing to the immune system being compromised by the presence of accumulated toxins. It has been found that even the paint used on the hulls of ships can add sufficient toxins to the oceans to cause widespread death of marine life. The paint contains **tributyl tin (TBT)** which prevents barnacles from sticking to the hull of vessels. The substance has been banned for use on small vessels but is still widely used on larger vessels. TBT is probably the most potent toxin deliberately introduced into the sea, as even a few nanograms in water can cause abnormal development such as female dog whelks developing male organs. However, the immunosuppression capabilities of the toxin could be one of the factors contributing to the widespread death of dolphins and other marine life. It was found, that marine mammals concentrate TBT in their tissues in concentrations of up to 10 parts per million.[18]

Marine pollution is a worldwide problem, particularly in industrialized or highly populated areas. In the Mediterranean, more than 500 million tonnes of sewage alone pour into the water every year. Sewage is not the only pollutant flowing into this sea, it is estimated that annually 120 000 tonnes of marine oils, 60 000 tonnes of detergents, 100 tonnes of mercury, 3 800 tonnes of lead, 1 million tonnes of crude oil and 3 600 tonnes of phosphates enter this sea. In 1985 the Mediterranean nations set themselves clean-up goals which were to be achieved by 1995, but none of these goals have been achieved.[19] If the wealthier nations of the world are struggling with clean-up goals, one wonders how the less fortunate are faring.

It is known that fish and shell-fish in particular, concentrate heavy metals such as mercury in their tissues, and these compounds can also be carcinogens. Already in 1953, cats and birds on the island of Minamata in Japan got the 'staggers' and died. Then the humans developed headaches, ataxia, fatigue, foetal deformities and mental abnormalities. Some 15 000 people were affected and at least 3500 died. A government investigation showed that the culprit was mercury salts that had been dumped in the river and had accumulated in the sediment of Minimata Bay. There the salts had become methylated and converted to methyl mercury, a highly toxic organic compound. Once this compound had found its way into the food chain, it was accumulated in the tissues of marine organisms, and biological accumulation led to high concentrations in tuna which in turn was consumed by the human population. A more recent episode involving mercury pollution can be found in the pollution of the river Rhine in Germany in November 1986, when a blaze in the giant chemical company Sandoz caused some 30 tonnes of mercury and pesticides to be washed into the Rhine. Only direct and targeted intervention by the industrialized European nations prevented this disaster from permanently destroying the delicate ecosystem of this river.

The TBT example illustrates the fact, that very minor concentrations of toxins can attain catastrophic proportions due to biological accumulation, not to mention the very high levels of pollutants in some areas. Humans that rely largely on animal products for their sustenance, will experience similar accumulations of toxic compounds as do the top carnivores in nature, and a reduction, or even avoidance of animal products can thus enhance the capacity to cope with disease.

Dairy products

Milk and dairy products are advertised as wonder foods that will supply all the nutrients required for healthy growth. The calcium levels in milk, in particular, are stressed as an essential component of the human diet, and the impression is created that a loss of this dietary source of calcium will lead to abnormal bone development. It is certainly true that dairy products are packed with nutrients, but this does not mean that the combination of nutrients is suited to human nutrition. Mother's milk is essential for infants, but then infants are specially designed to cope with this growth-promoting food. Prior to weaning the necessary enzyme systems needed for the digestion and assimilation of milk components are active, but they are progressively deactivated with age. The milk of other mammalian species also differs in composition from mother's milk, and this, together with the potential danger from ingested antigens, makes cows milk unsuitable for human consumption.

There is considerable resistance from industry, and even from the established scientific world, to the idea that dairy consumption is detrimental to health, but the evidence from recent scientific findings seems fairly conclusive with regard to this issue. Dairy consumption is being coupled with a host of diseases, and as consumption rises world-wide, so the evidence is becoming more and more conclusive. In the past, the detrimental effect of the consumption of dairy products may have been masked by the positive effects of other lifestyle choices such as higher consumption of grains, fresh fruits and vegetables with their high fibre content. Western diets have, however experienced a sharp increase in the consumption of animal products, including dairy products, with concomitant decline in the consumption of grains, legumes, fruits and vegetables, and this may explain the increase in the incidence of degenerative diseases in industrialized countries.

Lactose intolerance

Lactose, the sugar in milk, is broken down in the intestines by the enzyme **lactase**. Most people are able to digest lactose properly during infancy and early childhood, but as they grow older this ability declines. Approximately 75% of adults worldwide are lactose intolerant and those with the highest intolerance are native Americans and Asians and only slightly lower than these are the blacks, Jews, Hispanics, and southern Europeans. Lactose intolerance is lowest among northern Europeans and their descendants. In the US some 25% of Caucasians, 51% of Hispanics and 75% of all African Americans, Jews, and native Americans have insufficient levels of lactase to digest dairy products and 90% of Asian Americans are lactose intolerant.[20,21] It has been found that 90% of African people are lactase deficient, and in the case of the rural Zulu of South Africa it was found that they showed no change in blood glucose concentrations after ingesting 50 g of lactose.[22] When milk and dairy products are digested, **lactose** is broken down by the enzyme **lactase** into glucose and galactose (fig. 4.8).

The presence of lactose is a feature of mammalian milk, but the concentration of this sugar is normally geared to the needs of the species, as are the concentrations of all the other components of milk. In the case of humans, mother's milk does not only contain the essential nutrients that are required for growth and development, but also contains the bacterium **bacillus bifidus** that assists in the digestion of lactose. In cow's milk, however, the bacterial composition differs from that of human milk, and if cow's milk is fed to infants, this can interfere with the digestion of lactose. Moreover, human milk has a higher carbohydrate concentration (7%–7,5%) than cow's milk (4,5%–5%) and contains some 200 mmol/litre of lactose which makes it sweeter than cow's milk. The lower protein and higher carbohydrate content of human milk is also more suited to the needs of infants, because their growth rates are considerably lower than those of calves.

After the conversion of lactose to glucose and galactose, the available galactose is not utilized as such, but is converted to glucose in the liver by a series of steps requiring the initial presence of the enzyme **galactokinase**. The production of both the enzymes lactase and galactokinase declines with age, and the capacity to digest and utilize the products of lactose in adult life is thus curtailed. A deficiency in the enzyme lactase will result in fermentation of lactose by intestinal bacteria, which can result in abdominal distress such as the development of excessive gas, cramping, bloating, borborygmi (stomach rumbling), altered bowel habits and diarrhoea.[21] The severity of the symptoms depends on the quantity of lactose consumed and the level of intolerance.

Milk protein intolerance

A further problem with milk is encountered in the digestion of the milk protein **casein**. In comparison to human milk, cow's milk contains 300% more casein and more than double the amount of total protein. Casein and **β-lactoglobulin** are the two main proteins in milk and they are unique in that they contain a perfect blend of amino acids, which is precisely what is needed during early infant growth. Human infants, however, double their mass on average 180 days after birth, whereas cows achieve the same feat in only 47 days. Cow's milk is therefore geared to meet the rapid growth requirements of cows, but is not suitable for humans. Casein also naturally stimulates normal thyroid function in infants, and as the thyroid is involved in many developmental processes, including the development of the nervous system, casein from other mammalian species could have adverse effects on metabolic processes of infants particularly since a portion of the dietary casein can be absorbed undigested and serve as antigen.

As is the case with the enzyme lactase that digests lactose, the concentration of the enzyme **rennin**, that breaks down the casein, also declines with age in all mammals, and by the time milk teeth develop it is virtually non-existent in the human digestive tract. Without rennin, the digestion of casein has to be carried out by the normal proteolytic enzymes which are not as efficient in breaking down casein. The presence of casein in the diet of mammals has also been linked to elevated cholesterol levels and various degenerative diseases such as arteriosclerosis. Rabbits fed casein developed arteriosclerosis, but the

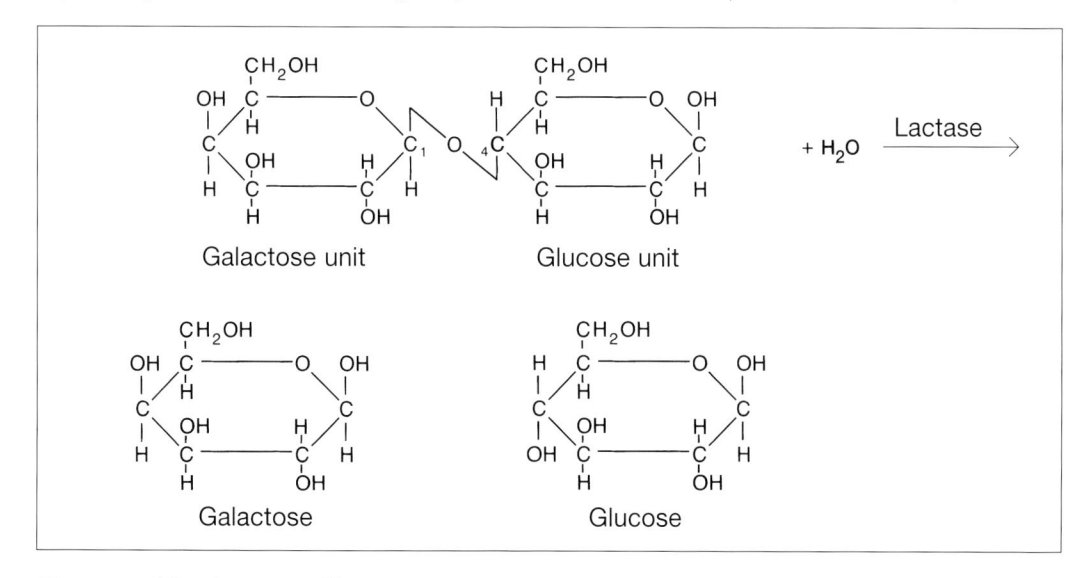

Figure 4.8. The digestion of lactose.

effect could be reduced if a plant protein source, such as soybean flour was introduced into the diet. This shows, that the amino acid pool produced by casein probably no longer meets the requirements of weaned or adult mammals. Casein also produced higher cholesterol levels than soy protein in a number of animal species, including rats, hamsters, guinea pigs, pigs, and monkeys. In humans, a reduction in cholesterol levels was also found if meat and dairy proteins were replaced by soy proteins.[23,24] Casein also seems to have an adverse effect on insulin secretion, thyroxine levels, gastrointestinal hormones and it has an adverse effect on calcium metabolism.

Calcium in dairy products

A matter which has received much media attention, is the calcium content of milk and dairy products. It certainly is true that dairy products do contain fair amounts of calcium, but a large proportion of the calcium in milk is combined with casein in the form of calcium caseinate. Dairy products are also not the only source of calcium available to humans, as grains, legumes, seeds, nuts and many vegetables are excellent sources of calcium. Moreover, fractional absorption of calcium from these sources is higher than from milk. A study done on whole-wheat products showed that fractional calcium absorption from whole-wheat bread exceeded the absorption of calcium from milk, ingested at a comparable load, in the same subjects.[25] Not only is the absorption rate of calcium higher from plant sources, but animal sources seem to cause calcium loss in view of the nature and the concentration of the proteins which they contain. Table 4.3 lists the calcium levels in some dairy products and plant foods.

Foods vary in their composition, and in the case of seeds, grains, beans and vegetables, there are considerable differences in calcium content of different varieties and in general, dark green vegetables are a good source of calcium. In addition to the foods listed above, almonds, sesame seeds, sunflower seeds, soybean products such as bean curd and soy flower, carob, chick peas, haricot beans, mung beans, garlic, parsley, watercress and dried fruits (especially figs) are good sources of calcium.

Calcium utilization is governed by complex processes, and the absorption, bone deposition and excretion of calcium is strongly influenced by other dietary components. It is well documented that increased protein consumption causes calcium loss in the urine,[27,28] and this is particularly true in the case of proteins from animal products.[29] An investigation into the effects of various protein diets on calcium retention showed that proteins from dairy products, such as cottage cheese, caused considerable calcium loss in the urine.[30] The culprit here seems to be casein, and other studies seem to corroborate this. In one study it was found that casein fed to weaning rats caused kidney calcification, an effect which was not observed if the protein came from another source.[31] If calcium losses exceed absorption, then a negative calcium balance exists, and calcium must be mobilized from bone in order to maintain plasma calcium levels in a dynamic state. This loss of calcium from bone can eventually lead to **osteoporosis**. It is, therefore, not surprising that osteoporosis seems more prevalent in countries where the consumption of dairy products is

Food	Serving	mg
Yoghurt, low fat	1 cup	415
Greens, collard	1 cup	400
Milk, low fat	1 cup	300
Greens turnip	1 cup	250
Chinese cabbage	1 cup	250
Greens, mustard tops	1 cup	200
Cottage cheese, low fat	1 cup	160
Broccoli	1 cup	150
Grains and pasta	1 cup	100–150
Bread	2 slices	100
Beans	1 cup	100

Table 4.3. Calcium levels in selected foods. (From reference 26)

high.[32,26] In table 4.4 the incidence of osteoporosis in various countries in relation to the consumption of proteins and dairy products is presented, and in figure 4.9, the relationship between dairy consumption and osteoporosis (expressed as hip fracture rate per 100 000 women) is presented.

Although dairy products are rich in calcium, paradoxically, it is apparent from the above data that the calcium from milk is not synonymous with healthy bone structure (see chapter 5 for more information on dairy free diets and osteoporosis). Moreover, calcium supplementation does not provide a solution for the dilemma, as countries, such as the United States, with the highest supplementation rates still have among the highest rates of osteoporosis. Not even in lactating women does calcium supplementation seem to have much of an effect in either white or black women. In one study on White, middle class women it was found that absorption of calcium from the intestines was not increased during supplementation compared to lactating women on low calcium diets. The calcium needs for milk production were met by decreased urinary excretion and increased bone resorption and not by increased intestinal absorption despite high calcium intakes.[33]

In a study on Gambian women similar results were obtained. Gambian women normally have a low calcium diet based largely on rice, millet, groundnuts and fish. This diet provides less than 300 mg/day of calcium which is considerably lower than current recommendations for lactating women. Increasing the calcium level threefold to bring it line with FAO/WHO recommendations had no discernable effect on breast milk calcium concentrations or on the maternal bone mineral content. This suggests that there was no benefit from increasing the calcium intake during lactation.[34] The women in the supplementation group had consumed a total of 0.26 kg (one quarter to one third of the whole-body calcium content) after 52 weeks, and showed significantly greater urinary calcium output (7% of the dose). As the bone mineral content did not change, the researchers concluded that the rest of the additional calcium was just not absorbed from the intestinal tract.[34] This study underlines the fact that calcium needs can be adequately met by even low calcium diets that contain no dairy products.

In our own laboratory we have consistently found that animals (sheep, rats, rabbits and vervet monkeys) fed animal proteins, particularly casein or dairy products showed significant increases in urinary calcium levels, compromised bone status, and in common with the other studies, reduced intestinal absorption. In a current study on vervet monkeys conducted at the Primate Unit of the Medical Research Council in South Africa two groups of

Country	Hip fractures (Rate/100 000 women)	Dairy food intake (g/day/person)	Protein intake (g/day/person)
United States	102	462	106
New Zealand	97	480	112
Israel	70	315	105
United Kingdom	63	455	90
Hong Kong	31	95	82
Singapore	15	113	82
South African blacks	5	10	55

Table 4.4. Correlation between osteoporosis, dairy food and protein consumption by countries. (Adapted from reference 26)

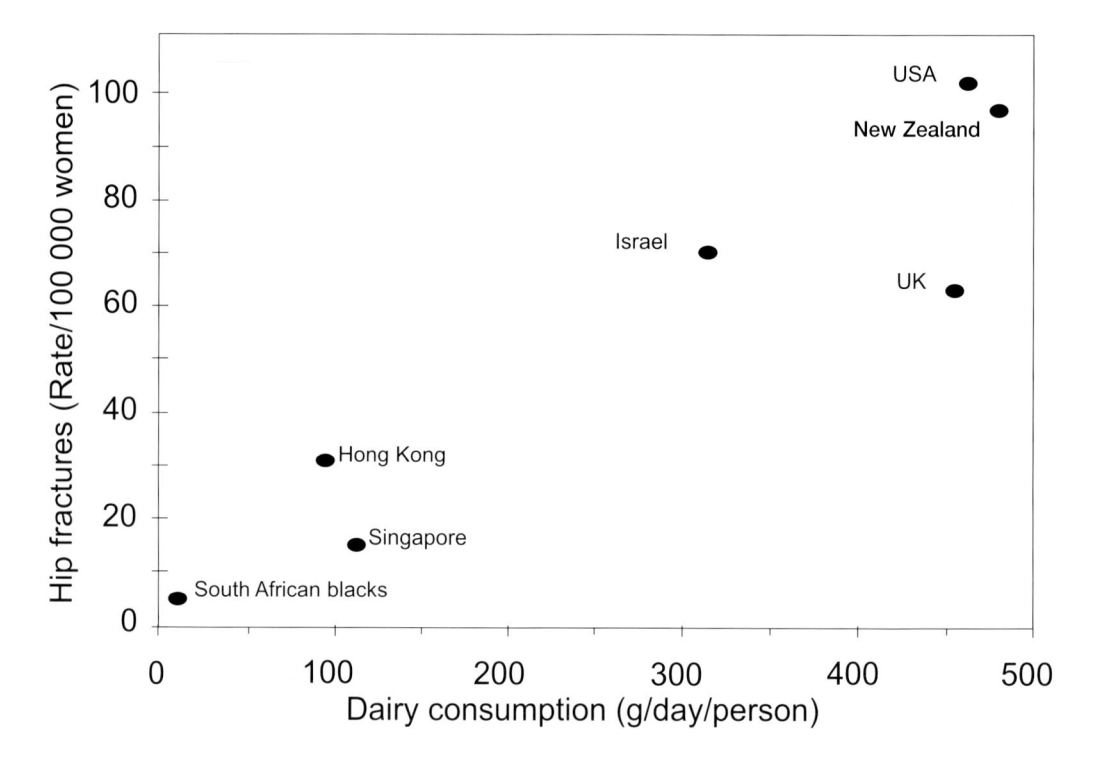

Figure 4.9 Correlation between osteoporosis and dairy food consumption by countries. (Adapted from reference 26)

monkeys were fed diets containing equivalent quantities of calcium, but one group received largely milk powder as protein source whilst the other group received kidney beans and maize as protein source. Stool calcium analyses showed that absorption of calcium was significantly lower in the dairy group than in the bean/maize group irrespective of whether they were on a high (17%) or low (8%) protein diet thus demonstrating the adverse effect of dairy products on calcium utilization.[35]

Dairy products and the immune system

Human milk not only contains less protein than cow's milk, but the distribution of proteins is also different. A group of proteins that are particularly important in this regard are the **immune globulins** which carry antibodies and are particularly numerous in the early milk known as **colostrum**. These globulins contain antibodies found in the mother's blood and transmit immunity to the newborn infant. When mother's milk or cow's milk is ingested, the system is capable of transporting these antibodies directly into the blood-stream via carrier systems, an ability that persists to a lesser extent even in adults. Human milk contains antibodies which differ from those found in cow's milk and when cow's milk is substituted for mother's milk, the immunoglobulins from the cow's milk will interact with the immune system and this can lead to an allergic reaction. Many allergies can primarily be attributed to milk, and will disappear when milk is removed from the diet.

Allergic disorders are a widespread health problem of particularly infants and young children in the developed world, and according to several population studies, the incidence and severity of these disorders has increased significantly of late.[36] Cow's milk is a major source of allergies and has been implicated in virtually all the common ailments of the respiratory tract. **Hay fever, sinusitis, chronic bronchitis, colds, ear infections** and even **asthma** can largely be ascribed to the intake of dairy products.[37,38,39] In addition to these ailments, children are prone to **diarrhoea, vomiting, constipation, colic, growth retardation, psychological disturbances, eczema** and asthma if fed cow's milk. Allergies need not immediately be apparent and can manifest later in life. Moreover, once an allergic reaction to a substance is manifested, greater sensitivity to other antigens is induced.[37] A causative factor in congestive diseases is the ability of dairy products to promote **mucus** formation, and milk, cheese, butter and cream are the most likely of all foods to promote the build up of mucus.

Cow's milk also causes colic in infants. The relationship between cow's milk and colic is well established, and in infants that are breast fed, but also receive cow's milk, colic is very common. Once cow's milk is removed from the diet, however, colic disappears in most cases.[40] Cow's milk allergy is frequently the first manifestation of allergy because the proteins in cow's milk are the first foreign antigens encountered in large quantities in infancy.[36] Allergy to cow's milk is most prevalent at the age of 1 year and has been reported in 2.8% of the general child population, but in infants with **atopic dermatitis** the incidence of cow's milk allergy is at least five times that figure.[36] Atopic dermatitis is a chronic eczematous skin disease which frequently begins in infancy and probably results from the repeated ingestion of allergins. This in turn leads to frequent scratching and the consequent trauma induced lichenified lesions. It has been established that casein from cow's milk causes an increased T-cell frequency and a specific T-cell-mediate immune response to casein can be found in the blood of adolescent and adult patients who suffer from milk-related exacerbation of atopic dermatitis.[40]

Cow's milk has been linked to the development of **insulin-dependent diabetes (IDD)**. IDD results from a chronic autoimmune process that can exist for years in a preclinical phase, with the classic manifestations of the disease (hyperglycaemia and ketosis) only occurring after most of the insulin-producing beta cells have been destroyed. There is evidence, that T-lymphocytes are a major contributor to the pathogenic process. In this regard, cow's milk has received much attention because people who were not breastfed or breastfed for only a short period of time are at increased risk of IDD. It is noteworthy, that 100% of newly diagnosed patients with IDD have antibodies to bovine serum albumin. Moreover, the pancreatic beta-cell proteins display substantial molecular cross-reactivity with bovine serum albumin from cow's milk. IDD can thus be an abnormal response to the foreign protein leading to an immune response to both bovine serum albumin and the pancreatic beta-cell protein.[41]

The findings by Cavallo et al [42] of peripheral blood T-cell reactivity to ß-casein in half their 47 patients with IDD adds weight to the cow's milk hypothesis.[43] There have been arguments for and against the cow's milk hypothesis, since IDD also occurs in infants that have never received cow's milk. However, it has now been conclusively shown that the antigens in cow's milk are transferred to the mother's milk if she consumes cow's milk. In a study done on Japanese women it was found that β-Lactoglobulin was transferred to the mother's milk because it is resistant to acid and enzymatic degradation and if taken orally is absorbed into the system.[44] Moreover, there have been reports of infants that are only breastfed and never received milk protein developing allergies to cow's milk, which was then alleviated when the mothers eliminated dairy products from their diets.[44]

Finally, the consumption of dairy products has been implicated in intestinal **ulcers**[45] and **cancer**. Milk consumption in particular has been positively correlated with prostate cancer,[5] and in an Italian case study, risk of breast cancer was positively associated with the intake of milk and dairy products.[46] For infants, the best food is mother's milk and cow's milk should be avoided at all costs. Mother's milk will ensure the normal development of infants at every level. It has even been established that the **intelligence quotients (IQ)** of children that were fed breastmilk are significantly higher than those of children that did not receive breastmilk even after adjustment for differences between groups, mother's education and social class.[47] For those that have become accustomed to the consumption of milk, the replacement of dairy products with legume, seed or nut milks and creams will provide a more than adequate alternative to milk.

Dairy products and infertility

The issue of a rise in infertility, particularly male infertility, has produced considerable controversy in scientific circles. More and more reviews have appeared in the scientific literature claiming a decline in semen quality which is being largely attributed to environmental factors such as exposure to oestrogens (dietary, pharmaceutical and environmental pollutants). It has been suggested that environmental factors, possibly acting in fetal and early neonatal life, may be responsible for the negative effects. Some researchers have claimed that the statistical methodology employed to determine the decline in semen quality was incorrect and that no real decline had taken place over the last decades. To investigate this claim, a group of researchers from the University Department of Growth and Reproduction and the Statistical Research Unit in Copenhagen Denmark, systematically reviewed the complete international literature on semen analysis since the 1930's using rigorous selection criteria and statistical analyses. They found, that linear regression of data weighted by the number of men in each study showed a significant decrease in mean sperm count from 113×10^6/ml in 1940 to 66×10^6/ml in 1990 ($p \leq 0.0001$) and in seminal volume from 3.40 ml to 2.75 ml ($p = 0.027$), indicating an even more pronounced decrease in sperm production than expressed by the decline in sperm density. They concluded, that there had been a genuine decline in semen quality over the last 50 years.[48]

The Danish study was subsequently also criticised with regard to the statistical methodology employed,[49] but the issue would still not come to rest. A group of researchers from the MRC Centre for Reproductive Biology in Edinburgh, on the strength of the arguments against the statistical methodologies employed, regrouped the data to account for the year of the donor's birth and found a similar decline in sperm concentration as reported by the Danish researchers,[50] and all the trends seem to point to a decline in the health of the male reproductive system.[51] It is true that a number of investigations, particularly with regard to the United States, have not shown a decline in semen quality,[52,53,54] but overall the evidence is overwhelming that reproductive health is on the decline. An analysis of semen quality among fertile men in Paris using sperm stored in the sperm bank, showed that between 1973 and 1992 there had been no decline in semen volume, but that sperm concentration, motility and the percentage of morphologically normal spermatozoa had declined significantly.[55]

Of interest is also an observation that some nations experienced a greater decline than others in terms of semen quality a notable example being the comparison between Finland and Britain, where it has been reported that the British men are less fertile than those from Finland.[56] Even in Finland, it has however been reported by researchers from the Forensic Department of the University of Helsinki, that the findings from post mortem analyses of two groups of men from 1981 and 1991 showed a dramatic decline in overall reproductive health. The researches reported that not only the number of men with normal spermiogenesis had declined by more than half, but the frequency of pathological disorders of the testes had increased.[57] The precise reason for the overall decline, as well as differences between nations in reproductive health have not been clearly established. The main argument revolves around environmental oestrogens,[58] but although this may be a contributing factor, even this hypothesis is still being considered as guesswork at this stage.[59] The strongest evidence for the oestrogen argument is that the sons of women who were given high doses of diethylstilboestrol in the first trimester of pregnancy to prevent spontaneous abortions, have a high incidence of reproductive abnormalities.[60] The main factors for male infertility are summarised in table 4.5.

Although male infertility has received so much attention of late, female infertility is even higher than that of males. One couple in 10 seeks medical help because of infertility and a 1982-85 multicentre study by the World Health Organization found that in 20% of cases the problem was predominantly male, in 38% the problem was predominantly female, in 27% abnormalities were found in both partners and in the remaining 15% no clear-cut cause of infertility was identified.[62] Although environmental pollutants and oestrogenic drugs may play a significant role in the decline in fertility, other factors, such as changes in diet, may be equally significant.

There have been significant changes in the consumption of animal products in Western societies over the last decades, and the consumption of dairy products in particular has increased dramatically. Fat consumption has also seen a significant increase in the past decades (see chapters 3 and 5) and these dietary changes have been associated with increased risk of degenerative diseases. Male

Pretesticular	Testicular	Post-testicular
Endocrine: Hypogonadotrophic Hypogonadism **Coital disorders:** Erectile dysfunction: Psychosexual Endocrine/neural/vascular Ejaculatory failure: Psychosexual Post genitourinary surgery Neural Drug related	**Genetic:** Klinefelter's syndrome Y chromosome deletions Immotile cilia syndrome **Congenital:** Cryptorchidism **Infective (orchitis)** **Antisperatogenic** agents: Heat Chemotherapy Drugs Irradiation **Vascular:** Torsion Varicocele **Immunological** **Idiopathic**	**Obstructive:** Epididymal: Congenital Infective Vasal: Genetic: cystic fibrosis Acquired: vasectomy **Epididymal hostility:** Epididymal asthenozoospermia **Accessory gland infection** **Immunological:** Idiopathic Post-vasectomy

Table 4.5. Aetiological factors in male infertility. (From reference 61)

prostate pathology has been linked to the consumption of dairy products,[5] and this led us to investigate the possible link between the consumption of dairy products and reproductive health. The study was conducted on vervet monkey at the Primate Unit of the MRC in South Africa, so as to get as a close a model to the human as possible. Twelve monkeys were divided into two groups of six individuals each and they were put on diets containing 17% protein. The one group received largely maize and legumes and the other group milk powder as protein source. In order to assess the impact of high and low protein concentrations, after an initial two month period the protein allocation was dropped to 8% from the respective sources and analyses were continued for an additional two month period. In this way the long- and short-term impact of the consumption of dairy products on reproductive health could be assessed. Already in the short-term, a significant decline in sperm quality, motility and concentration could be discerned, and these preliminary results were reported at the 6th International Congress on Cell Biology and 36th American Society for Cell Biology Annual Meeting held in San Francisco USA in 1996.[63]

When protein concentrations were high, the sperm concentrations between the two

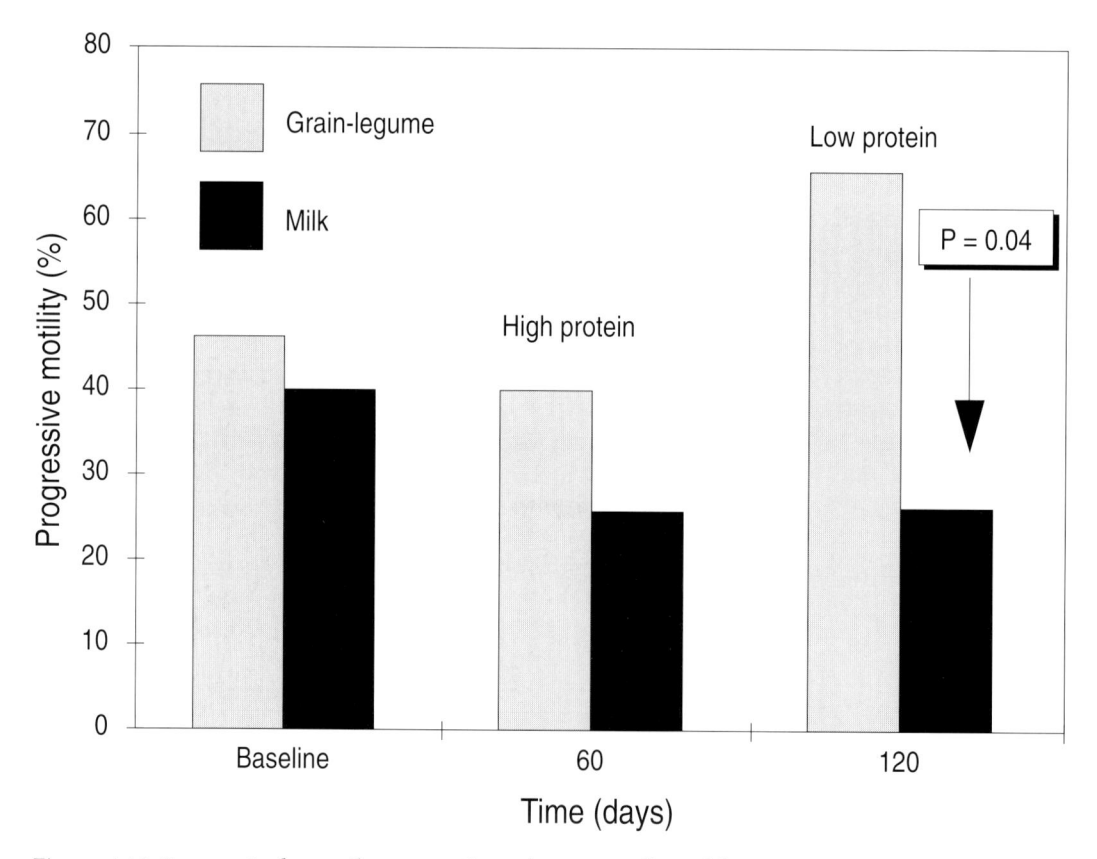

Figure 4.10. Progressively motile sperm of monkeys on milk and legume plus maize diets as protein source. (P = 0.04 verified via the Wilcoxin 2-sample Test) The baseline represents the status of the animals at the start of the experiment before the introduction of the new dietary regime. (From reference 35)

groups of monkeys were not significantly different, but progressive motility and the number of defective spermatozoa (particularly midpiece defects) increased. When protein concentrations were lowered to 8% crude protein, the group on dairy experienced a significant decline in sperm concentration, whilst the group on legume and maize showed no drop in sperm concentration and even showed an improved motility. Moreover, the number of defective spermatozoa also increased in the dairy group. In figures 4.10 and 4.11 the sperm progressive motility and the sperm concentration of the two groups of vervet monkeys is shown for the first four month period.

Animal products and foodborne illness

Foodborne illness is on the increase worldwide and in most cases animal products are implicated as the main source of infection. These infections may be mild, seriously debilitating, and can even be fatal, particularly in elderly people and infants. The contamination of the food is due to micro-organisms or their toxins, and is characterized by diarrhoea, vomiting or both, but can also involve other parts of the body as in the case of listeriosis (caused by **Listeria**) or botulism which is caused by toxins produced by the bacterium **Clostridium botulinum.** In the case of the latter, as little as 0,1 g of food in which this bacterium has grown can be seriously debil-

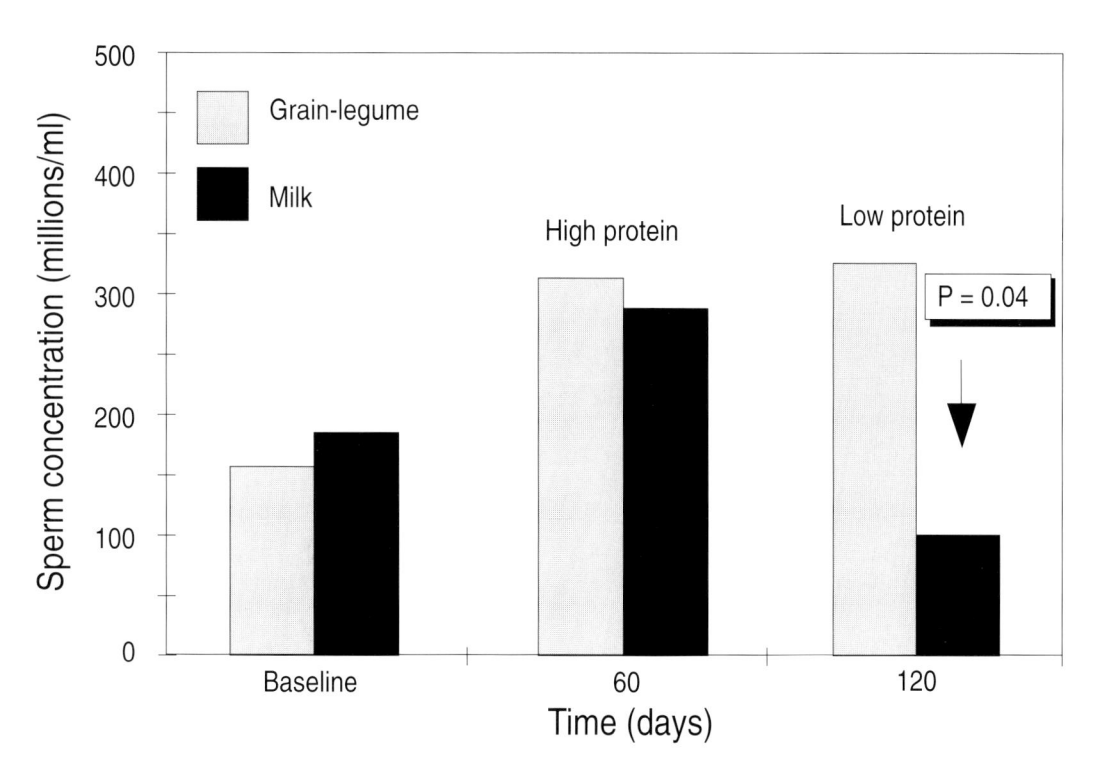

Figure 4.11 Sperm concentrations of monkeys on milk and legume plus maize diets as protein source. (P = 0.04 verified via the Wilcoxin 2-sample Test) The baseline represents the status of the animals at the start of the experiment before the introduction of the new dietary regime. (From reference 35)

itating, and in as many as 20% of cases botulism results in death. Most of the data pertaining to foodborne diseases is from the industrialized nations, but it must be borne in mind that the situation in poorer nations is probably worse.

The bacteria most often implicated with foodborne diseases are **Salmonella, Campylobacter, Listeria, Escherichia, Staphylococcus** and **Yersinia.**

Salmonella infections

Animals are the main source of this infection, but the infection can be spread from person to person. In the United States it is estimated that salmonellosis cases range from 790 000 to 3 690 000 per year, with as many as 7 041 deaths resulting from the illness.[64] In the last two decades there has been a steady increase in the number of reported cases, and in industrialised countries a dramatic increase seems to have occurred since the mid 1980's. In both the United States and Canada there has been a steady increase in salmonellosis and between 1975 and 1988 the incidence of notifiable diseases had more than doubled in these countries. Most outbreaks of the disease are associated with animal products such as eggs, cheese and improperly pasteurized milk. Between 1985 and 1989 there was also a steady increase in cases of Salmonella enteritidis in New England and the Mid-Atlantic states where there were 140 outbreaks (4 976 cases and 30 deaths) during this period in which eggs were associated with 65 of these outbreaks.[65]

Salmonella outbreaks in the UK have also been associated with infections in cattle and poultry, and increases in salmonellosis, since 1985 have been largely linked to a massive rise in cases caused by S. enteritidis attributed largely to poultry and hens' eggs (figure 4.12).[66] The eggs do not only become infected because of cracks in the shell, but they become contaminated because the ovarian tissue of the fowls is infected.

Prevention of contamination requires the co-operation of a wide variety of people from the breeders, veterinarians, epidemiologists, microbiologists and caterers, to every household cook. In view of this complexity it is difficult to control the spread of these diseases, particularly since transport and slaughter of animals increases the number of animals which carry Salmonella. In the UK the proportion of infected calves increases from 0,5% for calves leaving the farm to 36% after slaughter, whereas a US study found that in the case of pigs 7% are infected when they leave the farm, but 50% are infected after slaughter.[66]

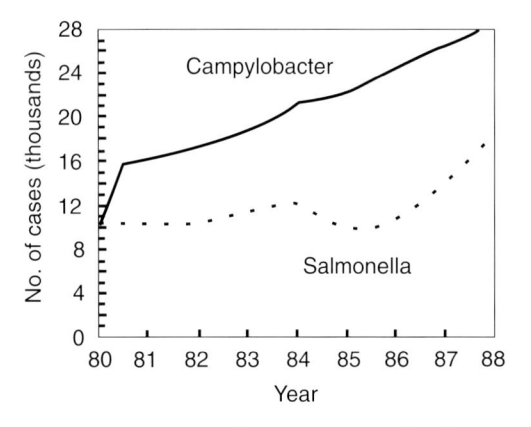

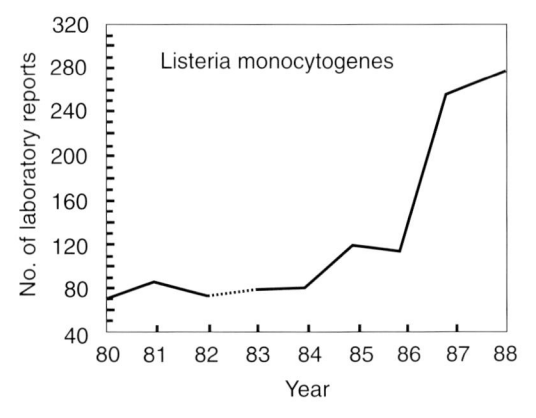

Figure 4.12. Cases of gastrointestinal infection due to bacterial contamination of food. (Adapted from reference 67)

Campylobacter infections

Campylobacteriosis is a common cause of sporadic disease associated mainly with poultry and milk. In Canada this micro-organism is responsible for more cases of infectious diarrhoea than is *Salmonella*, and in England and Wales it is the most common cause of this illness, with as many as 30 000 cases reported annually.[67] Figure 4.12 shows that the incidence of this infection in the UK has also increased dramatically since 1980. In third world countries however the situation is much worse, and in African populations campylobacteriosis is very common.

Listeria infections

Listeria infections are not nearly as common as those caused by *Salmonella* or *Campylobacter*, but in view of the serious nature of the symptoms caused by these infections, it is imperative that this organism be strictly controlled. *Listeria* causes a range of symptoms ranging from mild flu to chronic septicaemia. It can result in abortion, stillbirth or the birth of severely affected babies.[67] Listeriosis is caused by eating contaminated food, and in Canada it has claimed more lives than any other food-borne bacteria. The bacteria have been isolated from a wide range of dairy products such as milk, even pasteurized milk, chicken, and sea foods including fish. The bacteria have also been found in coleslaw and even black pepper. Bacterial contamination is also not uncommon in frozen and even pre-cooked chilled chicken.[68] In Spain, *Listeria* spp. were isolated from milk tanks on farms, and *Listeria monocytogenes* and *L. innocua* were detected in 2.56 and 1.73% of the samples. Moreover, milk contamination by *Listeria* appeared to be seasonal, with a higher incidence in autumn and winter than in spring or summer and interestingly, the incidence was also lower on mountain farms than in plateau farms.[69] Soft cheeses and pates are sometimes heavily infected and there has been a striking increase in disease cases in England and Wales since the mid-1980s (Figure 4.12) and also in North America where it was linked to "Mexican style" soft cheese. Outbreaks also occurred in Switzerland with more than 200 cases reported, and 91 deaths.[66] In South Africa there was an outbreak of listeriosis in Soweto which claimed the lives of 43% of the fourteen detected cases. In Soweto alone, between two and four cases of this disease are reported annually. *Listeria* is particularly troublesome because it can continue to grow at refrigeration temperature.

Escherichia coli infections

Some strains of *E. coli* can cause intestinal infections. In the US cases of haemorrhagic colitis, haemolytic uraemic syndrome, and thrombotic thrombocytopenic purpura have been reported since 1982. Animal products are again implicated in these infections, and milk and beef are the main sources of infection.[70] In May 1996, an epidemic of food poisoning rocked Japan, which the World Health Organization declared "unprecedented" in modern history. The outbreak started in Oku, a fishing village 180 km west of Osaka and spread to virtually every prefecture in Japan and effected more than 8000 people. The elderly and small children suffered most, and numerous deaths were reported. The infectious agent proved to be a particularly virulent strain (0157:H7) of *E.coli*. In this case, animal products were once again implicated. Since 1992 enterohaemorrhagic *E.coli* have become the most frequent causative agent of haemorrhagic diarrhoea in North America, and in Europe infections are also becoming more frequent. Unlike other *E. coli*, enterohaemorrhagic *E.coli* possess cytotoxic shiga-toxins which previously were known only in cases of *Shigella dysenteriae* infections.[71]

Yersinia infections

Milk and other animal foods are a source of *Yersinia enterocolitica* which can cause acute gastroenteritis. In Belgium, Canada, the Netherlands, Australia and parts of Germany, infections from this organism are as common as *Salmonella* infections, and children in particular are vulnerable. The organism can grow at temperatures as low as 0 °C and the increase in refrigeration practices may select for this organism.[67]

Other organisms

Staphylococcus aureus is becoming a frequent pathogen in hospital epidemics, and this is particularly alarming, since there is a limited number of drugs to which this bacterium is susceptible. It is feared that antibiotic strains of this species could lead to widespread hospital epidemics, should such strains become more common.[72] Other infectious micro-organisms that are transmitted by animal products include **Clostridium perfringens** which is found in meat. From 1986 to 1988 there has been a 46% reported increase of infected cases in the UK. A further organism is **Vibrio vulnificus** which occurs in oysters and has been implicated in infections in the U.S.A.[67]

Modern animal husbandry

Animal husbandry has numerous facets, and great changes in farming practices as well as an enormous expansion in the pharmaceutical industry, have changed the face of the animal-products industry over the past decades. Particularly the use of drugs has had a profound influence on animal husbandry. Drugs are not only used to curtail disease but they are also extensively used to stimulate growth, and this last factor has led to an unprecedented increase in the use of drugs.

Antibiotics

Antibiotics have had a profound effect on the agricultural sector, and today antibiotics are used extensively in animal husbandry. Antibiotics are not only administered to animals for the treatment of disease, but subtherapeutic doses of these antimicrobials are administered routinely for growth promotion in livestock and poultry production. Antibiotics are also used in wildlife and fish, and for the control of plant diseases and food spoilage. In the United States alone some 15 million pounds of antibiotics are administered to farm animals annually. The fact that animals grow faster when receiving subtherapeutic doses of antimicrobials serves as an incentive to farmers to administer these products, particularly since an added benefit is found in disease prevention. Although vehemently denied in some quarters, this practice is giving rise to a new generation of antibiotic-resistant microbes which can cause serious outbreaks of disease among humans. Infectious diseases account for millions of deaths annually, with respiratory infections, diarrhoeal diseases and tuberculosis accounting for the majority of these.

Drug-resistant bacteria have accounted for a steady increase in the incidence of human *Salmonella* infections,[73] and in 1983 an outbreak of *Salmonella* infection in the Midwestern states of the USA was actually traced to the farmyard from which the disease spread.[74] An epidemiologic investigation in Minnesota revealed that patients had eaten ground beef (hamburger) and that the meat had come from a farm lot where the cattle had been fed subtherapeutic quantities of chlortetracycline for growth promotion and disease prevention.

In outbreaks of gastrointestinal disease from drug-resistant bacteria, it is a common occurrence that infected patients had taken antibiotics for other diseases such as bronchitis, pharyngitis, otitis media (ear infection) or other non-diarrhoeal diseases prior to the onset of the gastrointestinal disease. This suggests that whilst patients are on antibiotics, and they consume foods infected with resistant bacteria, the destruction of the natural non-resistant intestinal bacteria offers some selective advantage to the drug-resistant varieties which then flourish and become pathogenic. The symptoms are normally diarrhoea, abdominal cramps, nausea and vomiting and in some cases chills, fever, and confusion. Furthermore, the disease is difficult to treat, as the bacteria will not respond to drugs in view of their antimicrobial resistance, and death can be the ultimate result, even in hospitals with all the necessary care facilities.

The fact that antibiotics are widely used in hospitals, accounts for the fact that outbreaks of antimicrobial-resistant bacterial infections are largely recorded in these institutions. Bitter rows have developed over this issue between governments and trade organizations. In Germany and Denmark the antibiotic **avoparcin**, which farmers inject into their livestock, was banned because of concern that antibiotic resistance could spread from the farmyard to hospitals. Brussels, on the grounds that the ban could interfere with free trade, declared the ban illegal. Avoparcin is similar to other antibiotics such as **vancomycin** and **teicoplanin** which are the only drugs available that kill methicillin-resistant *Staphylococcus aureus* (MRSA), which is becoming more and more prevalent in hospitals. Microbiologists were dismayed that the German studies had not been able to uphold the ban.[72] Sadly it is often the elderly or infants who succumb to the disease due to their weaker constitution.

In view of the widespread use of antibiotics in animal husbandry, the most common sources of contamination, by this new breed of antibiotic resistant bacteria, are poultry, cattle, calves, eggs and milk. In fact, in over two thirds of US outbreaks of multiple drug-resistant *Salmonella* infections with a definite source, the bacteria came from food animal populations, and the transmission of resistant bacteria to man, through the consumption of food animals, is thus not a rare event.[75] The World Health Organization has reported that resistant strains of *Salmonella typhimurium* have increased dramatically in many countries, and there was hardly any medication that was effective against the DT 104 strain of this species. In some European countries the total number of *Salmonella* infections has increased 20fold in the last decade and in Britain, where DT 104 was first isolated in 1988, the number of infections from this strain increase from 300 in 1990 to 3 500 in 1996. In Germany, the percentage of infections caused by this strain rose from ten to 18% within the year 1996 alone.[76]

Tetracyclines are the most commonly used antibiotics in feeding operations, and these drugs commonly occur in the animal products purchased from supermarkets and other stores. Contamination of foods with antibiotics may present various health hazards and can be strongly allergenic in sensitive individuals. A study on the occurrence of antibiotic residues and drug-resistant bacteria in beef and chicken tissues purchased from supermarkets in Hermisillo, Mexico, showed that 86% of beef samples were contaminated with streptomycin whilst other antibiotics were also prevalent. Chicken breasts sampled, likewise, showed high levels of contamination which exceeded FDA tolerance limits (Table 4.6).[77]

Antibiotic	Beef % Samples	Beef Range (ng/g)	chicken % Samples	chicken Range (ng/g)
Penicillin	–	–	–	–
Tetracycline	40	416–1920	23	480–1840
Streptomycin	86	96–800	93	80–1312
Chloramphenicol	12	256–1968	67	176–1008
Gentamicin	68	21–64	97	40–314

Table 4.6. Levels of antibiotics found in 50 beef and 30 chicken samples. (Adapted from reference 77)

Animal Products

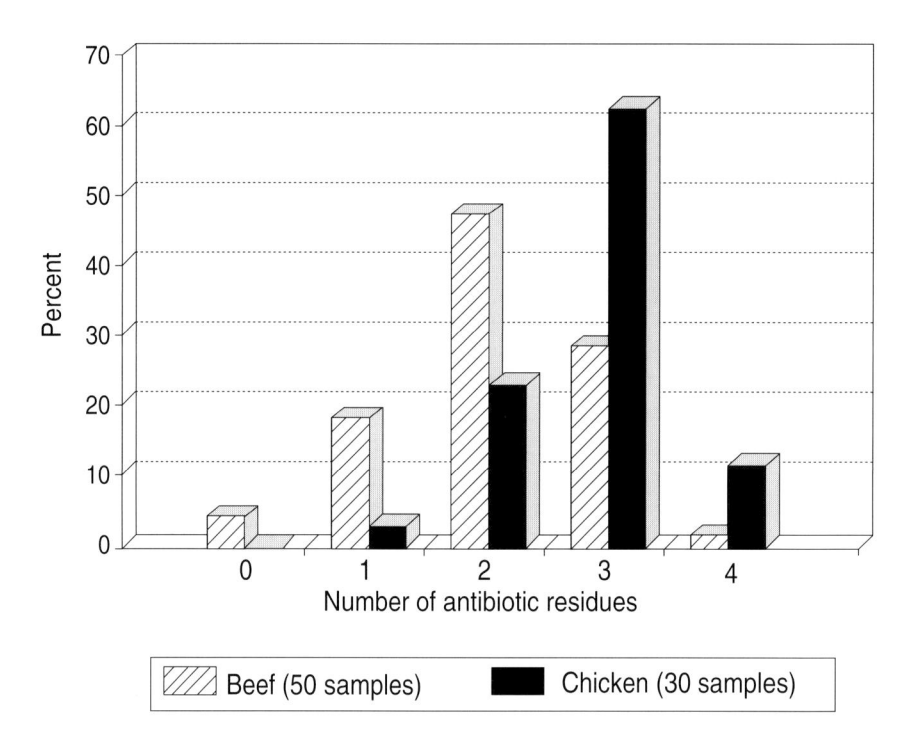

Figure 4.13. Number of antibiotics detected in beef and chicken samples. (Adapted from reference 77)

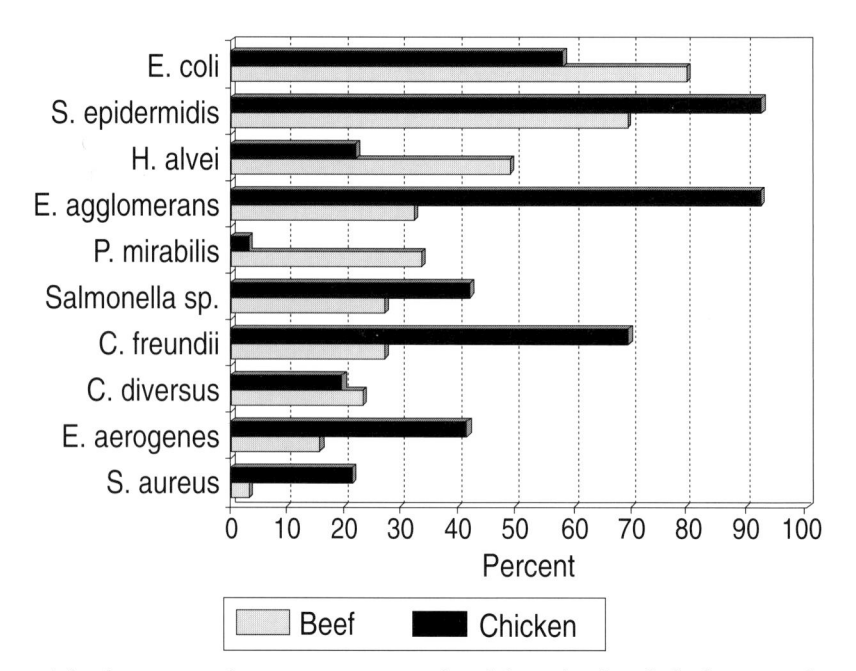

Figure 4.14. The frequency of microorganisms isolated from beef and chicken samples. (Adapted from reference 77)

In this study it was found that in more than 50% of the chicken and beef samples investigated, more than one antibiotic was present at the same time, and in some cases three or four different antibiotics had been administered to the animals simultaneously (Fig. 4.13).

The frequency at which the different microorganisms occurred in the samples varied, but a wide range of potentially pathogenic species was prevalent in both beef and chicken samples (Fig 4.14).

From table 4.7 it is evident that no penicillin was found in any of the samples investigated. The reason for this is that penicillin is no longer used subtherapeutically in these areas as it has become ineffective. Bacteria resistant to penicillin were however isolated from these tissues, showing that drug resistance persists beyond the time in which the drugs were used. Nearly all the bacteria isolated from the above mentioned tissues were resistant to penicillin, with high resistance to tetracycline and streptomycin also noted (Table 4.7).

In view of the current controversy surrounding the issue of antibiotic resistant bacterial strains, two questions seem vital at this stage:
1. Is the use of subtherapeutic doses on farms responsible for the increase in resistant strains?
2. What is the status regarding vancomycin resistance?

The argument by industry has been that subtherapeutic doses cannot enhance resistance, however, this does not seem logical as even low doses of antibiotics should provide a selective advantage to resistant strains. If indeed this is the case, then at least certain antibiotics should be banned for use in the animal husbandry industry. Vancomycin is a case in point, as vancomycin is the only drug that can kill methicillin-resistant *Staphylococcus aureus* which is causing hospital epidemics with alarming regularity.[72] To examine this issue, a project was jointly undertaken by the Departments of Zoology and Microbiology at the University of the Western Cape, in which chicken, pork, beef and milk samples were

Isolated organisms	% Resistance to									
	Penicillin		Tetracyclin		Streptomycin		Chloramphenicol		Gentamicin	
	Beef	Chicken	Beef	Chicken	Beef	Chicken	Beef	Chicken	Beef	Chicken
Escherichia coli	90	71	76	71	52	76	7	–	3	21
Staphyloc. epidermidis	100	38	45	38	32	19	6	–	9	–
Hafnia alvei	100	73	73	60	45	33	–	7	–	–
Enterobacter agglomerans	98	80	74	70	26	60	2	–	4	–
Salmonella sp.	100	75	57	80	38	38	5	50	–	–
Citrobacter freundii	100	63	86	75	46	63	–	–	–	–
Enterobacter aerogenes	100	50	52	75	43	25	14	25	10	25
Proteus mirabilis	100	60	50	100	75	38	–	5	–	–
Citrobacter diversus	100	57	73	43	36	29	–	–	9	–
Serratia liquefaciens	100	83	100	83	–	50	–	–	–	–
Morganella morganii	100	83	75	83	50	50	–	–	25	–
Staphylococcus aureus	91	–	75	–	36	–	–	–	–	–

Table 4.7 Antibiotic resistance in bacteria isolated from 50 beef and 30 chicken samples. (Adapted from reference 77)

tested for bacterial contamination and multiple antibiotic resistance in the greater Cape Town area. Animal bacterial samples were taken at abattoirs and at retail outlets, the rationale being that differences in resistance between the two groups of samples should pinpoint the source. Higher resistance levels in abattoir samples taken at the beginning of the slaughtering cycle would indicate that the resistance had emanated from the farm. The results for the chicken samples have thus far been evaluated, and are presented in table 4.8.

The results clearly show that a large proportion of the bacterial strains showed multiple antibiotic resistance, and in most cases the bacteria from the abattoir samples had a higher resistance to antibiotics than the retail samples thus indicating that the resistance route came via the farm. The very high resistance level displayed by most of the bacteria is certainly unsettling. Staphylococci were resistant to tetracycline and oxacillin but the percentage of abattoir isolates that displayed simultaneous resistance to both tetracycline and oxacillin was nearly double that of retail samples (69.6% versus 39.4%).Gram positive bacteria *(Staphylococcus)* are susceptible to vancomycin, and although resistance of *Staphylococcus* to vancomycin as well as methicillin was not very high, even the 7% resistance recorded in retail samples is cause for concern, considering that this is the only drug that can kill methicillin-resistant *Staphylococcus aureus*.[78]

Producers are required to observe a withdrawal period after administering antibiotics, prior to marketing their product. It is, however, not feasible to monitor all the meat that goes to market, and studies on swine have shown that producers do not adhere to the specified withdrawal times.[79] Antibiotic residues are even found in carcasses of cattle with no record of antibiotic treatment.[80] Even if they should adhere to these withdrawal times, it is doubtful whether this will be of much benefit, considering the fact that resistance has been maintained over years to antibiotics that are no longer in use. Besides the antibiotic problem, contamination of carcasses with antimicrobial agents and other dangerous compounds such as heavy metals, organochlorine compounds, organophosphorous compounds and growth stimulants, is now so widespread that methods are being devised to routinely monitor these contaminants in the interest of human safety.[81]

Additional growth promoters

Besides the addition of antimicrobials to promote growth, animal feed is also routinely spiked with hormonal growth promoters of which some may be carcinogenic. Hormone residues that have been isolated from beef include **trenbolone acetate, zeranol and stilbene diethylstilboestrol (DES), oestradiol, dienoestrol, hexaestrol, 17α-ethynyloestradiol, ketosteroids, testosterone, progesterone** and **progesterone acetate**, which

Antibiotic	*Salmonella* Abattoir	*Staphylococcus* Retail	*Staphylococcus* Abattoir	Enterobacteriaceae Retail	Enterobacteriaceae Abattoir	Total aerobic Retail	Total aerobic Abattoir
Tetracycline	96.6	79.5	90.5	54.2	100	34.8	90.7
Streptomycin	86.4	3.9	7.9	38.1	64.9	25	46.7
Gentamicin	5.1	–	–	5.1	1.8	1.5	4
Oxacillin	100	72.4	93.7	100	100	87.1	92
Vancomycin	100	7	14.3	100	94.7	62.1	36
Methicillin	100	14.1	17.5	100	100	71.2	64

Table 4.8. Percentage resistance of various retail and abattoir chicken isolates to six antibiotics. (From reference 78)

are all used as anabolic steroids to promote weight increase. To promote lean meat production, animals are fed **β-agonists**, a group of drugs that convert fats to fatty acids and stimulate the formation of proteins, to promote rapid weight gain. In addition in some countries growth hormone is administered and even genetically-engineered hormones are used, such as **PST**, which is used to promote lean meat production in pigs. Some of these growth promoters, such as **clenbuterol**, are banned, but there is a healthy black market trade in these growth-promoting drugs as shown by the clenbuterol scandal in 1996 when German authorities found that the drug was being used on more than 40 calf fattening farms in Nordrhein-Westfalen and consequently prohibited the slaughter of 2400 calves and arrested a veterinary drug dealer. In a further case around the county of Gütersloh, calves were found with the banned antibiotic Chloramphenicol.[82]

Farm animals today are often treated as commodities, like inanimate consumer goods. They are frequently housed in unhealthy environments and fed virtually anything that will promote growth and increase profits, even though the long-term effect on the health of the animals or the human consumer is not known. In large chicken hatcheries the chicks never see sunlight, but are subjected to low-intensity light for close on 24 hours per day. The lights are switched off only for approximately 15 min each day so that the chickens can get used to darkness, lest they panic during a power failure and cause production losses. Animals are cramped together to limit their movements and energy expenditure, because growth and mass increase are the paramount criteria that are taken into account when designing these facilities. New breeds of chickens are selected for growth performance with virtual disregard for all other parameters. In the past, a free range chicken could be assumed to consume approximately 17 kg of feed to grow to a market mass of 1.5 kg. Today, some breeds utilise only 3.5 kg to achieve the same mass increase, and this in only six weeks. The chickens are geared for rapid growth, but their other systems are severely compromised. The cardiovascular system, internal organs and immune systems are poorly developed so that extreme care must be taken not to induce stress or exposure to infectious bacteria lest they die before reaching market size.

Farm animals are fed carcass meal, fish meal, edible plastic, sewage, petro-chemical residues and excrement. On some farms veritable food chains have been set up where chicken manure, from battery chickens, is fed to the sheep and cattle, and dead chicks and unhatched eggs in turn are the feed items used in the piggery. In the chicken industry, the slaughter offal such as entrails, legs and heads are often dried, ground and recycled as feed , thus effectively turning the chickens into cannibals. Moreover, the chickens are routinely manipulated with a host of growth stimulating, antimicrobial and digestibility enhancing drugs.

Prion diseases

Prions cause a group of animal and human neurodegenerative diseases which are now classified together because of their etiology and pathogenesis. The infectious agent is not a virus, nor does it contain DNA sequences, it is a brain protein which has undergone modification. Prion proteins are thus thought to exist in two forms, the benign Prion protein (PrP^c) and the infectious 'scrapie form' (PrP^{Sc}).[83,84] The normal Prion protein consists of strands of amino acids twirled into helices whereas in the infectious form the amino acid strands are flattened into β-sheets which can cause transmissible dementias. Transmissible dementias are degenerative conditions associated with neuronal loss, and neuronal vacuolation or spongiform (spongy) changes. Furthermore, the changes are accompanied by the accumulation of the abnormal proteinase-resistant prion protein known as PrP^{Sc} which has undergone posttranscriptural changes, and the ensuing disease is thus termed a **prion disease**.

Prion disease is becoming a high-profile public health issue, particularly since the **Bovine Spongiform Encephalitis (BSE)** or "mad cow's disease" epidemic rocked Britain. Beginning in 1986, this previously unknown prion disease decimated the beef industry in Britain and it has been proposed that some 160 000 cattle were affected. The infectious agent was probably transferred to the animals by routinely feeding them meat and bone meal dietary supplements. Carcass meal is predominantly prepared from animals that have died of disease, or animals that have been condemned at the abattoir as unfit for human consumption. The carcass meal and excrement is heat-sterilized to kill the bacteria, but recently chemical sterilization has become the method of choice in many countries, as it is cheaper. Since 1988 the feeding of dietary protein supplements derived from sheep or cattle offal has been banned in Britain and it is argued, that this step has brought the epidemic under control. The incidence of reported cases has indeed declined since the peak was reached in 1992 (figure 4.15).

Spongiform encephalopathies are transmissible dementias, and occur in man as **Creutzfeldt-Jacob disease (CJD), Gerstman-Straussler syndrome**, and **kuru**. In other animals it occurs as **scrapie** in sheep and **transmissible mink encephalopathy** in ranch mink. In the UK alone some 75 000 people per year die demented, of which 50% have **Alzheimer's disease** and 2% have Creutzfeldt-Jacob disease.[86] The latter disease is characterized by a sudden onset of disease, with rapid progression through dementia and death within a year.[87] Economic pressures led to initial denials that consumption of BSE contaminated beef could lead to Creutzfeldt-Jacob disease, but in 1996, after a decade of ministerial denials the British

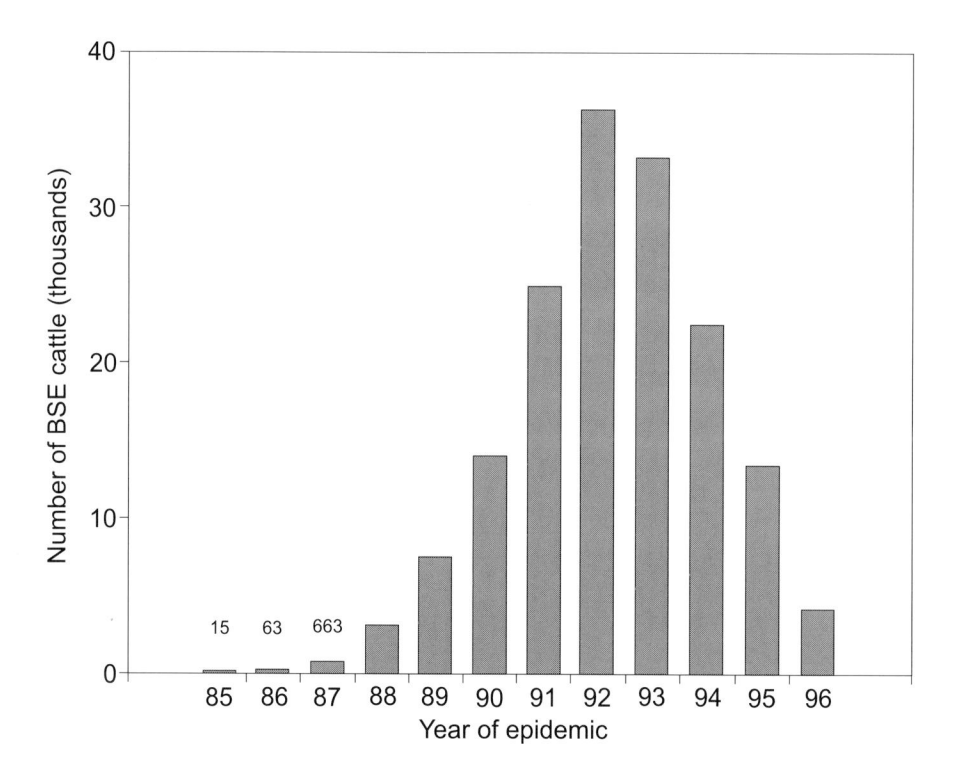

Figure 4.15. The number of bovine spongiform encephalopathy cases reported in Great Britain during the epidemic. (Adapted from references 83, 85)

Government reluctantly admitted the link between the two.[88,89] Since this time, European governments have reacted strongly, banning British beef[90] and even slaughtering thousands of head of cattle to restore consumer confidence. In Switzerland the government subsidized the slaughter of 230 000 cows born before 1 December 1990 to restore faith in Swiss beef.[91]

Prior to the admission that there was a link between BSE and CJD it was argued, that cross species contamination was not possible and that one could not contract the disease from eating contaminated food. However, instances of exotic animals in captivity with transmissible dementias have been linked to consumption of meat and bone meal, and instances in domestic cats in the UK are assumed to be due to BSE-infected offal in cat food.[92] In early 1996 it was recognized that the new variant of CJD that was affecting 12 young persons in the UK had been transmitted via BSE contaminated beef. The experimental transmission of the disease by inoculating macaques (Old World monkeys) with BSE infected brain homogenate proved that cross species transmission was possible,[93,94] and it is now even well established that transmission occurs between infected cows and their calves thus raising questions about the future of the epidemic.[95,96,97]

It has been argued, that what happened in Britain is but the tip of the iceberg, and that major epidemics could erupt worldwide. Thousands of Europeans could be unknowingly infected with the disease and could die, and even in the US some researchers feel that the conditions which led to the UK outbreak can lead to similar events in the USA.[98] Statistics already suggest, that BSE is now Europe-wide and by May 1996 Switzerland had reported 211 cases of BSE, Eire 125, France 18, Portugal 30, whilst a total of 71 706 tonnes of British meat and bone meal and 33 424 breeding bovines have been exported to EU member states from 1985 to 1990.[99] Even if infection of new animals ceases, it has been predicted that between 15 000 and 24 000 new cases of BSE would occur between 1996 and 1999.[100]

Mycotoxins

Regulations regarding animal feeds are not as stringent as those regarding food for human consumption, and feed that is contaminated with **mycotoxins** can be a further source of disease if fed to farm animals. Mycotoxins are toxins produced by fungi, and contaminated foodstuffs is a major problem in most tropical and subtropical countries. Aflotoxins are fungal toxins produced by *Aspergillus flavus*, *A. parasiticus* and *Penicillium puberculum*, and constitute a serious worldwide problem. Aflotoxins contaminate peanuts, nuts, rice, grains, soya beans, peas and sorghum seeds, all of which can end up as animal feed. Aflotoxins AFM and AFM_2 are hydroxylated metabolites of the aflotoxin AFB and AFB_2, which are the most potent liver carcinogens in rats, producing 100% incidence of liver tumours in rats at a dosage of 95 µg/kg. These aflotoxins have been found in liver, milk, blood and kidneys of animals fed aflotoxin-contaminated feeds.[12] Orchatoxin-A, another potent carcinogen, is produced by *Penicillium*, and has been found in cereals and meat products at levels of 1035 µg/kg.

Contamination of the animals does not end at the farmyard, but continues in the slaughterhouses of the world. Abattoirs are concerned with speed rather than the well-being of the animals, and stress and terror are endemic.[74] Carcasses are contaminated by faecal bacteria when they come into contact with ruptured intestines or fall on the ground. Because of contamination with the faecal bacteria *Yersinia enterocolitica*, *Campylobacter* spp., *Salmonellae* and *Aeromonas hydrophila,* as well as residues of veterinary drugs and mycotoxins, it has even been suggested that carcasses be decontaminated by radiation to combat the health hazards.[101]

Genetic engineering

Genetically engineered livestock is expected to revolutionize the agricultural industry. It is envisaged that animals can be made to grow faster and to incorporate changes in fat composition so as to be more suitable for human dietary needs. Gene transfers have been carried out on laboratory animals, but have also recently been extended to domestic animals. Most studies have centred around growth-regulation, as studies in mice have shown that gene transfers of bovine, ovine, rat or human growth-hormone genes can almost double the rate of growth in mice. Transgenic farm animals already include chickens, cows, pigs, sheep, rabbits and fish. Human, Bovine and rat growth-hormone genes have been transferred to pigs, but the mortality rates in these animals is high. Leaner meat has been produced in transgenic pigs, but at a price.

Transgenic animals suffer from a variety of pathological changes which shorten their lifespan. In pigs it was found that the animals were lethargic, and suffered from lameness, uncoordinated gait, protruding eyeballs and thickened skin. Moreover, they suffered from gastric ulceration, severe synovitis, degenerative joint disease, pericarditis and endocarditis, cardiomegaly, parakeratosis, nephritis and pneumonia.[102] The risk of disease from contaminated animal products today is indeed something to consider. In the past the major concerns revolved around infectious diseases and parasitic and viral infections. This risk still exists today, but additional risk factors have been added through modern animal husbandry.

Modern technology has also had its effect on plant foods, with gene transfers being currently in vogue. The long term effects of these manipulations are also not known and these products may also be viewed with some degree of scepticism. However, man has to eat, and if a choice has to be made between manipulated plant or animal foods, the consumption of plant foods would certainly be associated with lower risks of contracting diseases. A diet free from animal products, and concentrating on a variety of fresh whole foods will supply excellent nutrition and will at the same time protect against many of the modern ills associated with Western diets. Such a diet need not, and indeed should not, be less attractive than a diet based on animal products. A little ingenuity with emphasis on variety will provide an exciting, healthy lifestyle.

References

1. Parkin, D.M. et al. 1992. In: Bingham, S.A. Epidemiology and mechanisms relating diet to risk of colorectal cancer. *Nutrition Research Reviews.* (1996), 9:197–239.

2. Bingham, S.A. 1996. Epidemiology and mechanisms relating diet to risk of colorectal cancer. *Nutrition Research Reviews*, 9:197–239.

3. Muir, C. et al. 1987. In: Bingham, S.A. Epidemiology and mechanisms relating diet to risk of colorectal cancer. *Nutrition Research Reviews* (1996). 9:197–239.

4. Armstrong, B. and Doll, R. 1975. Environmental factors and the incidence and mortality from cancer in different countries with special reference to dietary practices. *International Journal of Cancer*. 15:617–631.

5. Snowdon, D.A. 1988. Animal product consumption and mortality of all causes combined, coronary heart disease, stroke, diabetes and cancer in Seventh-day Adventists. *Am. J. Clin. Nutr.* 48:749–53.

6. Snowdon, D.A., Phillips, R.L. 1985. Does a vegetarian diet reduce the occurrence of diabetes? *Am. J. Public Health* 75: 507–12.

7. Mc Burney, M.I., Horvath, P.J., Jeraii, J.L., Van Soest, P.J. 1985. Effect of in vivo fermentation using human faecal inoculum on the water holding capacity of dietary fibre. *Br. J. Nutr.* 53: 17–24.

8. Ames, B.N and Gold, L.S. 1990. Too many rodent carcinogens: Mitogenesis increases mutagenis. *Science* 249: 970–971.

9. Bone, E., Tamm, A., and Hill, M. 1976. The production of urinary phenols by gut bacteria and their possible role in the causation of large bowel cancer. *Am.J.Clin.Nutr.* 29:1448–1454.

10. Cummings, J.H., Hill, M.J., Bone, E.S.,

References

Branch, W.J., Jenkins, D.J.A. 1979. The effect of meat protein and dietary fibre on colonic function and metabolism. II Bacterial metabolites in feces and urine. *Am. J. Clin. Nutr*. 32: 2094–1011

11. Obana, H., Hori, S. and Kashimoto, T. 1981. Determination of polycyclic hydrocarbons in marine samples by high-performance liquid chromatography. *Bulletin of Environmental Contamination and Toxicology* 26: 613–620.

12. Tricker, A.R. and R. Preussmann. 1990. Chemical food contamination in the initiation of cancer. *Proc. of the Nutritional Society* 49: 133–144.

13. Bingham, S.A. 1988. Meat, starch and non-starch polysaccharides and large bowel cancer. *Am.J. Clin. Nutr*. 48: 762–7.

14. Sugimara, T. 1985. Carcinogenicity of mutogenic hetero-cyclic amines formed during cooking process. *Mutation Research* 150: 33–41.

15. Overvik, E., Kleman, M., Berg, I., Gustafsson, J.A. 1990. Influence of creatine, amino acids and water on the formation of the mutagenic heterocyclic amines found in cooked meats. *Carcinogenesis* 10 (12) 2293–2301.

16. Bartsch, H. and Montesano, R. 1984. Relevance of nitrosoamines to human cancer. *Carcinogenesis* 5: 1381–93.

17. Bingham, S.A., Pignatelli, B., Pollock, J.R.A., Ellul, A., Malaveille, C., Gross, G., Runswick, S., Cummings, J.H., and O'Neill, I.K.O. 1996. Does increased endogenous formation of N-nitroso compounds in the human colon explain the association between red meat and colon cancer? *Carcinogenesis*. 17 (3): 515–523.

18. F. Pearce. 1996. Dead dolphins contaminated by toxic paint. *New Scientist*. 13 January 1996.

19. F. Pearce. 1995. Dead in the water. *New Scientist*. 4 February, 1995.

20. Editorial. 1991. Lactose intolerance. *Lancet*. 338:663–664.

21. Levine, B. 1996. Most frequently asked questions about lactose intolerance. *Nutrition Today*. 31 (2) March/April 1996.

22. O'Keefe, S.J.D., O'Keefe, E.A., Burke, E., Roberts, P., Lavender, R. and Kemp, T. 1991. Milk-induced malabsorption in malnourished African patients. *Am.J.Clin.Nutr*. 54:130–5.

23. Carroll, K.K. 1991. Review of clinical studies on cholesterol-lowering response to soy protein. *J.Am.Diet.Assoc*. 91:820–827.

24. Van der Meer, R., Beynen, A.C. 1987. Species-dependent responsiveness of serum cholesterol to dietary protein. *J.Am.oil. Chem.Soc*. 64:1172–1177.

25. Weaver, C.M., Heany, R.P., Martin, B.R., Fitzsimons, M.L. 1991. Human calcium absorption from whole-wheat products. *J.Nutr*. 121:1769–1775.

26. Blank, R.P., Diehl, H.A., Ballard, G.T., Melendez, R.C. 1987. Calcium metabolism and osteoporotic ridge resorption: A protein connection. *J.Prosthetet.Dent*. 58:590–595.

27. Howe, J.C. 1990. Postprandial response of calcium metabolism in postmenopausal women to meals varying in protein level/source. *Metabolism*. 39:1246–1252.

28. Kitano, T., Esashi, T., Azami, S. 1988. Effect of protein intake on mineral (calcium, magnesium, and phosphorus) balance in Japanese males. *J.Nutr.Sci.Vitaminol*. 34:387–389.

29. Kok, D.J., Iestra, J,A., Doorenbos, C.J., Papapoulos, S.E. 1990. The effect of dietary excesses in animal protein and sodium on the composition and the crystallization kinetics of calcium oxalate monohydrate in urines of healthy men. *J.Clin.Endocrinol.Metab*. 71:861-867.

30. Howe, J.C. 1985. Effect of dietary protein, calcium and phosphorus on calcium metabolism in humans. In Kies C. (ed): Nutritional Bioavailability of calcium. Washington, DC, American Chemical Society., pp 125–139.

31. Greger, J.L., Krzykowski, C.E., Khazen, R.R., Krashok, C.L. 1987. Mineral utilization by rats fed various commercially available calcium supplements or milk. *J.Nutr*. 117:717.

32. Bailie, I.E. 1987. Osteoporosis and 'affluent diet'. *Hospital practice*. April 15, p16.

33. Specker, B.L., Vieira, N.E., O'Brie, K.O., Ho, M.L., Heubi, J.E., Abrams, S.A., Yrgey, A.L. 1994. Calcium kinetics in lactating women with low and high calcium intakes. *Am.J.Clin.Nutr*. 59: 593–9.

34. Prentice, A. Jarjou, L.M.A., Cole, T.J., Stirling, D.M., Dibba, B., Fairweather-Yait, S. 1996. Calcium requirements of lactating Gambian mothers: effects of a calcium supplement on breast-milk calcium concentration, maternal bone mineral content, and urinary calcium excretion. *Am.J.Clin. Nutr*. 62:58–67.

35. Johnson, Q. 1997. The effect of dairy consumption on reproductive health and other parameters of vervet monkeys. Ph.D. dissertation. (In prep)

36. Isolauri, E. 1996. Studies on Lactobacillus GG in food hypersensitivity disorders. *Nutrition Today. Suppl.* 31(6) November/December 1996

37. Buisseret, P.D. 1978. Common Manifestation of Cow's milk Allergy in Children. *Lancet.* Vol.1 Feb. 11 p 304–305.

38. Gerard, J.W. 1967. Milk Allergy: Clinical Picture and Familial Inudience. *Canadian Medical Association Journal* Vol 97 Sept 23 p 780.

39. Murray, A.B 1986. Infant Feeding and Respiratory Allergy. *Lancet* Vol.1 Mar. 6 p 497.

40. Werfel, T., Ahlers, G., Schmidt, P., Boeker, M., Kapp, A., Neumann, C. 1997. Milk- responsive atopic dermatitis is associated with a casein-specific lymphocyte response in adolescent and adult patients. *J.Allergy Clin.Immunol.* 99:124–133.

41. Ellis, T.M., and Atkinson, M.A. 1996. Early infant diets and insulin-dependent diabetes. *Lancet* 347:1464–1465.

42. Cavallo, M.G., Fava, D., Monetini, L., Barone, F., Pozilli, P. 1996. Cell-mediated immune response to β-casein in recent-onset insulin-dependent diabetes: implications for disease pathogenesis. *Lancet.* 348:926–928.

43. Harrison, L.C.. 1996. Cow's milk and IDDM. *Lancet.* 348:905–906.

44. Fukushima, Y. Kawata, Y., Onda, T., Kitagawa, M. 1997. Consumption of cow milk and egg by lactating women and the presence of ß-lactoglobulin and ovalbumin in breast milk. *Am.J.Clin.Nutr.* 65:30–35.

45. Jakobson, I., Lindberg, T. 1978. Cow's milk as a cause of infantile colic in breast-fed infants. *Lancet.* August 26, 1978. pp 432–439.

46. Truelove, S.C. 1961. "Ulcerative colitis provoked by milk". *British Med. J.* 1:154–165.

47. Lucas, A., Morley, R., Cole, T.J., Lister, G., Leeson-Payne, C. 1992. Breast milk and subsequent intelligence quotient in children born preterm. *Lancet.* 339:261–264.

48. Carlsen, E., Giwercman, A., Keiding, N. Skakkebaek N.E. 1992. Evidence for decreasing quality of semen during past 50 years. *BMJ* 305:602–613.

49. Farrow, S. 1994. Falling sperm: fact or fiction? *BMJ* 309:1–2.

50. Irvine, D.S. 1994. Falling sperm quality. *BMJ* 309:476

51. Skakkebaek, N.E., Keiding, N. 1994. Changes in semen and the testis. *BMJ* 309:1316–1317.

52. Fish, H., Goluboff, E.T., Olson, M.S.T., Feldshuh, J., Broder, S.J., Barad, D.H. 1996. Semen analyses in 1 283 men from the United States over a 25-year period: no decline in quality. *Fertility and Sterility* 65 (5):1009–1014.

53. Paulsen, C.A., Berman, N.G., Wang, C. 1996. Data from men in greater Seattle area reveals no decline downward trend in semen quality: further evidence that deterioration of semen quality is not geographically uniform. *Fertility and Sterility* 65 (5):1015–1020.

54. Mc Carthy, M. 1996. US studies find no decline in sperm counts. *Lancet.* 347:1319–1502.

55. Auger, J., Kunstman, J.M., Czyglik, F., Jouannet, P. 1995. Decline in semen quality among fertile men in Paris during the past 20 years. *N. Engl. J. Med.* 332:281–285.

56. Joffe, M. 1996. Decreased fertility in Britain compared with Finland. *Lancet.* 347:1519–1522.

57. Ärzte Zeitung. 1997. Immer mehr Männer mit Spermiogenese-Störung. *Ärzte Zeitung* 15. Januar. 1997.

58. Sharpe, R.M., Skakkebaek, N.E. 1993. Are oestrogens involved in falling sperm counts and disorders of the male reproductive tract? *Lancet.* 341:1392–1395.

59. The Lancet editorial 1995. Male reproductive health and environmental oestrogens. *Lancet.* 345:933–935.

60. Stillman, R.J. 1982. In utero exposure to diethylstilboestrol: adverse effects on the reproductive tract and reproductive performance in male and female offspring. *Am. J. Obstet. Gynecol.* 142:905–921.

61. Kretser, D.M. 1997. Male infertility. *Lancet.* 349:787–790.

62. World Health Organization. 1987. Towards more objectivity in diagnosis and management of male infertility. *Int. J. Androl.* 79 (Suppl): 1–53.

63. Johnson, Q. Veith, W.J., van der Horst, G. Seier, J. 1996. The impact of dietary protein on testosterone production and sperm quality in male vervet monkeys. Abstract H160. 6th International Congress on Cell Biology & 36th American Society for Cell Biology Annual Meeting, San Francisco, December 11, 1996.

64. Talami, R., La Vecchia, C., Decartli, A., et al. 1984. Social factors, diet and breast cancer in a northern Italian population. *Br.J.Cancer.* 49: 723–9.

65. Todd, E. 1990. Epidemiology of foodborne illness: North America. *Lancet.* 336:788–790.

66. Waittes, W.M and Arbuthnott, J.P. 1990.

References

Foodborne illness: an overview. *Lancet*. 336: 722–725.

67. Cooke, E.M. 1990. Epidemiology of foodborne illness: U.K. *Lancet*. 336:790–793.

68. Varabioff, Y. 1990. Incidence and recovery of listeria from chicken with pre enrichment techniques. *Journal of Food Protection*. 53(7):555–557.

69. Gaya, P., Saralegui, C., Medina, M., Nuez, M. 1996. Occurrence of Listeria monocytogenes and other Listeria spp. in raw Caprine milk. *J.Dairy Sci.* 79:1936–1941.

70. Smith, H.R., Rowe, B., Gross, R.J., Fry, N.H., Scotland, S.M. 1987. Haemorrhagic colitis and vero-cytolyxin-producing Escherichia coli in England and Wales. *Lancet*. 1. 1062–65.

71. Ärzte Zeitung 1997. Gegen EHEC-Infektionen gibt es noch immer keine spezifische Therapie. *Ärzte Zeitung* 13. Januar. 1997.

72. Coghlan, A. 1996. Animal antibiotics 'threaten hospital epidemics'. *New Scientist*. 27 July 1996.

73. Ryder, R.W., Blake, P.A., Murlin A.C., et al. 1980. Increase in antibiotic resistance among isolates of Salmonella in the United States, 1967–75. *J. Infec. Dis.* 142:485–91.

74. Holmberg, S.D., Osterholm, M.T., Senger, K.A., Cohen, M.L. 1984. Drug-resistant Salmonella from animals fed antimicrobials. *New Eng. J. Med*. 311(10):617–622.

75. Holmberg, S.D., Wells, J.G., Cohen, M.L. 1984. Animal-to-Man Transmission of Antimicrobial-Resistant Salmonella: Investigations of U.S. Outbreaks, 1971–1983. *Science* 225 No 4644: 833–835.

76. Ärzte Zeitung 1997. Zahl resistenter Salmonellen nimmt dramatisch zu. *Ärzte Zeitung* 14. Januar. 1997.

77. Vazquez-Moreno, L., Bermudez, A., Langure, A., Higuera-Ciapara, I., Diaz De Aguayo, M., Flores, E. 1990. Antibiotic Residues and Drug Resistant bacteria in Beef and Chicken Tissues. *J. Food Science* 55(3):632–344, 657.

78. Manie, T. Khan, S., Brösel, V.S., Veith, W.J., Gouws, P.A. 1998. Antimicrobial resistance of bacteria isolated from slaughtered and retail chicken in South Africa. *Lett. Apl. Microbiol.* (in Press).

79. Salisbury, C.D.C., Chan, W., Patterson, J.R, Mac Neil, J.D., Kranendonk, C.A. 1990. Case report: an investigation of chlortetracycline and oxytetracycline residues in suspect swine-slaughtered in Manitoba, Canada, October 1987 to March 1988. *Food additives and contaminants*. 7(3):369–373.

80. Eriksen, J.O. 1990. Antibiotic contamination via the veterinary surgeon as a possible cause of detection of residues in carcasses. *Dansk Veterinaertidsskrift* 73(17):911–916.

81. Kluge-Berge, S. 1989. Monitoring for contaminants in carcasses as contaminated with heavy metals, organochlorine compounds, organophosphorous compounds, antimicrobial agents, growth stimulants. *Norsk. Veterinaertidsskrift* 101(1):30.

82. RIDA News. Edit. R-Biopharm GmbH. IV/96

83. Prusiner, S.B. 1996. Molecular biology and pathogenesis of prion diseases. TIBS 21:482–487.

84. Riek, R., Horneman, S., Wider, G., Billeter, M., Glockshuber, R., Wüthrich, K. 1996. NMR structure of the mouse prion protein domain PrP(121-231). *Nature*. 382:180–182.

85. Anderson, R.M., Donelly, C.A., Ferguson, N.M., Woolhouse, M.E.J., Watt, C.J., Udy, H.J., MaWhinney, S., Dunstan, S.P., Southwood, T.R.E., Wilesmith, J.W., Ryan, J.B.M., Hoinville, L.J., Hillerton, J.E., Austin, A.R., Wells, G.A.H. 1996. Transmission dynamics and epidemiology of BSE in British cattle. *Nature* 382:779–788.

86. Editorial. 1990. Prion disease spongiform encephalopathies unveiled. *Lancet*. 336:21–22.

87. Will, R.G. and Mathews, W.B. 1984. A retrospective study of Creutzfeldt-Jacob disease in England and Wales 1970-79. I: Clinical features. *J.Neurol.Neurosurg.Psychiatry*. 47:134–40.

88. Masood, E. 1996. 'Mad cow' scare threatens political link between food and agriculture. *Nature*. 380:273–274.

89. Nature 1996. Lessons from BSE for public confidence. *Nature*. 380:271.

90. Butler, D. 1996. Slow release of data adds to BSE confusion. *Nature*. 380:370.

91. Klaffke, O. 1996. Swiss cull to meet fears of BSE. *Nature*. 383:289.

92. Smith, P.G., Cousens, S.N. 1996. Is The new variant of Creutzfeldt-Jakob Disease from mad cows? *Science* 273:748.

93. Lasmézas, C.I., Deslys, J.P., Demalmay, R., Adjou, K.T., Lamoury, F. Dormont, D., Robain, O., Ironside, J., Hauw, J.J. 1996. BSE transmission to macaques. *Nature*. 381:743–744.

94. Aguzzi, A. 1996. Between cows and monkeys. *Nature*. 381:734–735.

95. Skegg, D.C.G. 1996. Sacred cows, science and uncertainties. *Nature*. 382:755–756.

96. Masood, E. 1996 BSE transmission data pose dilemma for UK scientists. *Nature*. 382:483.

97. Wise, J.1996. Scientists find low level transmission of BSE. *BMJ* 313:317.

98. Kluger, J. 1997. Could mad-cow disease spread further? *Time*. January 27, 1997.

99. Butler, D. 1996. Statistics suggest BSE now 'Europe-wide'. *Nature*. 382:4

100. Stekel, D.J., Nowak, M.A., Southwood, T.R.E. 1996. Prediction of future BSE spread. *Nature*. 381:119.

101. Skovgaard, N. 1989. Future prospects for meat inspection. Possibilities and trends. *Dansk Veterinaertidsskrift* 72(5):241–249.

102. Pursel, V.G., Pinkert, C.A., Miller, K.F. et al 1989. Genetic engineering of livestock. *Science*. 244:1281–87.

Chapter 5
The vegan-vegetarian Lifestyle

To most people in the industrialized world a vegetarian lifestyle conjures up images of carrots and lettuce leaves, but nothing could be further from the truth. Vegetarian diets can be very satisfying indeed, as underscored by most of mankind that has subsisted for much of human history on vegetarian or near-vegetarian diets. Even in this modern age, the vast majority of the people who inhabit this planet subsist on a largely vegetarian diet.[1] A prime example are the Hunzas of the Himalayas who are known for their disease-free society and longevity of life. The Tarahumara Indians of Mexico are also renowned for their stamina and vibrant health, yet both these tribes subsist on largely vegetarian whole-food diets.[2] Vegetarian lifestyles are becoming more and more popular, and many people are adopting the vegetarian diet for reasons of health, religious beliefs, philosophical considerations or environmental convictions. However, not all the vegetarian practices dictated by some of these convictions are equally beneficial, and some of them, particularly those dictated by religious or metaphysical beliefs, can place severe restrictions on the utilization of certain foods. Moreover, some groups, in addition to following restrictive diets, shun the expertise of nutritional science and the medical profession, and run the risk of suffering malnutrition and associated diseases.

Vegetarians can be divided into various categories, depending on the range of foods which are included in the diet.

Vegan vegetarians: Avoid all animal products

Lacto vegetarians: Include dairy products in their diet

Lacto-ovo-vegetarians: Include dairy products and eggs in their diet

As discussed in the previous chapter, dairy products should, if possible, not be included in the human diet, and the other animal products also have their health risks, particularly in view of modern husbandry practices and the rising incidence of animal food-borne diseases. However, a diet that excludes all animal products might seem restrictive, and indeed can be, if certain criteria are not met. The more restrictive one's diet the greater the chance of developing deficiencies and nutrient-deficiency related diseases. Risks will increase if single plant food regimes are adopted such as diets consisting only of fruit or only of legumes or only of cereals. The higher diet levels of the **Zen macrobiotic diet** are, for example, made up entirely of cereals, and cases of scurvy, anaemia, hypo-proteinaemia, hypocalcaemia and even death from malnutrition have resulted from this lifestyle.[3,4]

Vegan vegetarian diets must be well planned, and special attention must be given to nutrients which occur in low levels or are absent from plant foods. Moreover, pregnant or lactating women and infants and growing children also need specific dietary consideration. However, if due consideration to these points is given, a total plant-based diet can supply all our dietary needs. At this point it can be emphasized again that a variety of plant foods, incorporating grains, nuts, seeds, legumes, fruits and vegetables, will supply ample nutrients for healthful living. Nutritionists often express scepticism as to the adequacy of a vegetarian diet, and their main concerns revolve around adequacy of proteins, calcium, iron, riboflavin and vitamin B-12.

If combinations of cereals and legumes are used, protein-deficiency is extremely unlikely, and numerous studies have proved not only the adequacy, but even the superiority of plant proteins over those of animal origin.[3,5] Indeed, the reverse is true in that it is difficult not to exceed recommended protein allowances on a varied vegan diet. It is only when calorie needs are not met that the body will preferentially utilize proteins as an energy source, and this may result in deficiencies. Such conditions are mostly found in populations where malnutrition is a common phenomenon. Regarding the other nutrients listed, **all** these nutrient requirements can be met by plant foods, except for vitamin B-12, but this can be supplied through fortified soybean milk, nutritional yeast grown on a B-12 medium, or through supplementation.[6,7] Even without supplementation, reports of vegans suffering from vitamin B-12 deficiency are extremely rare (for a more detailed discussion of this issue, see chapter 6).

Vegan dietary practices

Vegan diets in general are lower on calories than omnivorous diets, and as a result vegans are normally slimmer than their omnivorous counterparts. It was found that vegetarians weigh some 8 kg less than meat eaters who in turn are, on average, 5–7 kg overweight.[3] The lower weight of vegetarians has distinct health advantages in that slim people fall into lower risk categories regarding cardiovascular diseases and cancer.[8,9] Obviously the body requires a minimum intake of energy to stay alive, and the number of calories required varies with sex, size and body weight. Adults require some 1 000–1 700 calories per day at rest (basal metabolic rate or BMR) whilst activity increases the energy expenditure. The average energy consumed per day is 2 000 calories for women and 2 700 for men, whereas heavy manual labour or sporting activity can increase the requirements to as much as 4 000 calories per day. The vegan diet has a lower fat and protein content and a higher carbohydrate content than most other diets, and particular attention must be paid to energy intake as the energy supply from fat is some 9,4 kcal/g, whereas carbohydrates and proteins supply only 4,2 and 4,3 kcal/g respectively.

Vegetarian dietary patterns for adults

Food guides in general are useful in teaching, but the average person will not pay much heed to them unless he can be educated to do so. The vegetarian tribes of the world also do extremely well without the use of dietary charts and lists of recommended daily allowances (RDA). The diets that have been established in these tribes have, however, arisen over time and have been practised for generations, whereas Western societies must rediscover simple wholesome eating practices. Moreover, there are so many so-called health foods and metaphysically inspired health notions, that the health-food industry has become a veritable minefield of misinformation. Under these circumstances it is prudent to make a thorough investigation of the issue, and not to avoid the voice of science.

In general the Western societies adhere to the **Basic-Four nutritional guide** which correlates adequate nutrition with regular intake of the four basic food types: Dairy products, breads and cereals, fruits and vegetables and meat. It is interesting that even this Basic-Four Food Guide was found to be lacking in vitamin E, vitamin B-6, magnesium, zinc and iron.[10] In the past, these four food groups were depicted as of equal importance, and the plate was divided into four quarters each with one of these food groups. This Basic-Four diet has recently come under attack from health circles, but intensive lobbying by the meat and dairy industry has managed to keep it at least partially afloat in the minds of the general public. In the past American school children were taught that a healthy diet included meat every day, but now the US government has recognised that a vegetarian diet can be healthy. In 1992 the USDA issued a revised recommendation in which the **"food pyramid"** was used for the first time. It was now suggested that grains and cereals form the bulk of the diet, vegetables and fruits were suggested as next in importance followed by animal product and finally fats, oils and sugars which were to be used sparingly. The 1996 guidelines are a further advance on this, and the inclusion of vegetarianism as a healthy alternative may almost be considered bold. The 1996 guidelines state *"Most vegetarians eat dairy products and eggs and, as a group, these lacto-ovo-vegetarians enjoy excellent health"*. The guidelines, however still warn against a strict vegan diet and supplementation of iron, zinc, and B-vitamins is suggested.[11] The change of heart comes from an overwhelming body of evidence that the consumption of animal products is a health risk, and it can be expected that more changes in lifestyle will be recommended in the future. Already, Michael Jacobson, executive director of the "Centre for Science in the Public Interest" criticized the US government for not coming out more strongly against meat in the 1996 guidelines.[11] Vegan vegetarians need different guidelines to those commonly accepted in Western societies, and they need to plan their eating regimes carefully, nevertheless a balanced vegan lifestyle is not only possible, but can indeed be desirable in terms of health.

Ovo-lacto- and lacto-vegetarians have less of a problem in meeting caloric needs than do vegan vegetarians, and that is why the safety of lacto-ovo-vegetarian eating patterns is normally emphasized in dietetic recommendations, whilst specialized dietary planning is recommended for vegan type diets.[6,12] The energy component of ovo-lacto-vegetarian diets is boosted by the animal fats included in these diets and is therefore not to be regarded as a positive aspect of these diets. Vegan vegetarians must plan diets that will compensate for the omission of dairy products, by ensuring that they include adequate quantities of high energy foods in their diets, which must also meet all the other basic needs of the body. Provided this is done, it has been shown that a vegan diet can provide all the body's needs and can be followed without fear. A number of suggested vegan diet patterns have been analysed, and it was

Number of servings	Food groupings	Serving size
1	Legumes, nuts, seeds, including nut butters	1/2 cup legumes or 2 tbsp. nuts or seeds
2	B-12 fortified vegetable protein (e.g. Soy milk)	1 cup or 1 item
3	Vegetables, including green leafy vegetables	1 cup raw, 1/2 cup cooked
4	Fruits (fresh, dried or juice)	1 fruit, 1/2 cup juice, tbsp. dried
5	Grains and breads (whole grains)	1 slice bread or 1/2 cup cooked

Table 5.1. Chaij-Rhys diet plan for adult vegans. (From ref. 6 and 13)

found that the diet suggested by Selma Chaij-Rhys came closest to satisfying daily nutritional needs of adults.[7,16] In addition this diet uses a simple numerical formula and starts off by using grains, fruits, nuts and vegetables, and adds vegetable-protein foods fortified with vitamin B-12, such as fortified soy milk or simply a B-12 supplement. The numerical formula used in this diet guide is the 1-2-3-4-5 pattern, to help the user remember the number of servings to be used in each food category per day (Table 5.1).

This eating pattern will supply more than double the RDA of iron, particularly as the high vitamin C content will enhance the utilization and absorption of non-haem iron.[14] Riboflavin and niacin needs are also met. The pattern, however, falls short in protein and energy, particularly in men, but the use of a larger serving size would help to bridge the energy gap. In women the Chaij-Rhys diet plan will supply adequate nutrition in all the nutrients with the exception of calories. Again a somewhat larger serving will cater for all the needs, including energy needs.

To satisfy protein needs, correct food combinations are essential, as various plant-protein sources complement one another. This issue will be discussed more fully in chapter 7, but an example can be given here to illustrate the point. Legumes are high in lysine but low in the sulphur-containing amino acids methionine and cystine, and the combination of legumes with grains, which are high in methionine and threonine and low in lysine, will provide an excellent protein.[15] To achieve a proper amino-acid balance is thus not nearly as complicated as it sounds, and the ordinary peanut butter sandwich will supply complete proteins as it is a combination of a grain (wheat) and a legume (peanuts).

Dietary patterns for pregnant and lactating mothers

Vegetarian women are on the whole more health-conscious than non-vegetarians and will tend to adjust their diets to meet the demands of pregnancy or lactation. Pregnant women have greater energy needs, but the relative increase in energy needs is small compared to the greater need for certain vitamins and minerals (Fig. 5.1).

This data suggests that the choice of energy-rich foods during pregnancy must also include adequate concentrations of vitamins and minerals. Nutrients that need particular attention during this period are vitamins D and B-12, calcium, iron and zinc. Fortified soy milk is a good way of obtaining these nutrients, particularly B-12, as deficiencies of this vitamin have been reported in cases of breast-fed infants whose mothers were vegans.[17]

Dietary patterns that supply satisfactory quantities of nutrients for pregnant women are the Seventh-day Adventist Dietetic Association plan for pregnant women.[6] This plan requires four protein servings of nuts, seeds or legumes, four soy milk servings, six grain or cereal servings, and eight servings of vegetables or fruits per day.[18] The Chaij-Rhys plan does not supply sufficient nutrients to cater for the increased demands of pregnancy, even if an additional serving is added in each category of food,[6] but if more fortified soy milk is added in addition to the increased number of servings, then nutrient levels should satisfy the additional demands experienced during pregnancy or lactation. In countries where fortified soy products such as soy milk are not readily available it is advisable to take supplements or to add vitamin D and B-12 to homemade soy milk. Finally it is strongly recommended that one minimizes the use of empty-calorie foods such as refined foods, and concentrate on whole foods. Additionally, it goes without saying that substances and foods that are detrimental to health, such as alcohol, tea and coffee, should be avoided at all costs during pregnancy.

Dietary patterns for infants and young children

Children have smaller stomachs than adults and they have higher needs for nutrients per unit weight, therefore diets that are appropriate for adults can indeed be deficient for young children. Children under three years can accommodate only 200-300 ml food at each meal, and a high-fibre, low-calorie diet will put them at risk in view of their inability to consume sufficient quantities to meet their needs. Restrictive dietary regimes should again be avoided, and there must be a shift to more high-energy foods in order to sustain normal development. Again, variety is the watchword, and single-plant food diets, such as an exclusively fruitarian diet, would not supply sufficient nutrients for normal development.

Mother's milk is the best food there is for infants. It is not advisable, if it can be helped, to substitute mother's milk for the milk of other animals, as the composition of milk varies from species to species. Human infants are designed to drink human milk and a demand-type breast-feeding schedule would go a long way in meeting the infants' needs, failing this, one should ensure that infants consume adequate quantities per meal as dictated by their age. The composition of mother's milk will also vary with the mother's diet, but it can be said that good wholesome food will make good wholesome milk. On the whole, the breast milk of vegetarians contains fewer environmental contaminants and additives than does the milk from omnivores,[19] and it has been found that the vegetarian infant can thrive if care is taken to supplement iron, B-12 and vitamin D intake.

When the transition from breast-feeding to table foods is made, care must again be exercised not to follow restrictive diets as followed by some groups such as Zen macrobiotics, Black Hebrews and Rastafarians. These diets are normally schooled around a few grains, vegetables and fruits in addition to milk made from grains. They are often deficient in calories and proteins as well as numerous minerals and vitamins, particularly vitamins D and B-12. Such diets have led to numerous hospitalizations for malnutrition, and have been responsible for the deaths of a number of children.[15,20,21]

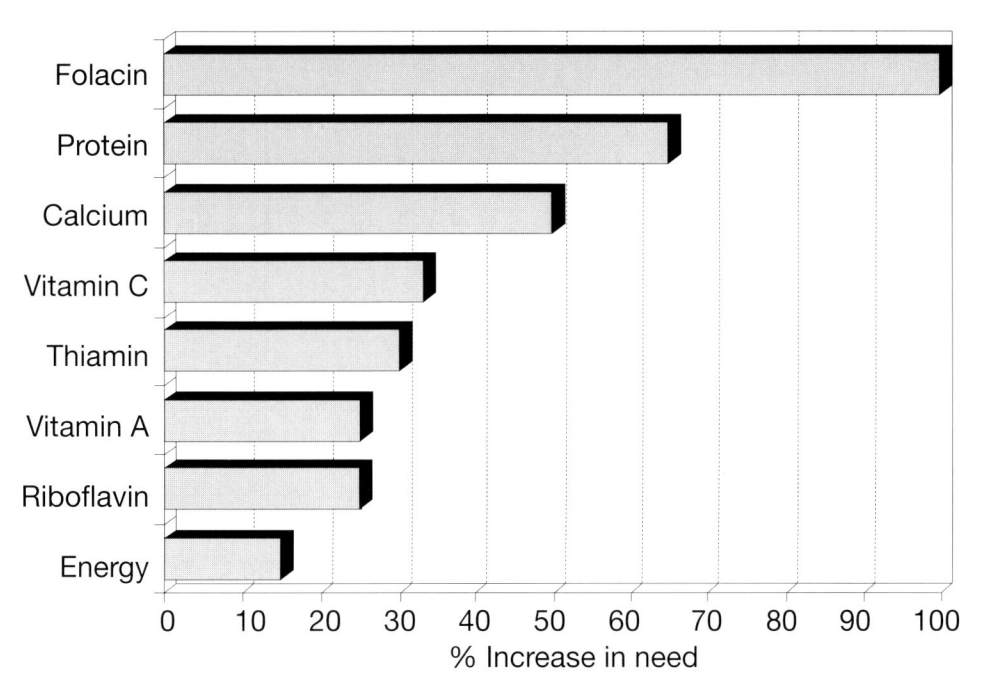

Figure 5.1. Percent increase in dietary needs during pregnancy. (From reference 15)

Some grains such as maize, increase up to six times in volume when cooked as a porridge, thus drastically reducing the energy content per unit-volume. Porridges in general will not supply sufficient energy for small children, and increased intake of cereals, nut butters, avocados, dried fruit spreads and legumes is recommended whilst limiting the amounts of fruits, vegetables and porridges (gruels).[15,22,23] Nut butters such as almond, brazil, cashew, peanut, pecan and walnut butters or sesame-chick-pea butter, can be given to toddlers whilst avocado can also be served even to infants.[22] Avocados are a rich source of numerous nutrients including fat, copper, potassium and riboflavin, and in view of their fat content they also supply more energy per unit mass than other fruits. Care must also be taken to choose combinations of grains and legumes or nuts and seeds to satisfy the amino acid requirements of vegan children. Furthermore, weaned children should receive vit. D and B-12 fortified soy milk or nut milk, particularly in areas where exposure to the sun is limited. Bearing these points in mind, it has been shown that vegan diets can support normal growth and development.[24] In table 5.2 a diet plan for young vegan children is presented.

The nutritive value of the diet plan for vegan children supplies sufficient nutrients to meet the demands of growing children, and can be substantially increased by more liberal servings. The nutritive value of the above diet plan is presented in figure 5.2.

As stomach capacity increases a gradual shift to adult eating patterns can take place. Preschoolers should still receive greater portions of energy-rich foods and foods high in Ca, Zn, Fe, plus supplementation of vitamin D and B-12.[25] Furthermore, it is important to ensure a good mix of plant-protein sources. A whole-food diet, comprising legumes, grains, nuts, seeds, fruits and vegetables (inclusive of the leafy green varieties) together with fortified soy milk will have children brimming with health. If wholesome eating practices have been adopted in the family and care is taken to supply the special needs of younger children, then there is no need for concern. Furthermore, it is not necessary to cook separate meals for younger children, but merely to ensure that the relative portions that children obtain are geared to their needs.

Parents tend to enforce their own eating habits onto their children and might insist that the child eats more of the vegetables or fruits than of the nut-grain-legume dishes which the child needs for growth. Moreover, children also have a natural tendency to consume more of the energy-rich foods, and this should not be discouraged as long as it does not lead to the exclusion of the other essential foods. Healthful eating patterns should be established early, and if parents are concerned about the health and well being of their vegan children, then a *"do as you please"* attitude should not be adopted. However, having said this, it is also important that flexibility should be maintained and extremes avoided. Eating should be a pleasure, not a burden, and mealtimes should be something to look forward to. There should be a relaxed atmosphere at the table, conducive to good digestion, and children should not feel pressurized because parents hold very rigid, or fanatical views on nutrition.

A study done on British vegan children showed that the average energy intake was less than the recommended daily allowance for British children in general, particularly in the 2–4 year age group. But this is not uncommon, as many non-vegetarian children fail to meet the RDA. The average nutrient density, however, was higher for vegan diets for most nutrients, with the exception of calcium and fat, when compared to the average UK diet. The children tended to be lighter than the average, but normal in terms of their blood formation, educational and physical development. Vegan diets have received a bad press because of a few inappropriate diets, but appropriate vegan diets will rear healthy children. Moreover, there is no evidence that either intellectual function or physical stamina are adversely affected by a well-planned vegan diet.[24]

Food group	Approximate serving size	Daily servings per age		
		6 months – 1 yr	1 – 4 yr	4 – 6 yr
Bread	1 slice	1	3	4
Cereals (enriched)	1 – 5 tbsp	1/2 (finely ground)	1	2
Fats	1 tsp	0	3	4
Fruits:				
Citrus	1/4–1/2 cup	0	2 (juice)	3
Other	2–6 tbsp	3 (pureed)	2 (chopped)	3
Protein foods	1–6 tbsp	2 (cooked and sieved)	3 (chopped)	3
Vegetables				
green leafy or deep yellow	1/4–1/2 cup	1/4 (cooked and pureed)	1/2 (chopped)	1
other		1/2 (cooked and pureed)	1 (chopped)	1
Soy milk (fortified)	1 c	3	3	3
Miscellaneous				
brewers yeast	1 tbsp	0	1	1
molasses	1 tbsp	0	1	1
wheat germ	1 tbsp	0	optional	optional

Cereals:	Include commercial varieties of breakfast cereals and enriched rice, millet, macaroni, brown rice, wheat berries, dry oats and granola.
Other fruits:	Include avocado, apple, peach, banana, pear, berries, grapes as well as dried fruit spreads made with dried peaches, apricots, raisins and figs.
Protein foods:	Include nuts, nut butters, peanut butter, legumes, miso, seed butters and tofu. (Nuts and seeds should be ground for toddlers.)
Green leafy or deep yellow vegetables	Include carrots, green peppers, brocoli, spinach, endive, escarole and kale.

Table 5.2 Diet plan for young vegan children. (From reference 22)

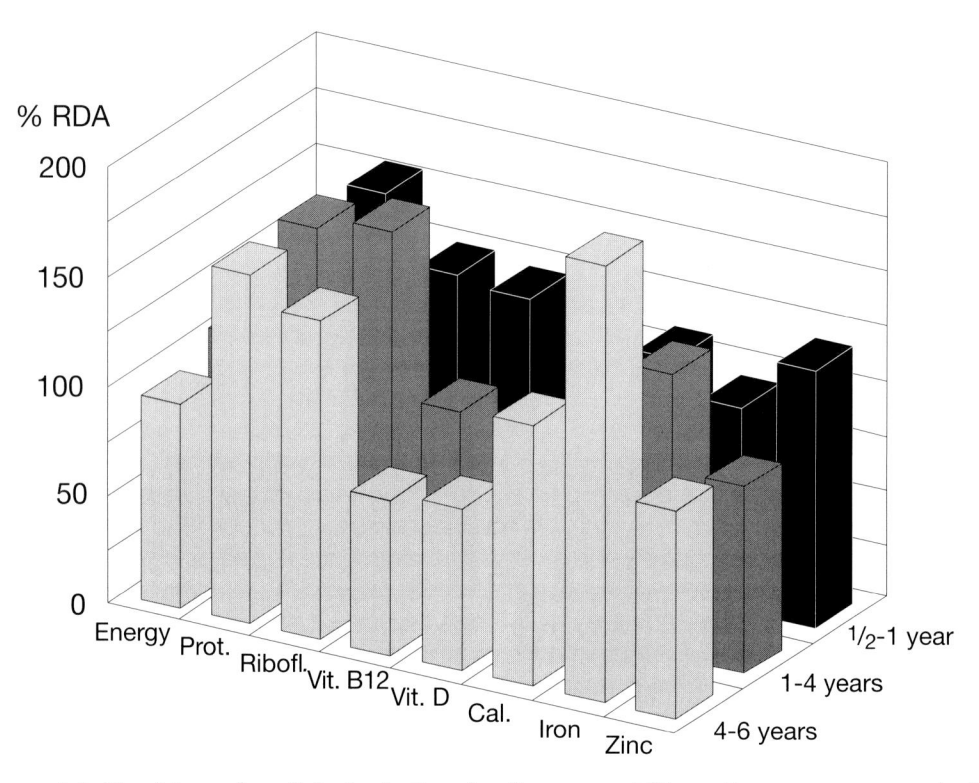

Figure. 5.2. Nutritive value of the basic diet plan for vegan children. Energy content can be increased with more liberal servings, B12 content can be improved by increased supplementation, vit. D by exposure to sunlight or supplementation and zinc content by the addition of wheat germ or supplementation. (From reference 22)

Adolescents and young adults

Adolescents have greater needs for energy, protein, Ca, P, Fe, Zn and vitamin A because of the rapid growth during this stage.[15] Besides catering for the higher protein and energy needs, care should be taken that the diet includes green leafy vegetables or other foods rich in calcium. Supplementation to augment supplies of B-12 and zinc are also recommended for this stage.

Energy requirements

Energy requirements depend largely on lifestyle, but tend to vary between 1 800 calories per day for a sedentary to mildly active individual to in excess of 3 500 calories per day for intensely active individuals. Vegan vegetarians need to consume a greater proportion of high energy foods such as grains, legumes, seeds, nuts and energy rich fruits and vegetables than do non-vegans. Non-vegan vegetarians tend to have a higher fat intake than vegans, because of the consumption of dairy product and eggs, and this makes it easier for them to meet their energy demands. The consumption of these animal fats and proteins, however puts them in a higher risk category in terms of degenerative diseases. Normally, the natural cravings of the system will ensure that sufficient energy-rich foods are consumed, particularly by active people, but when there are changes in lifestyle it may be useful to calculate what the body's needs are in order to put one's mind at rest.

To calculate the daily number of calories required for one's particular lifestyle, it is necessary to know what one's **BMR (Basal Me-**

Activity	Multiple of BMR
Chair-bound or bed-bound	1.2
Seated work with no option of moving around and little or no strenuous leisure activity	1.4–1.5
Seated work with option or requirement to move around and little or no strenuous leisure activity	1.6–1.7
Standing occupation such as housewife or shop assistant	1.8–1.9
Strenuous occupation or highly active leisure activities	2.0–2.4
For significant amounts of sport or strenuous leisure activity (30-60 min 4-5 times per week) in addition to the above lifestyle	Add 0.3
Cyclists in the Tour de France, or athletes in rigorous training (not a level for a permanent lifestyle!)	3–4

Table 5.3. The multiple of BMR associated with various activities. (From reference 26)

tabolic Rate) is, and the **multiple of BMR** associated with a particular lifestyle. The BMR is the energy expended while lying awake but completely still and the multiple of BMR is the factor by which BMR must be multiplied in order to account for other daily activities such as walking etc. The "Dunn Clinical Nutrition Centre" in Cambridge UK, recently collated measurements from all over the world in order to estimate the multiple of BMR associated with various activities. These are summarised in table 5.3., and the formulas for calculating the BMR are presented in table 5.4.

Using the data above, it is now possible to calculate the total energy needs per day. First calculate the BMR using the formulae in table 5.5 and multiply it by the appropriate "multiple of BMR" from table 5.4.

Example:
A housewife aged 35 and weighing 55 kilograms
BMR = (8.3 x 55) + 846 = 1302
Multiple of BMR for a housewife = 1.8
Total calories required = 1302 x 1.8 = 2345

To convert to kilojoules, multiply this figure by 4.2.

Health aspects of the vegetarian diet

Vegetarians have a lower incidence of degenerative diseases than do non-vegetarians, and as the foundations for many of these diseases are already laid in childhood,[27] it is prudent to establish good eating habits early on in life.

The vegetarian lifestyle has often been met with suspicion, if not outright scorn, but in

Equations for estimating BMR (Weight must be measured in kilograms)	
Men	
18–29 years	(15.1 x Weight) + 692
30–59 years	(11.5 x Weight) + 873
60 + years	(13.5 x Weight) + 487
Women	
18–29 years	(14.8 x Weight) + 487
30–59 years	(8.3 x Weight) + 846
60 + years	(10.5 x Weight) + 596

Table 5.4. Equations for calculating BMR. (From reference 26)

recent times the positive effects of a vegetarian lifestyle have come to be recognized. More research has been done on vegetarianism in the past two decades than in the entire history of the human race, and thorough reviews of the relevant literature exist.[28] Of all the vegetarian groups studied, the World Health Organization made special mention of the Seventh-day Adventists as they, on different occasions have received special notice because of their low number of heart attacks, cancer and other diseases related to lifestyle.[29] Seventh-day Adventists generally, though not exclusively, follow a vegetarian lifestyle, with all types of vegetarianism represented. They also avoid alcohol and smoking, which makes them an ideal study group and probably accounts for the fact that mortality rates for lung cancer are only 20% of those of the general populace, whereas the low figures for throat cancer (5%), bladder cancer (28%) and cirrhosis of the liver (13%) are probably also as a consequence of the avoidance of these commodities. Mortality is also down for most other diseases, and with the exception of breast cancer (72%), digestive tract cancer (65%), ovarian cancer (61%) and heart attacks and angina (55%), the mortality for most other diseases is less than 50% of that of the general populace.[5,28,30,31,32,33,34,35,36]

In view of the strong correlation between the consumption of dairy products and eggs with some of the types of cancers listed above, it is not surprising, that those who's lifestyles where more vegetarian, or tended towards the vegan lifestyle, had lower age specific mortality rates than those whose lifestyles tended towards omnivorous diets.[37] Numerous studies, on vegetarianism in general, have shown that it is not only the longevity of life that is extended in vegetarians, but that the quality of life is also improved. This is because many of the common diseases that plague mankind are less prevalent among vegetarians than among their omnivorous counterparts.

Vegetarianism and obesity

The body mass of vegetarians in general, and vegans in particular, is closer to the desirable level than the body mass of non-vegetarians.[37] People with a body mass 20% above optimal are considered to be at a significantly greater risk of mortality or morbidity (contracting a degenerative disease) than people with normal, or slightly under normal weights.[38] The level of obesity can also be assessed by measuring the waistline. A measure of more than 35 inches (78,9 cm) for women and 40 inches (101,6 cm) for men indicates obesity. As percentage overweight is not the easiest parameter to work with, and waistline measurements can be arbitrary, obesity is usually expressed in terms of **body mass index (BMI)**. Clinical obesity is defined as a BMI which is greater than 30. Desirable BMI would be in the range 20–25. BMI can be calculated as follows:

Equation for calculating BMI
$$BMI = \frac{Weight\ (kg)}{Height \times Height\ (m)}$$

Obesity is on the increase in affluent societies, and can be ascribed to changes in lifestyle. The reasons for obesity are multifactorial, but increased consumption of fatty foods, overeating and more sedentary lifestyles are the main reasons sited for this phenomenon. Since the last world war, the British population has shown an increase of 3 BMI units in weight and the average adult is now 10 kg heavier at an equivalent height than five decades ago. Since the mid 1980's, the number of clinically obese people has doubled in the UK,[39] and figures for the USA are similar, with 33.4% of the adult population being obese and one in ten 12- to 19-year olds are significantly overweight.[40,41] The changes in fat consumption relative to carbohydrate consumption in the UK are presented in figure 5.3.

Studies have shown, that a high fat-carbohydrate ratio in the diet is associated with obesity.[42] The old notion that overweight people should cut down on carbohydrates is thus not true, they should cut down on fat in the diet. In fact, data compiled from over 11 600 Scottish men and women showed that the groups consuming the most sugar had the lowest level of obesity, and this can be ascribed to the lower fat intake associated with a high carbohydrate intake.[39] However, not all people on a high fat diet become obese, and there must be other reasons as well as to why some are more prone than others to becoming obese. Nevertheless, a reduction in fat consumption can lead to the desired weight loss in obese people without undue restrictions in the amount of food consumed. It is the change in the ratio of fats to carbohydrates that induces the weight loss. Studies on the effect of reduced fat diets have shown that if the percentage fat in the diet is reduced to between 15% and 20% then weight loss follows in obese people even if their overall consumption remains the same.[39]

Obese people are up to three times more likely to die prematurely than lean people, and the most likely conditions from which they may suffer are heart attacks, strokes, and some forms of cancer. Many studies have shown that obesity is associated with increased risk of **hypertension, insulin resistance** and **diabetes, hypertriglyceridaemia** reduction in the levels of **HDL-cholesterol** and increases in the levels of **LDL-cholesterol** as well as other diseases such as **gout, gallstones, renal failure, infertility** and degenerative joint diseases such as **arthritis**. Moreover, obese individuals also tend to suffer more frequently from **psychological problems** and **depression**. Obese women are at a greater risk of contracting **endometrial cancer**, whereas in obese men the risk of **prostate cancer** is increased.[38] In fact the risk

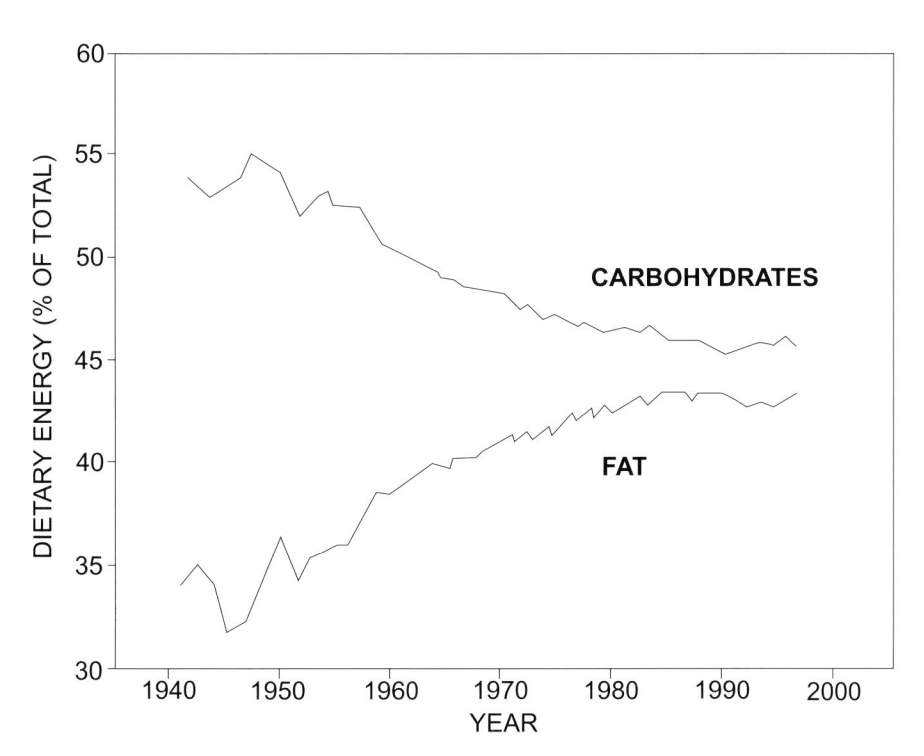

Figure 5.3. Changes in carbohydrate and fat incorporation in the diet over time in the UK. (From references 39)

of cancer in general is increased, and the incidence of **breast, colon, rectum, kidney, cervix, ovary, thyroid and gallbladder cancer** is higher in obese than in normal people.[43] The issue is however complex, as fat intake and detrimental habits such as smoking and drinking cloud the issue. A study on 750 000 men and women showed that the effect of obesity seems to differ between the sexes. Men who are within 10% of their ideal body mass had the lowest risk of contracting colon, prostate and kidney cancers, whereas women who were 10–20% below the average weight for age and height had lower incidences of colon, breast, uterus, gallbladder, ovary, cervix and kidney cancer.[44]

The distribution of body fat is also significant in determining the level of risk. Abdominal obesity is more dangerous than gluteal-femoral (upper thigh and buttocks or **pear-shaped**) obesity. In women the effect of an increased Waist-to-hip ratio (commonly referred to as **apple-shaped**) has been positively linked to cancer. Increased levels of upper body or abdominal fat have also been related to hypertension and diabetes. Moreover, in some cases it seems probable that the distribution of body fat is of greater significance in increasing the risk of disease, than is the degree of obesity.[38]

Adipose tissue increases the levels of **oestrogens**, and increased levels of these hormones have been associated with cancer, particularly of the breast. Pre-menopausal women who are vegans or are on a low-fat vegetarian diet, have lower levels of oestrogens and their menstrual cycles are also shorter by 1–2 days.[45] Western diets lead to raised levels of oestrogen in general and this has been associated with cancer. Breast cancer rates are lower in countries where vegetarian diets are commonly consumed.[28] The issue is complex, and the causes of cancer are multifactorial. Nevertheless, it has been established that a vegetarian diet offers protection against specific cancers, and colon cancer rates in vegetarians are lower than in non-vegetarians.[46] **Secondary bile acids** have been linked to intestinal tumour formation, and here again vegan vegetarians have the lowest ratio of secondary to primary bile acids.[47] Furthermore, cell proliferation, a factor correlated with tumour growths and development,[48] is lowest in the colon of vegetarians.[28]

The dangers of undernutrition

The Body Mass Index (BMI), is the most convenient indicator of chronic undernutrition. As noted previously, a desirable BMI would be in the range 20–25, but low BMI values also impact negatively on health. In India, individuals with a BMI lower than 16 had a mortality rate of 32.3/1000/year compared with 12.1/1000/year in individuals with a BMI greater than 18.5. Figure 5.4 shows the relationship between low BMI's and fathers not working because of illness. Women suffer even more than men in this regard.

Whilst it is true, that high fat intakes can lead to obesity, fat intake should be regulated to maintain a desirable BMI. Moreover, fat intakes that are desirable for adults may be totally inappropriate for infants and growing children. Fears that fat consumption in children may lay the foundation for cardiovascular disease, cancer and other degenerative diseases in adulthood, may have been premature, as there is no convincing scientific data to support this claim. The fact is, children need more fat in their diets than adults.[51,52] Vegan vegetarians on a whole food low fat diet should monitor their children to ensure that they receive adequate quantities of fat in the diet. This can be achieved by selecting whole foods with a high fat content such as nuts, seeds, avocado, olives and high fat legumes. Spreads and nut or seed creams and milk can be used liberally by children whereas adults may need to restrict the intake of large quantities of these foods. The key lies in monitoring one's BMI, and using foods with a high fat content to maintain body weight at an optimum. Children on vegan diets need not and should not look like undernourished children.

At a recent symposium of the American Institute of Nutrition, the following point of view found substantive support: 1) Providing adequate energy and nutrients to ensure adequate growth and development remains the most important consideration in the nutrition of children. 2) During preschool and childhood years, nutritious food choices should not be eliminated or restricted because of fat content. During early adolescence, an energy intake adequate to sustain growth should be emphasised, with gradual lowering of fat intake. Once linear growth has stopped, fat intake at the level recommended for adults is appropriate. 3) Food patterns that emphasise variety and complex carbohydrates and include low-fat choices are appropriate for children. 4) Physical activity and healthy eating are important lifestyle habits for children. They conclude that from the age of two until the end of linear growth there should be a transition from the high-fat diet of infancy to one with no more than 30% of calories from fat and no more than 10% of energy from saturated fat.[52]

Diabetes mellitus

Diabetes has two forms: **Insulin Dependant Diabetes** or **Type I Diabetes** which normally develops early on in life as a consequence of the destruction of insulin-producing cells in the pancreas. **Non-Insulin Dependant Diabetes** or **Type II Diabetes** which usually develops later on in life. In Type II Diabetes, the pancreas produces insulin, but production is impaired. This disease is positively correlated with lifestyle and obesity in particular. Individuals with a BMI of 30 are seven times more likely to develop Type II Diabetes than are non-obese people. Individuals with a BMI of 42 have 42fold increase in risk (Figure 5.5).[53]

Diabetes mellitus is another disease that

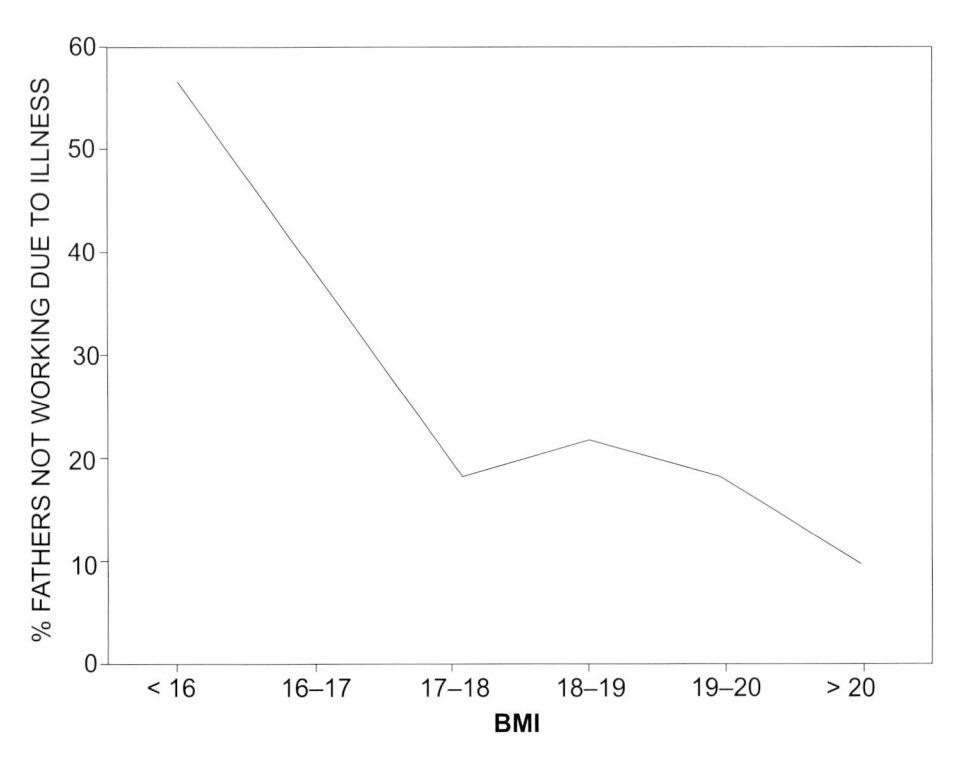

Figure 5.4. Relationship between BMI and fathers not working due to illness in Bangladesh. (Adapted from references 49 and 50)

occurs less frequently among vegetarians than among non-vegetarians. An American study showed that Seventh-day Adventists (who follow mainly a vegetarian lifestyle) are only half as likely to develop this disease than the American population as a whole.[54] The fact that vegetarians in general consume more complex carbohydrates in the form of whole foods, and thus have a more gradual release of glucose from the intestinal tract, is one of the factors which affords protection against hyperinsulinism and glucose surge associated with a diet of refined foods. Vegetarians, and vegan vegetarians in particular are less likely to be obese, and this affords further protection, particularly, since a Scandinavian study showed that even moderate obesity was associated with a 10-fold rise in the risk of diabetes, and this risk increased substantially with more severe obesity.[38,55]

Cardiovascular disease

The evidence that vegetarians have lower blood pressures than non-vegetarians is impressive. This is even true if the non-vegetarian group consist of non-smokers, though abstinence from alcohol may also help to keep the blood pressures of vegetarians lower than that of non-vegetarians.[56] The increase in blood pressure with age is also significantly less in vegetarians than in non-vegetarians. Furthermore, blood pressures of vegan vegetarians are slightly lower than those of ovo-lacto vegetarians, being some 5-8mm Hg lower in the vegans.[57] When 250 g/day of lean beef was fed to 21 strict vegetarians it was found that systolic blood pressure increased significantly by the third week, but diastolic blood pressure was not significantly affected. Furthermore, plasma cholesterol levels rose by 19% during the meat period but returned

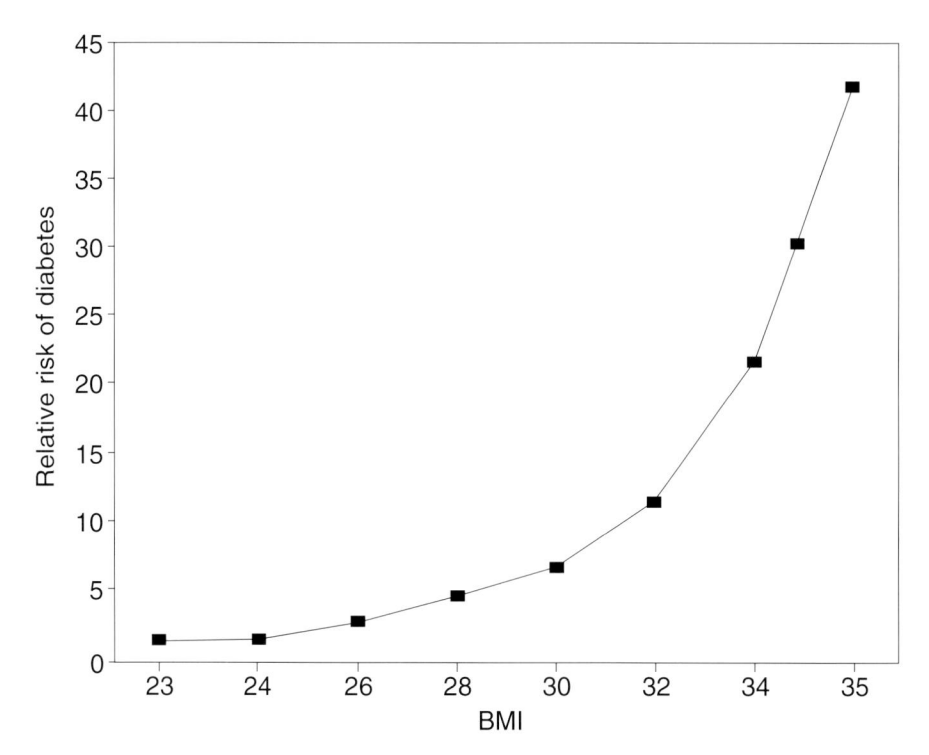

Figure 5.5. Increase in relative risk of contracting diabetes with increase in BMI. (Adapted from ref. 53)

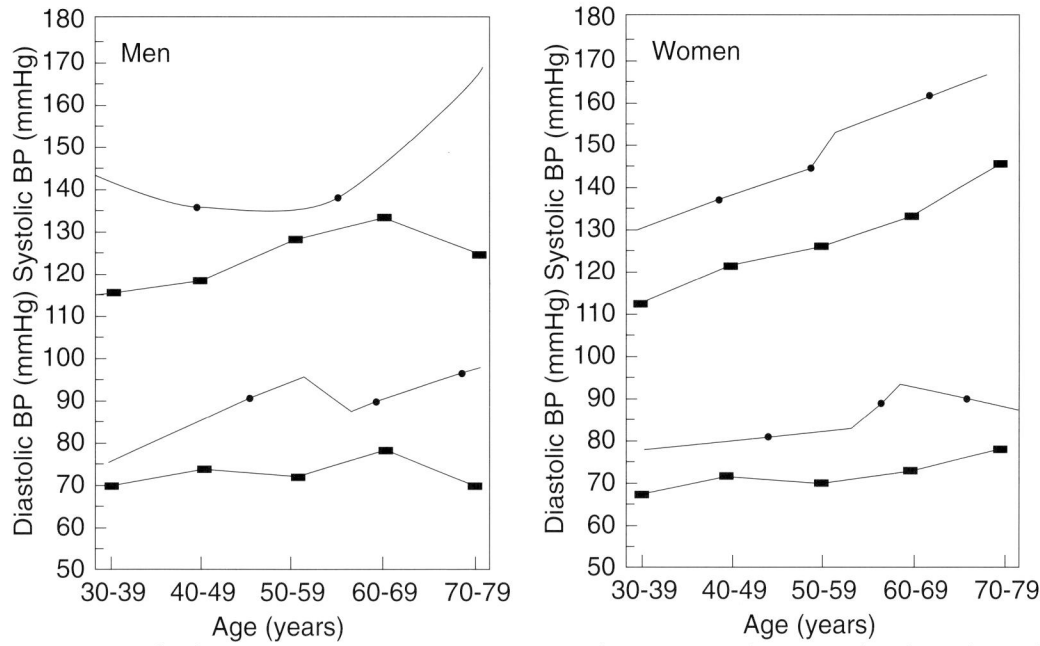

Figure 5.6. Blood pressure in vegetarians (squares) and omnivores (dots). Results of systolic and diastolic pressures for men are shown on the left and those for women on the right. (Adapted from reference 59)

to normal after ten days on the vegetarian diet.[57] It has been shown that increase in blood pressure cannot be attributed to the presence of meat protein, so some other factor must be responsible for the observed blood pressures of vegetarians.[58] Considering that even a small reduction in systolic blood pressure (5 mm Hg) can substantially reduce the number of major coronary events, it is not surprising that vegetarians are less likely to suffer heart attacks, resulting from cardiovascular disease, than their omnivorous counterparts.[37,59] In figure 5.6 a typical blood pressure profile of vegetarians and non-vegetarians is shown.

Osteoporosis

Calcium loss from bone causes osteoporosis which is particularly prevalent in postmenopausal women. In a comparative study between 1600 ovo-lacto-vegetarians and omnivorous women in Michigan USA it was found that the vegetarians had only 18% loss of bone mineral by age 80, whereas closely paired omnivores had 35% loss of bone mineral.[60] High-protein diets cause calcium loss in the urine,[61] and evidence suggests that the rates of osteoporosis are higher in Western countries than in developing countries where diets tend to be vegetarian. The higher rate of calcium excretion may also be a reason for the observed higher incidence of kidney stones in affluent Western societies than in vegetarian or semi-vegetarian societies.

In a study carried out on merino rams, in which fifty weaned (100 day old) rams were divided into five groups of ten and fed diets containing either 20% plant protein (gluten-grain) or a mixed ration consisting of 12% plant and 8% animal protein (fishmeal and bloodmeal as is standard practice in the animal husbandry industry) it was shown that the addition of animal protein to the diet severely compromised bone development, although weight gain and food consumption did not differ significantly between the two groups.[62,63,64] Increased protein consumption enhanced calciuresis and resulted in significant limb skewness. The limb skewness could not be ascribed to osteopenic bones and compared with animals consuming lower protein rations, the **bone mineral density (BMD)** and **vertebral trabecular bone volume (TBV)** of animals fed high protein diets were significantly increased. In animals consuming higher protein diets, skeletal radiology and quantitative bone histology revealed no evidence of bone turnover as would be expected in animals which are in negative calcium balance. The ratio of Calcium: Phosphorus in the bone was inversely correlated with increased protein intake and resulted from an increase in phosphorus content of bone while the amount of bone calcium was unaffected. Bone density was thus not a good indicator of bone strength, as sheep with the highest BMD were worst affected by limb deformity.

A comparison between those sheep receiving the highest protein rations (20% plant protein vs. 20% protein of which 12% was of plant origin and 8% of animal origin) showed that the addition of animal protein significantly impaired bone development. The group receiving animal protein showed a significant increase in calciuresis (fig. 5.7 a), had a higher BMD (fig. 5.7b), increased limb deformity (fig. 5.7c) and had a lower calcium to phosphorus ratio (fig. 5.7d) than those receiving plant proteins. This study shows, that the common practice of measuring BMD as an indicator of bone strength and the risk in terms of osteoporosis, is not necessarily sound. Other factors, such as qualitative

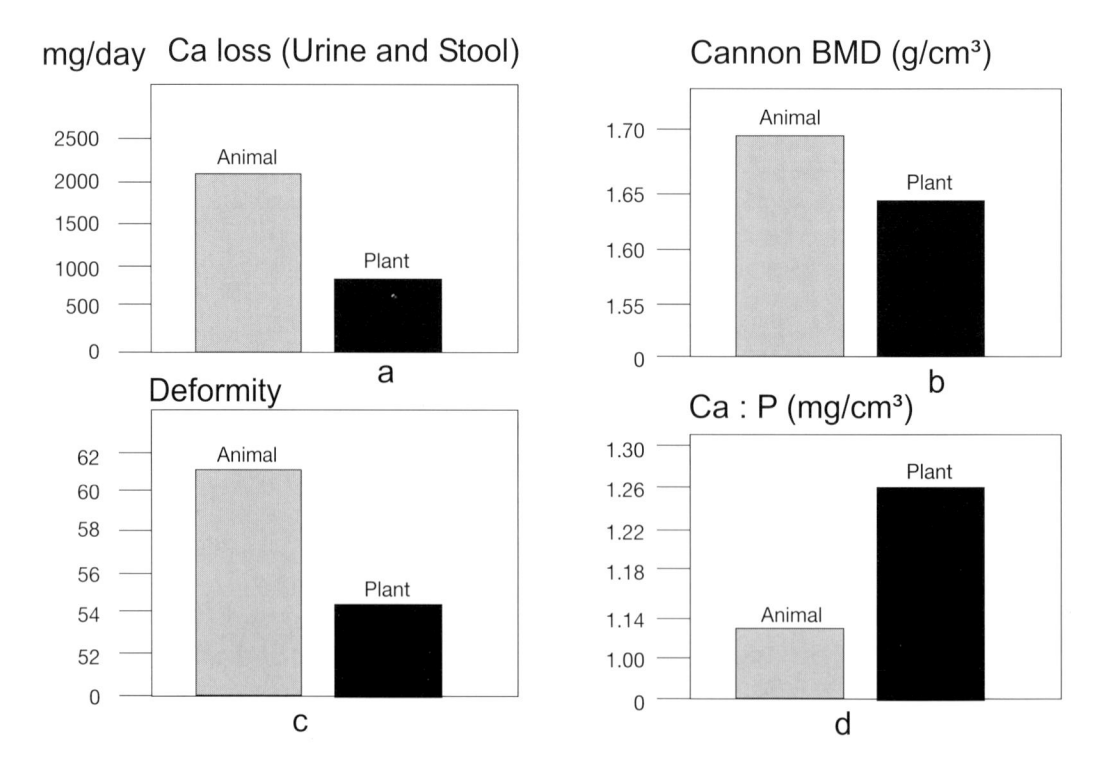

Figure 5.7. Change in parameters reflecting bone mineral status in merino rams fed diets containing only plant proteins (20% plant protein) and mixed proteins (12% plant and 8% animal). Units for deformity are arbitrary units in which 50 represents normal straight legs and 100 would repesents legs bent at a 90° angle. (From reference 64)

micro-architectural abnormalities, and not mere bone loss, may underlie the skeletal deformities induced by increased protein consumption, particularly animal proteins.

Preliminary results in follow up studies on rats, rabbits and vervet monkeys, using the milk protein **casein** as animal protein source, and comparing it with plant protein (soya), show the same trend in all the groups studied. In our modern society the notion exists that dairy products are essential for maintenance of calcium levels and prevention of osteoporosis. Vegan diets are often criticized on the grounds that they will lead to severe calcium depletion. In fact there is no evidence that this is the case and if anything, the reverse is true, as indicated by current research findings. Moreover, osteoporosis is more prevalent in Western countries where an abundance of milk is consumed than in countries where vegan diets are more common.[28] There is also no clear evidence that dietary calcium supplementation will slow the rate of bone loss in postmenopausal women, a position also held by the US department of Health and Human services.[65]

Rheumatoid arthritis

Obesity once again plays a role in the prevalence of this disease, and vegetarians in general are advantaged over non-vegetarians in that they tend to have lower body masses. Many claims have been made that vegetarian diets will cure arthritis, but these claims could not be readily substantiated.[28] It is known that most patients with rheumatoid arthritis benefit from a short period of fasting, but in most cases there is a relapse as soon as food is reintroduced. However, a recent study showed that a vegan diet, which also excluded citrus fruit, salt, refined sugar, strong spices, tea, coffee and alcohol substantially reduced the negative symptoms of this debilitating disease, and this improvement was maintained even if the patients were gradually reintroduced to dairy products.[66] The change from an omnivorous to a vegetarian diet causes a considerable change in the fatty-acid profile of the serum phospholipids,[67] and these changes can stimulate the production of prostaglandins and leucotrienes, which can counteract inflammatory activity.

At this point a word of admonition might be in order. The vegetarian lifestyle is not to be regarded as an instant cure for all the ills that prevail in industrialized societies. Unfortunately, some over-enthusiastic groups have made such claims in the past, and the impression is created that the vegetarian lifestyle is not only an alternative lifestyle, but a substitute for commonly accepted medical norms. Nevertheless, from the evidence it is clear that the vegetarian lifestyle offers a healthy, satisfying alternative to the commonly accepted diet of the industrialized world. Moreover, a number of studies have shown that properly conducted vegetarian diets, including vegan diets, fare well when they are compared in terms of their adequacy of nutrients, to non-vegetarian diets.[68] What is more, these diets were found to be exemplary and, more in line with dietary recommendations than were diets of omnivores.

In closing it is important to remember that variety should be the watchword in any vegetarian diet, and if the simple rules are adhered to then one can adopt this lifestyle with complete peace of mind.

References

1. American Dietetic Association. 1980. Position paper on the vegetarian approach to eating. *Am. Diet.Assoc.* 77:61–69.

2. Balke, B., Snow, C. 1965. Anthropological and physiological observations on Tarahumara endurance runners. *A.J.Phys. Anthropol.* 23: 293–301.

3. Register, U.D. and Sonnenberg, L.M. 1973. The vegetarian diet. *J.Am.Diet.Assoc.* 62: 253–261.

4. Council on Foods and Nutrition. 1971. Zen Macrobiotic diets. *J.A.M.A.* 218:397.

5. Snowdon, D.A. 1988. Animal product consumption and mortality of all causes combined,

coronary heart disease, stroke, diabetes and cancer in Seventh-day Adventists. *Am. J. Clin. Nutr.* 48: 739–48.

6. Mutch, P.B. 1988. Food guides for the vegetarian. *Am. J. Clin. Nutr.* 48:913–9.

7. Nieman, D.C. 1988. Vegetarian dietary practices and endurance performance. *Am.J.Clin.Nutr.* 48: 754–61.

8. Beil, L. 1988. Lean living. *Science News* 134: 142–143.

9. Butrum, R.R., Clifford, C.K., Lanza, E. 1988. NCI dietary guidelines: rationale. *Am. J. Clin. Nutr.* 48: 888–95.

10. King, J.L., Cohenour, S.H., Corruccini, C.G. Schneeman, P. 1978. Evaluation and modification of the Basic Four Food Guide. *J.Nutr.Educ.* 10:27–9.

11. Kleiner, K. 1996. Life liberty and the pursuit of vegetables. *New Scientist.* 13 January, 1996

12. Michigan Department of Public Health. 1980. Basic Nutrition facts. Lansing, M.I.: MD PH (MDPH publication) H-808.

13. Chaij-Rhys, S. 1980. A diet pattern for total vegetarians. *Adventist Rev.* 157: 1014–4.

14. Smith, M.V. 1988. Development of a quick reference guide to accommodate vegetarianism in diet therapy for multiple disease conditions. *Am.J.Clin.Nutr.* 48;906–9.

15. Jacobs, C. and Dwyer, J.T. 1988. Vegetarian children appropriate and inappropriate diets. *Am.J.Clin.Nutr.* 48:811–8.

16. Johnston., P.K. 1988. Counseling the pregnant vegetarians. *Am.J.Clin.Nutr.* 48:901–5.

17. Davis, J.R., Goldenring, J, Lubin, B.H. 1981. Nutritional vitamin B-12 deficiency in infants. *Am.J.Dis.Child.* 135:566–7.

18. Heath, P.K. ed. 1983. Diet manual including a vegetarian meal plan. Loma Linda, LA. Seventh-day Adventist Dietetic Association.

19. Hergenrather, J., Hlady, G., Wallace B. 1981. Pollutants in breast milk of vegetarian. *N.Engl.J.Med.* 309:792.

20. Ward, P.S., Drakeford, J.P., Milton J. 1982. Nutritional rickets in Rastafarian children. *Br.Med.J.* 285:1242–3.

21. Van Staveren, I.B., and Dagnelli, P. 1988. Food consumption, growth and development of Dutch children fed on alternative diets. *Am.J.Clin.Nutr.* 48:819–21.

22. Truesdell, D.D. 1985. Feeding the vegan infant and child. *J.Am.Diet.Assoc.* 85:837–40.

23. Robson, J.R.K. 1974. Zen macrobiotic problems in infancy. *Pediatrics.* 53:326–9.

24. Sanders, T.A.B. 1988. Growth and development of British vegan children. *Am.J.Clin.Nutr.* 48:822–5.

25. Vyhmeister, I.B., Register, U.D., Sommenberg, L.M. 1977. Safe vegetarian diets for children. *Pediatr.Clin.North.Am.* 24:203–10.

26. Dunn Clinical Nutrition Centre. 1995. How much energy do you need? *FEEDback* Newsletter for Nutrition Research Volunteers. (5) Spring 1995

27. Newman, W.P., Freedman, D.S., Voors, A.W. et al. 1986. Relation of serum lipoprotein levels and systolic blood pressure to early arteriosclerosis: the Bogalusa Heart Study. *N.Engl.J.Med.* 314:138–44.

28. Dwyer, J.T. 1988. Health aspects of vegetarian diets. *Am.J.Clin.Nutr.* 48:712–28.

29. WHO Report of a study group. 1990. Diet, nutrition, and the prevention of chronic diseases. WHO Technical Report Series 792.

30. Kahn, R.H., Phillips, R.L., Snowdon, D.A., Choi, W. 1984. Association between reported diet and all cause mortality: twenty-one year follow up on 27 530 adult Seventh-day Adventists. *Am.J. Epidemiol.* 119: 775–87.

31. Philips, R.L. 1980. Cancer among Seventh-day Adventists. *J.Environ.Path. Toxicol.* 3:157–169.

32. Schultz, T.D.. Leklem, J.E. 1983. Dietary status of Seventh-day Adventists. *J.Am.Diet.Ass.* 83:27–33.

33. Berkel, J., De Waard, F., 1983. Mortality pattern and life expectancy of Seventh-day Adventists in the Netherlands. *Int.J.Epidemiol.* 12:455–459.

34. Snowdon, D.A., Philips, R.L., and Fraser, G.E. 1984. Meat consumption and fatal ischemic heart disease. *Preventive Medicine.* 13:490–500.

35. Fonnebo, V. 1985. The Tromso heart study: Coronary risk factors in Seventh-day Adventists. *Am.J. Epedimol.*122:789–793.

36. Mills, P.K., Annegers, J.F., Philips, R.L. 1988. Animal product consumption and subsequent fatal breast cancer among Seventh-day Adventists. *Am. J. Epidemol.* 127:440–453.

37. Fraser, G.E. 1988. Determinants of ischemic heart disease in Seventh-day Adventists: a review. *Am. J. Clin.Nutr.* 48:833–836.

38. Pi-Snyder, X.F. 1991. Health implications of obesity. *Am.J.Clin.Nutr.* 53:1595S–1603S.

39. Prentice, A.M. 1995. Are all calories equal? In. Weight Controll. Ed. Richard Cottrell, Chapman & Hall, London.

40. Kuczmarski, R.J., Flegel, K.M., Campbell, S.M., Johnson, C.L. 1994. Increasing prevalence

References

of overweight among US adults: The National Health and Nutrition Examination Surveys 1960 to 1991. *J. Am. Med. Assoc*. 272:205–211.

41. Nutrition today newsbreaks. 1995. Shape-Up America programme launched. *Nutrition Today*. 30 (1) January/February 1995, p. 5.

42. Hill, J.O., and Prentice, A.M.1995. Sugars and body weight.*.Am.J.Clin.Nutr.* 62 (supplement), 178S–194S.

43. Albanes, D. 1987. Caloric intake, body weight, and cancer: a review. *Nutr.Cancer*. 9:199–217.

44. Lew, E.A. and Garfinkel, L. 1979. Variations in mortality by weight among 750 000 men and women. *J.Chronic.Dis.* 2:563–76.

45. Hill, P., Chan, P.L., Cohen, L.A, Wyder, E.L., and Kuno K. 1977. Diet and endocrine related cancer. *Cancer*. 39:1820–6.

46. Phillips, R.L., and Snowdon, D.A. 1983. Association of meat and coffee use with cancers of the large bowel, breast and prostate among Seventh-day Adventists: preliminary results *Cancer. Res.*[Suppl] 45:2403–8.

47. Turjiman, N., Goodman, G.T. Jaeger, B., Nair, P.P. 1984. Diet, Nutrition intake and metabolisms in populations at high risk for colon cancer: metabolism of bile acids. *Am.J.Clin.Nutr.* 4:937–41.

48. Ames, B.N. and Gold, L.S. 1990. Too many rodent carcinogens: Mitogenesis increases mutagenesis. *Science*. 249:970–971.

49. Scrimshaw, N.S. 1996. Nutrition and Health from Womb to Tomb. *Nutrition Today*. 31 (2) March/April 1996.

50. James, W.P.T., Ferro-Luzzi, A., Waterlow, J.C., 1988. Definition of chronic energy deficiency in adults. Report of a working party of the International Dietary Energy Consultative Group. *Euro.J.Clin.Nutr.* 42:969–81.

51. Olson, R.E. 1995. The folly of restricting fat in the diet of children. *Nutrition Today* 30 (6). November/December. pp. 234–244.

52. Nutrition Today Newsbreaks. 1995. Fat in the diet of children. *Nutrition Today* 30 (3) May/June 1995. p. 100.

53. Dunn Clinical Nutrition Centre. 1995. Obesity damages your health. *FEEDback* Newsletter for Nutrition Research Volunteers. (6) Autumn 1995

54. Snowdon, D.A. and R.L. Phillips. 1985. Does a vegetarian diet reduce the occurrence of diabetes? *Am. J. Public Health* 75: 507–12.

55. West, K.M. and Kalbfleish J.M. 1971. Influence of nutritional factors on prevalence of diabetes. *Diabetes*. 20:99–108.

56. Gruchow, H.W., Sobocinski, K.A., Barbgoriak, J.J. 1985. Alcohol nutrient intake and hypertension in U.S. adults. *J.A.M.A.* 253: 1567–70.

57. Sacks, F.M. and Kass E.H. 1988. Low blood pressure in vegetarians: effect of specific foods and nutrients. *Am.J.Clin.Nutr.* 18:795–800.

58. Margetts, B.M., Beilin, L.J., Armstrong, B.K. 1988. Vegetarian diet in mild hypertension effects of fat and fiber. *Am. J. Clin. Nutr*. 48:801–5.

59. Beilin, L.J., Rouse, I.L., Armstrong, B.K., Margetts, B.M, and R. Vandongen. 1988. Vegetarian diet and blood pressure levels: incidental or causal associated. *Am.J.Clin.Nutr.* 48:806–10.

60. March, A.G., Sanchez, T.V., Michelsen, O., Chaffee, F.L., and Fagal, S.M. 1988. Vegetarian lifestyle and bone mineral density. *Am.J.Clin.Nutr.* 48:837–41.

61. Femel, M.B. 1988. Calcium utilization: effect of varying level and source of dietary protein. *Am.J.Clin.Nutr*. 48:880–3.

62. Brand, T.S., Johnson, Q., Frank, F., Veith, W., Conradie, R., Hough, F.S. 1997. The influence of dietary crude protein intake on bone and mineral metabolism in sheep. (Submitted to *Osteoporosis International*).

63. Johnson, Q., Veith, W., Conradie, R., Hough, S., Brand, T.S., Frank, F., Aalbers, J. 1997. Dietary crude protein and the occurrence of bone abnormalities in sheep. The effect of crude animal and plant protein source. (In prep).

64. Johnson, Q., Veith, W.J., Brand, T., Frank, F. 1993. The effect of elevated dietary protein concentrations on calciuresis and its implications for osteochondrosis in sheep. XV International Congress on Nutrition, Adelaide, Australia.

65. U.S. Department of Health and Human Services 1984. Osteoporosis consensus conference. Bethesda M.D. National Institutes of Health.

66. Kjeldsen-Kragh, J., Haugen, M., Borchgrevink, C.F., Laerum, E. et.al. 1991. Controlled trial of fasting and one-year vegetarian diet in Rheumatoid arthritis. *Lancet*. 338:899–902.

67. Phinney, S.D., Odin, R.S. Johnson, S.B., Holman, R.T. 1990. Reduced archidonate in serum phospholipids and cholesteryl esters associated with vegetarian diets in humans. *Am.J.Clin.Nutr.* 51:385–95.

68. Carlson, E., Kipps, M., Lockie, A., Thomson, J.A., 1985. A comparative evaluation of vegan vegetarian and omnivore diets. *J.Plant Foods*. 6:89–100.

Chapter 6
Additional dietary components and hazards

Concern is often expressed as to the adequacy of vegetarian diets, particularly in relation to their ability to supply sufficient micronutrients. In this section the vitamin and mineral status of vegetarians will be briefly discussed, and we will take a look at the role of food additives, alcohol, and the consumption of alkaloid-rich beverages in nutrition.

Vitamins and Minerals in vegan diets

To this day, vegetarian diets are considered to be deficient in many ways. Invariably the negative issues raised are protein, vitamin A, vitamin B-6, vitamin B-12, vitamin D, iron, zinc and calcium adequacy. Omnivorous diets, on the other hand, are regarded as exemplars of dietary adequacy, and the impression is created that without adequate consumption of at least dairy products, serious dietary shortages will arise. Modern research has, however, shown that most of these assumptions are incorrect, and the reverse may indeed be true. Most vegetarian diets fare well when they are compared in their adequacy with dietary patterns of non-vegetarians. Vegans, vegetarians and wholefood omnivores whose diets were compared with those of the general public, were found to be exemplars of balance, variety and moderation. Also they were more in line with current dietary recommendations for nutrient intakes than were omnivorous diets.[1]

The explosion of knowledge in the last decades has made mankind acutely aware of all the possible dietary shortages which may arise. The fear of deficiency diseases, together with the inroads made by manufacturers of dietary supplements has led to a large-scale increase in intake of dietary supplements. However, dietary deficiencies in vitamins and minerals will only arise if impoverished diets are followed or if stress and disease place additional demands on the system. It is possible to exist without vitamin and mineral supplementation (as has mankind for much of its existence), a fact that has also been recognized by health organizations.[2]

Most people in the Western world consume huge quantities of vitamins and minerals in the form of supplements, and it has been found that a very real danger of potential toxicity exists in some of these cases. Supplement use is greater in females than in males, and the data suggests potentially harmful levels of vitamins A, C and E were being consumed, with some people consuming up to 275 000 IU/day of vitamin A. This is 55 times the Recommended Dietary Allowance (RDA). It was also found that more than 50% of people who consumed mineral supplements exceeded the RDA of iron, zinc and calcium whilst many consumed more than five times the RDA for calcium and iron.[3] Excessive mineral intake can also impact negatively on health.[4] Nevertheless, moderate dietary supplementation has its place, particularly in the case of children, and in cases where research has indicated that additional vitamins might be required. A detailed analysis of the vitamin and mineral composition of specific foods will be presented in chapter 7, and only those micronutrients which are of special interest to vegetarians will be discussed here.

Vitamin A

The World Health Organisation (WHO) estimates that 40 million children in the world suffer from vitamin A deficiency, but the incidence varies greatly from region to region. Approximately 350 000 infants and young children become blind annually because of vitamin A deficiency, and 70% of these die within one year.[5] In a number of supplementation studies carried out in affected areas, it was found that there was on average a 33% reduction in mortality after supplementation, even though some studies reported no effect.[6] Vitamin A (**Retinol**) is one of the fat-soluble vitamins, and it has a variety of functions. Vitamin A is one of the recognized anticancer vitamins in view of its antioxidant properties, but it also affords protection against infectious diseases, is essential for the formation of eye pigment, plays a critical role in growth and bone remodelling, maintenance of a healthy skin and epithelia, such as those of the respiratory tract and gastrointestinal tract, and it also plays a role in spermatogenesis and embryonic development.[7] The need for vitamin A is increased in adolescents, and pregnant women require some 25% more vitamin A than non-pregnant women.[8,9]

Preformed vitamin A is found only in animal sources as it is usually associated with lipids, but **provitamin A (ß-carotene)**, the original source of retinol, is found in plant pigments. Vitamin A concentrations in the literature are normally given in International Units (IU). One IU is the equivalent to the biological activity of 0.3 µg of retinol or 0.6 µg of β-carotene. In 1974 the food and Nutrition Board of the US National Research council decided to replace the IU with the Retinol Equivalent (RE), as this measure accounts for the absorption and conversion of carotene to retinol. The equivalents of this unit are:

1 RE = 1 µg retinol (3.33 IU)
1 RE = 6 µg beta carotene (10 IU)
1 RE = 12 µg other carotenoids (10 IU)

It thus takes six times more ß-carotene than retinol to meet the bodies needs, but on a vegan diet with plenty of fruits and vegetables, there is virtually no possibility of suffering from a vitamin A deficiency. In fact, oversupply can be a real danger especially in cases where large doses are taken as supplements. In its final state (as retinol) vitamin A is toxic, and taking more than the recommended amount will lead to hypervitaminosis A the symptoms of which are fatigue, nervousness, headaches, dizziness and decalcification of bones. Vitamin A is poorly supplied in most meat dishes with the exception of liver, some fish and dairy products. RDA of vitamin A for adults is 1 000 RE/day for men and 800 RE/day for women. Vitamin A is moderately unstable and it is destroyed by heat, light, exposure to oxygen and acids. Diets rich in cooked animal products are thus not the best source of vitamin A. Provitamin A is, however, well retained in cooked vegetables, and a varied diet which includes pigmented fruits (particularly red and yellow) and green and yellow vegetables will supply ample vitamin A. Deficiency diseases in poor countries can be ascribed to a lack of fruits and vegetables in the diet and the fact that the diets of the underprivileged consist largely of grains which on the whole are poor suppliers of vitamin A.

Vitamin B-6

Vitamin B-6 is the name for three compounds that are precursors for this vitamin (**pyridoxine, pyridoxal** and **pyridoamine**). Pyridoxal phosphate functions as a co-enzyme and it plays an important role in many enzyme reactions. Vegan vegetarians may have a lower vitamin B-6 status than the general public because certain factors in plants may influence the bio-availability of this vitamin. The presence of certain fibre types in the diet may inhibit the uptake of vitamin B-6. Some investigations show that the addition of cooked wheat-bran can reduce the bio-availability of the vitamin by 17% or less.[10]

However, the presence of cellulose, lignin or pectin has little effect on the absorption of vitamin B-6. Another factor which seems to affect the bio-availability of the vitamin is the presence of pyridoxine glucoside which is found in some plant foods, particularly the crucifers (cabbage family), and which can substantially reduce the availability of vitamin B-6. Finally the processing of foods also impacts on the availability of vitamin B-6. Thermal processing reduces the availability from animal products, and processing foods with a high vitamin C content has the same effect.[11]

Good plant sources of vitamin B-6 include whole grains, legumes and green leafy vegetables. In view of the factors that influence the availability of the vitamin, it is advisable to follow a varied whole-food diet. Whole foods are rich in fibre, and such a regime would eliminate the need for added bran. If care is taken to prepare vegetables in waterless cookware or by steaming, then the loss of vitamins through leaching will also be reduced to a minimum. Variety is, however, the most important watchword, and if practised, then there is no need for the elimination of any foods which may on occasion interfere with the uptake of vitamin B-6.

Vitamin B-12

Vitamin B-12 (**cobalamin**) is a complex molecule that contains the minerals cobalt and phosphorus. The vitamin is an important co-enzyme required for the metabolism of carbohydrates, proteins and fats. It functions together with folacin and plays an important role in DNA synthesis and the maturation of red blood cells. Severe vitamin B-12 deficiency can result in pernicious anaemia and can lead to irreversible neurological deterioration.

Plants do not produce vitamin B-12 and neither do animals. The vitamin is produced by bacteria, and animals thus obtain their supply from their intestinal bacteria, or from eating the flesh of animals. The bacteria that produce vitamin B-12 are very sensitive to acid and so they are confined to intestinal regions that have a low acidity. For ruminants there is thus no problem, as the rumen contains an alkaline medium and ample bacteria which can produce the vitamin. In non-ruminant plant eaters such as rodents and rabbits, the bacteria that produce vitamin B-12 are mainly confined to the posterior portions of the intestinal tract where absorption of the vitamin is minimal. They solve this problem through the phenomenon known as coprophagy (eating one's own excreta), and thus satisfy their vitamin B-12 demands. Carnivores, in turn, obtain their supply of vitamin B-12 from the stored vitamin in the flesh of animals, but they also prefer to eat the rumen content of their prey, which is rich in nutrients, including vitamin B-12.

The human digestive tract also contains the bacteria which produce vitamin B-12, but these bacteria are again largely confined to the colon, where absorption is minimal or non existent because of the absence of the intrinsic factor required for its absorption. The bacteria are there, and B-12 is produced in the colon as was proved by correcting vitamin B-12 shortages with extracts of human stools.[12] Short of coprophagy, there is thus no other way of obtaining vitamin B-12 but through the diet. As plants do not produce vitamin B-12 (although there is evidence that some plants may produce small amounts), the vegan vegetarian can only obtain this vitamin from food that is contaminated with bacteria, or from the small amounts which are available from the intestinal bacteria. Vegan vegetarians have a high consumption of fibre, and as a consequence, they have higher concentrations of bacteria in the lower portions of the small intestine where B-12 can still be absorbed because of a high enough concentration of the necessary intrinsic factor.[13] The bacterial flora in the mouth can also contribute to the vitamin B-12 requirements of vegans.[13] The more alkaline the diet, the higher the intestinal bacterial concentration will be, and great care should thus be taken to ensure proper food combinations and to consume correct proportions of alkaline to acid forming foods.

The requirements for vitamin B-12 are extremely low, and nobody needs more than 1 mg/day. It has even been found that doses as low as 0.1 mg/day could reverse symptoms of deficiency.[14] Moreover, vitamin B-12 is reabsorbed very efficiently from bile and thus has the longest reserve capacity of all vitamins, and this explains why it takes up to 20 years to run out of vitamin B-12 after one stops consuming it. In cases of disturbed absorptive capacity, mostly because of intestinal infections or a reduction in the production of the intrinsic factor required for the absorption of vitamin B-12 it will however take only 3 years to run out of vitamin B-12.[14] The production of the intrinsic factor is normally impaired when portions of the stomach have been operatively removed, or if there is an infection of the stomach mucosa (gastritis). This probably explains why cases of vitamin B-12 deficiency are rarely reported in the literature.[8] Vegan vegetarians need thus not panic over the issue, but they should be aware of the possible shortages which may arise, particularly in small children, and should supply the lack in the form of a supplement or foods fortified with cobalamin. Fortified soy milk or vitamin B-12 fortified nutritional yeast are possible sources for this purpose. It is important to ensure sufficient dietary B-12 in the case of infants that are breast fed, as B-12 reserves will decline over time in mothers that breast feed if reserves are not maintained.[13] For peace of mind in this regard, it would be prudent to have a serum analysis done to determine the concentrations of B-12 in the blood, as this is the most accurate way of determining B-12 status.

When purchasing fortified foods or supplements, it is important to note that the product contains cobalamin, and not some analogue of the vitamin. Most of the claims of B-12 content on products are incorrect, as the analysing techniques used do often not distinguish between analogues and the active B-12 which is cobalamin. Fermented soy foods, such as tempeh, also do not contain vitamin B-12, and neither does Spirulina, which is often sold in health shops as a source of vitamin B-12.[14] Spirulina may even make matters worse because it contains analogues which may interfere with normal absorption of cobalamin.

Vitamin D

Vitamin D is really a pro-hormone, and its active form is the hormone **1,25-dihydroxycholecalciferol** [$1,25(OH)_2D_3$]. The two compounds with vitamin D activity are **ergocalciferol (vitamin D_2)** and **cholecalciferol (vitamin D_3)**. Vitamin D_2 is found in ergot, a fungus growth on cereals, and vitamin D_3 is formed when the skin is exposed to sunlight. The vitamins are also found in yeast and the oil of fishes. Vitamin D is fat-soluble, and requires the presence of bile salts in order to be absorbed from the intestines. Vitamin D is essential for the absorption and transport of phosphorus and calcium, and it promotes normal bone mineralisation. Deficiencies result in malformation of the bone structure in growing children, a condition known as **rickets**.

Since vitamin D does not occur in plants per se, it is possible to develop shortages of this vitamin if exposure to the sun is minimal. Vegans living in sunshine-poor areas should thus provide some form of supplementation to children and infants in particular. Nutritional rickets may occur in infants if the nursing mothers are themselves deficient in vitamin D.[8] It is therefore, advisable for nursing mothers, in sunshine-poor areas, to also take a vitamin D supplement. Margarines are normally fortified with vitamin D, but if oils and margarines are avoided, then supplementation through tablets seems desirable in sunshine poor areas.

Iron

Iron deficiency is the most widespread nutrition problem in the world today. According to the WHO the incidence of iron deficiency in developing countries is 26% for men, 42% for women, 46% for school-age children and 51% for children 0 to 4 years of age.[6] Iron is essential for the formation of haemoglobin and shortages will lead to anaemia. Iron, together with zinc and copper is also essential for maintaining immunocompetence. Deficiencies in either of these minerals will lead to increased susceptibility to infectious illnesses.[15] An early symptom of iron deficiency is chronic tiredness, whereas dizziness, breathlessness, interference with body temperature regulation and constipation are further warning signs. In infants, iron-deficiency anaemia has been shown to delay psychomotor development and impair the cognitive performance, and deficiency in mothers during pregnancy increases maternal mortality, prenatal and perinatal infant loss and premerturity.[6]

Iron can enter into the body in two forms, **nonhaeme iron** and **haeme iron**. All the iron in plant foods is in the form of nonhaeme iron, whereas in animal tissues three fifths of the iron is in the form of nonhaeme iron and two fifths is in the form of haeme iron. Haeme iron is more readily absorbed than nonhaeme iron, and this has prompted the concern that vegetarians may suffer from iron deficiency. The RDA for iron is 10 mg/day for men and 18 mg/day for women in their childbearing years. In a recent survey of the relevant literature it was found that adult menstruating women need to absorb 2,84 mg/day of iron and, as only a fraction of the dietary iron is absorbed, this would require a dietary intake of 18,9 mg/day. Teen-age girls would require a somewhat higher intake of 21,4 mg/day. However, many factors, such as the type of contraceptive used and the type of diet consumed, impacted on iron requirements.[16]

Most vegetarians living in Western countries have less iron deficiencies than might be expected from the type of iron which they consume. One of the reasons for this phenomenon is that nonhaeme iron absorption is enhanced by other factors in the vegetarian diet. Vitamin C intake in vegetarians is normally high, and this enhances the uptake of iron, and can counteract the effect of absorption inhibitors such as phytate which acts as a chelator of iron. The mineral content of plant foods is often high, and this can also offset the effects of inhibitors. Black tea also contains high concentrations of inhibitors, which impact negatively on iron absorption and avoidance of this beverage is thus advisable. A further factor which can lead to inadequate iron absorption is a high calcium level in the diet.[17] Finally it can be said that a vegetarian whole-food diet can supply all the iron requirements, provided a varied diet is followed, which includes a regular consumption of iron-rich foods as outlined in chapter 7.

Calcium (See also calcium in dairy products in chapter 4)

Calcium is the most abundant mineral in the human body. It is essential for a host of physiological functions and for the normal growth and development of the skeletal system. One of the most misrepresented issues in human nutrition is the issue of calcium, and some of these issues have already been discussed. In chapter 1 the negative impact of high protein, particularly animal-protein diets, on calcium absorption and storage was discussed, and in chapter 4 the availability of calcium from dairy products was also investigated. It was shown that most diets in affluent societies are directly responsible for calcium loss from bone, and that distinct correlations exist between the consumption of dairy products and the incidence of osteoporosis. High-protein diets cause calcium loss in the urine, and animal proteins pose a greater risk than plant proteins.[18,19,20,21,22] The reason for this is that sulphate (a product of protein metabolism) excretion is linked to calcium excretion.

High sodium diets also cause calcium loss via the urine as do diets rich in chloride.[23] Calcium homeostasis is best achieved by a balanced relationship between macro- and micro-nutrients. Dietary excesses of anions seem to inhibit absorption of calcium, and dietary excesses of cations seem to cause calcium loss. Affluent diets and diets rich in animal products are usually high in sodium and can thus account for substantial calcium loss in the urine. In contrast, whole-food programmes will provide a superb relationship between the macro and micro nutrients, and will curtail the loss of urinary calcium. Some investigators have found that phytic acid (found in grains and legumes), may impact negatively on calcium absorption, but this issue has not yet been satisfactorily resolved as other investigators did not find similar results.[23] Grains, legumes, nuts, some seeds and dark green vegetables, are excellent sources of calcium, and if care is taken to regularly include these calcium-rich foods in the diet, then concern for calcium deficiencies is unwarranted.

Zinc

The significance of zinc in the diet has only recently been appreciated. Zinc forms an important component of many enzymes known as **metaloenzymes**, of which many participate in the digestion and assimilation of nutrients. Zinc is also essential to the proper function of the endocrine system because it forms a structural component of the hormone receptor system.[24] Moreover, zinc plays a role in the synthesis of RNA and DNA, and is essential for the proper functioning of the immune system.[15]

Most dietary guidelines will recommend the consumption of animal products as a source of zinc, but it has been found that, as in the case of calcium, the high protein content of diets rich in animal products impacts negatively on zinc availability.[23,25] Incomplete hydrolysis of casein, the protein in milk, also inhibits the uptake of zinc.[23] As in the case of calcium, phytate, found in grains and legumes, may inhibit the absorption of zinc, but this may be partially offset by the protein composition of these foods. Finally, it seems as if the toasting of foods renders the protein-phytate mineral complexes less digestible and leads to lower mineral availability.[26]

A vegetarian whole-food diet will supply more zinc than an omnivorous diet. Legumes and seeds have a relatively high zinc content ranging from 2.7–3.2mg/100g, and grains are also rich in zinc. The bran and the germ of wheat are the main storage area of zinc in grains and contain an average of 9.8 and 14.3 mg/100 g respectively.[27] It is better to obtain zinc from whole foods, however, than from added bran and wheat-germ, as the high fibre content of such fortified meals will make the zinc less available. Vegetables and fruits are relatively low in zinc content, emphasizing the need for a varied diet which, beside fruits and vegetables, includes grains, seeds and legumes. The zinc content of selected plant foods is presented in table 6.1, and values for some animal products are given for comparison.

Food additives

Food additives are substances which are added to food, but are not commonly regarded as food. These substances can be added at any stage of the manufacturing process and affect the keeping quality, texture, appearance, odour, acidity or alkalinity and the consistency of the food. **Colorants, antioxidants, preservatives, emulsifiers** and **stabilizers** as well as numerous miscellaneous additives such as **sweeteners, solvents** and **improving agents** fall into the category of food additives. In most countries their use is extensive, and they are controlled by comprehensive legislation. In the following discussion a brief overview of some commonly used additives is given, with discussions on their impact on health. It is not the intention to create the impression that all food additives are bad, or that the various legislative bodies permit the use of food additives without due consideration for the well-being of the consumer. However, a great deal of controversy surrounds the use of some of these substances, and the current scientific literature provides sufficient evidence for circumspection in their use.

The 1984 UK food act does not include vitamins and minerals, that are added to foods to fortify them, as additives, and neither are herbs and spices, hops, salt, yeast or yeast extracts, the products of food protein

Food item	Zinc content (mg/100 g)	Food item	Zinc content (mg/100 g)
Animal products		**Legumes**	
Beef (lean, raw)	4.2	Beans (common, dry)	2.8
Beef (lean, cooked)	5.8	Beans (common, boiled)	1.0
Chicken (cooked, drained)	4.8	Beans (Lima, raw)	2.8
Chicken (Breast meat, raw)	0.7	Beans (Soya, raw)	3.5
Chicken (Breast meat, cooked)	0.9	Beans (Soya, cooked)	1.2
Chicken (drumstick, cooked)	2.5	Cowpeas (blackeye, raw)	2.9
Liver (beef, cooked)	5.1	Cowpeas (blackeye, cooked)	1.2
Liver (chicken, cooked)	3.4	Lentils (raw)	3.1
Pork (lean, cooked)	3.8	Lentils (cooked)	1.0
Milk (whole)	0.4	Peanuts (roasted)	2.9
Milk (evaporated)	0.8	Peanuts (butter)	2.9
Grains		Peas (green, raw)	0.9
Corn (whole, yellow or white)	2.1	**Fruits**	
Corn (sweet, cooked)	0.4	Apples	0.05
Oats (rolled, dry)	3.4	Bananas	0.2
Oats (rolled, cooked)	0.5	Peaches	0.2
Popcorn (popped)	4.1	**Vegetables**	
Rice (brown, raw)	1.8	Cabbage (raw)	0.4
Rice (brown, cooked)	0.6	Cabbage (cooked)	0.4
Rice (white, cooked)	0.4	Carrots (raw)	0.4
Wheat (whole, hard)	3.4	Carrots (cooked)	0.3
Wheat (whole, soft)	2.7	Potatoes (raw)	0.3
Wheat (flour, whole)	2.4	Potatoes (cooked)	0.3
Wheat (bran, crude)	9.8	Spinach (raw)	1.5
Wheat (germ, crude)	14.3	Tomatoes (raw)	0.2

Table 6.1. The zinc content of selected foods. (Adapted from reference 27)

hydrolysis or autolysis, starter cultures, malt or malt extracts, air or water regarded as additives. Finally, substances that are in foods as a consequence of crop management or animal husbandry do also not fall under the regulations controlling food additives. This last category thus excludes substances such as pesticides, fumigants, sprout depressants, veterinary medicines and substances that are added to the feed of animals. In table 6.2 the European Community categories of food additive are listed and the table also contains information on the stage of functionality of the additives.

An extensive body of legislation guides the use of food additives on national and international levels. The international evaluation of the safety of Food Additives is undertaken by the Joint FAO/WHO Expert Committee on Food Additives (JECFA) which also develops specifications on the purity of these substances. In recent times there has been an increase in public awareness of the potential health effects of the thousands of food additives which are utilized by the food industry, but unfortunately sufficient information to make informed judgements on their safety is often lacking. The safety of additives is mostly assessed from long-term feeding trials, where additives are fed to experimental animals in doses which exceed those to which humans would generally be subjected, and the ADI (acceptable daily intake) is then determined. Although new compounds are subjected to this type of testing before they can be used as food additives, many substances that were in use prior to the new regulations, are used without knowledge of their potential toxicity. In the USA these compounds are listed, under a special clause, on the GRAS (Generally Regarded as Safe) list of food additives.

The conventional methods of testing for toxicity are directed mainly at pathology, and effects on reproduction, embriotoxicity, tetragenicity and mutagenicity are normally assessed. There are, however, other criteria, which are equally as significant in determining the safety of food additives, which are not as readily resolved by conventional trials, and these include functional defects such as be-

EC listing	Functional during processing	Functional in the final product
Colourants	Aerating/foaming agents	Antimicrobial agents
Preservatives	Antifoam agents	Antioxidants
Antioxidants	Catalysts	Colours and colour modifiers
Emulsifiers	Clarifying/flocculating agents	appearance control/noncolour
Thickeners	Colour control agents	Flavour and flavour modifiers
Gellig agents	Freezing/cooling agents	Moisture control agents
Stabilisers	Oxidising/reducing agents	Nutrients
Flavour enhancers	pH control/modifying agents	pH control agents
Acids	Release/antistick agents	Sequestrants
Acidity regulators	Sanitysing/fumigating agents	Surface tension control agents
Anticaking agents	Seperation/filtration aids	Sweeteners
Modified starch	Solvents/carriers/	Texture/consistency control agents
Sweeteners	encapsulators	Firming agents
Raising agents	Washing/surface	Leavening agents
Antifoaming agents	removal agents	Masticatory substances
Glazing agents		Propellants
Flour treatment agents		Stabilizers and thickeners
Firming agents		Texturizers
Humectants		
Sequestrants		
Yeast nutrients		
Foam stabilisers		
Enzymes		

Table 6.2. List of food additives as defined by the EC and classification on the basis of their technical effects. (Adapted from references 28 and 29)

havioural abnormalities and effects on the intelligence. Moreover, it is often difficult to pinpoint the levels of exposure to food additives, particularly as new products appear and old ones are replaced at rates which make long-term assessment difficult.[30] The quantities of food additives which may be added to foods are only prescribed for certain categories of additives, and in the case of colorants, emulsifiers, stabilizers, solvents and most miscellaneous additives, there are mostly no prohibitions as to the amounts of these substances which may be used in foods, although their use may be restricted to certain categories of foods.

Maximum daily ingestion of some food additives has been estimated to be up to 100 mg/day of azo colours, 50 mg/day of non-azo colours, 200 mg/day of antioxidants and 1g/day of benzoate products.[31] It is, therefore not surprising that adverse effects, ascribed to food additives, are being reported more and more in the literature. Interest in this topic was stirred when Finegold, the paediatric allergist, who alleged that many children suffering from hyperactivity and minimal brain dysfunction were actually sensitive to certain constituents in their diet, singled out synthetic food colours and flavourant as being among the chief offenders.[32] Finegold came under much criticism, but a large body of current research shows that his assertions cannot be summarily rejected.[33] Much of the criticism revolves around the relatively low doses of additives to which humans are exposed, compared to clinical trials which take place in the laboratories. It must, however, be remembered that in clinical trials the animals are subjected to one agent at a time, whereas humans are subjected to numerous additives simultaneously. Moreover, laboratory rats are fed high-fibre diets, whereas modern Western diets are very low in fibre, and it has been established that low-fibre diets greatly magnify the toxic effects of colorants and other additives. Beside Finegold's assertions, a surprising number of the symptoms associated with food allergies have been reported, and some of these are summarized in table 6.3.

Artificial and natural colorants

Colorants are used to make the food more acceptable to the consumer, but since many adverse reactions to artificial colorants have been reported, many of these have been banned in some countries and natural colorants are being used more frequently. In the UK some foods are not permitted to contain added colorants, namely raw meat, game, poultry, fish, fruit or vegetables, tea, coffee, condensed or dried milk, cream and certain types of bread. Bread, cheese and butter may contain a restricted number of dyes, and raw meat may be coloured with the basic dye **me-**

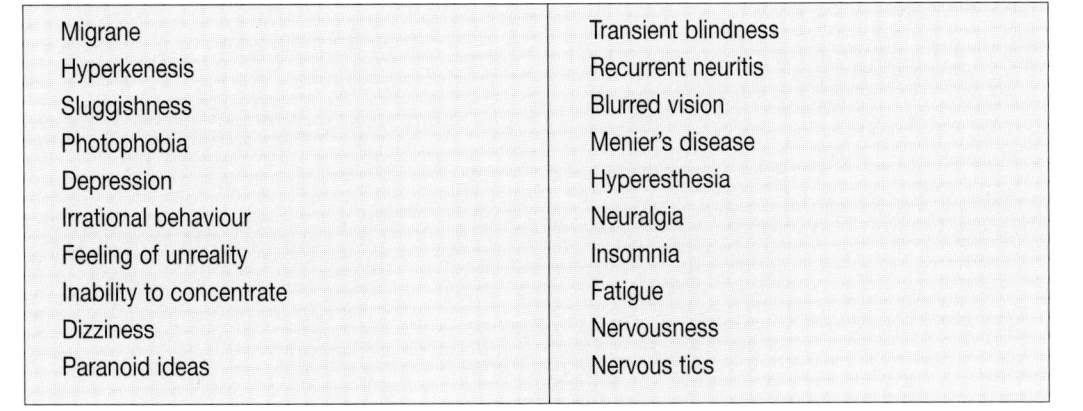

Migrane	Transient blindness
Hyperkenesis	Recurrent neuritis
Sluggishness	Blurred vision
Photophobia	Menier's disease
Depression	Hyperesthesia
Irrational behaviour	Neuralgia
Feeling of unreality	Insomnia
Inability to concentrate	Fatigue
Dizziness	Nervousness
Paranoid ideas	Nervous tics

Table 6.3. Neurobehavioural reactions attributed to food allergy. (From reference 33)

thyl violet. Allergic reactions or intolerant responses have been reported for most of **azo dyes** used as food colorants, and in some countries (Norway) they have been banned. In other countries, including Sweden, Finland, Austria, Greece and Japan, their use has been severely restricted. Nevertheless, azo dyes are still used extensively throughout the world in spite of the reported health hazards.

Some of the more common azo colours include **amaranth** (red), **azorbin** (red), **brilliant black**, **sunset yellow** (yellow), **carmousine** and **tartrazine** (yellow), most of which are potential allergens as demonstrated in their potential to induce histamine release by leucocytes of normal and urticaria patients.[31] A similar, though reduced potential, was also demonstrated for **non-azo colours** such as **quinoline yellow**, **green S** and **indigo carmine**. Colorants have been shown to induce **asthma, rashes, hay fever, blurred vision** and **tummy upsets**. Moreover their role in inducing **hyperactivity** and other behavioural disorders in children has been clearly established. In one study, a group of children on an additive-free diet, were given a cookie containing a blend of eight food colours. Within three hours after the ingestion of the cookie some of the children showed impaired perceptual-motor performance and increased hyperactive behaviour with the greatest effect being on the youngest individuals.[33,34] Impaired learning ability is another negative response to colorants, and some children develop a short attention span, whine and tend to throw tantrums.[33]

Azo compounds have also been reported to effect aggregation of platelets, and to have an inhibitory effect on both prostaglandin synthetase and thromboxane activity, though these claims have been challenged. Tartrazine in particular has been implicated in cases of acute urticaria angio-oedema, eczema, asthma, nausea and migraine attacks by impacting on the immune system.[35,36] Some of the **caramels**, particularly **ammonia caramel**, have been shown to have lymphocyte depressing effects, and the orange/red colorant **canthaxanthin**, which is used to obtain artificial browning, has been found to produce crystalline deposits on the retina. Another red colorant, **erythrosine**, has been shown to affect thyroid function and may have oncogenic and carcinogenic effects. Concern about these issues has prompted a reduction of the ADI and NEL (no effect level) for most of these compounds.[37] In the USA the colorant **amaranth** and **ponceau 4R** (red) are also banned.

Natural food colours are becoming increasingly popular, and the main classes are the carotenoids, beetroot extract, anthocyanins, riboflavins, cochineal, chlorophylls and naturally coloured foods such as paprika, turmeric, saffron, and sandalwood together with extracts of these materials. Though sensitivity to natural colorants is considerably lower than artificial colorants, in some cases they may also elicit a negative response. Overall it can thus be said that avoidance of food colorants can only be of advantage to the consumer.

Antioxidants

Antioxidants are added to oils and fats to prevent rancidity and normally this is best achieved when mixtures of antioxidants are used for this purpose. **Natural antioxidants** include some vitamins (particularly **vitamin E** and **ubiquinols**) and some phenolic compounds occurring in foods, especially spices. Most regulatory bodies permit the use of various gallates such as **butylated hydroxyanisole (BHA)** and **butylated hydroxytoluene (BHT)** in dairy products and fats. Some directives also regard **calcium disodium EDTA** as an antioxidant for use in salad dressings and mayonnaise. BHA and BHT are used mainly for the protection of unsaturated fats and oils as well as baked goods, cereals, nuts (particularly walnuts), milk powder and in dehydrated potato products such as potato chips and snacks.

The safety of these synthetic antioxidants has been questioned lately,[38] and in the case of BHA sufficient evidence for carcinogenicity in experimental animals has been found to prompt changes (but not withdrawals) in the recommended usage of this compound.[37,39] BHA has been shown to produce hyperplasia and/or tumours in the forestomach of rats, mice and hamsters.[37] BHT, on the other hand, has been shown to have adverse effects on thyroid function, and haematological studies have also revealed that some, but not all, species show haemorrhaging effects and/or reduction in prothrombin index.[38] Some evidence also exists for a carcinogenic effect of BHT, as demonstrated by two recent Danish and Japanese studies.[37]

The natural antioxidants, such as the tocopherols (vitamin E) and ubiquinols have a cyclic nucleus and a hydrocarbon tail, and the antioxidant properties are produced by the cyclic nucleus of these molecules. When these compounds form part of the membrane systems of cells, the orientation in cell membranes is, however, accomplished by the other components of the molecules. Synthetic antioxidants contain only the fragments which ensure the antioxidant properties of the compounds, and this may be the source of their destructive and perturbative action on cell membranes and can explain their toxicity.[40] Natural antioxidants can be very effective, and research has shown that they can compete with the synthetic varieties.[41]

Emulsifiers and stabilizers

Emulsifiers are used to disperse tiny globules of one liquid in another so that they will stay mixed. Their use has made it possible to market oil-containing foods, such as peanut butter and margarines, that will not separate and so are instantly usable. Emulsifiers are used extensively in the baking industry to help increase volume and to effect the fineness of the grain. Stabilizers and thickeners are used to bind together solids and liquids so that they will not separate. They are used in ice-cream, many cake and pudding mixes, cheese spreads, salad dressings, soups and many others too numerous to mention.

Most commercial stabilizers and thickeners are pure plant extracts, and the use of **plant gums** for this purpose, is quite extensive. Gums are extracted from seaweed, trees and seeds, while **cellulose derivatives** are obtained from wood pulp and cotton. The seaweed extracts include **agar, algin, carrageenan** and **furcellaran**. The tree gums include **arabic, ghatti, karaya, larch** and **tragacanth**. Then there are still extracts of seeds which include **guar**, and extracts from the carob bean, and finally the commonly used cellulose derivatives are **methylcellulose, carboxymethyl-cellulose** and **hydroxypropyl-methylcellulose**. The most commonly used natural emulsifier is **lecithin** which is obtained from soybeans and other vegetable oils, but synthetic **mono-, di- and triglycerides** are also extensively used. Synthetic stabilizers and emulsifiers are used extensively in the baking and dairy industry, and in the UK the permitted substances include **stearyl tartrate, complete glycerol esters, partial glycerol esters, partial polyglycerol esters, propylene glycol esters, monostearin sodium sulphoacetate, sorbitan esters of fatty acids** and their **polyoxyethylene derivatives, cellulose ethers, sodium carboxymethyl cellulose** and **acetic** and **tartaric acid esters of mono- and diglycerides**. Some of these compounds are suspected to be carcinogens, and approval for the use of some of the polyoxyethylene compounds has been withdrawn in some countries.

Solvents

Solvents are used to dissolve raw materials and concentrates and they are also used to incorporate flavours, oils, colours, antioxidants and vitamins into foods. Many of the compounds used are considered to be health risks, and the use of some of these compounds has been banned in some countries. In the UK, solvents are categorized as carrier solvents, extraction solvents and processing solvents. The list of permitted solvents in the UK is presented in table 6.4. The list is extensive, and raises questions as to the desirability of consuming foods treated in this way, particularly since some are suspected of having carcinogenic properties.

Preservatives

Preservatives are used to prevent the growth of mould, or as antimicrobials. Food preservation is a very old industry, and since ancient times food has been preserved by drying, smoking or by the addition of salt or sugar. Today, food preservation has become a huge industry, and beside the ancient methods, canning, bottling and refrigeration are extensively used to preserve foods. With the expansion of the chemical industry, however, the use of synthetic organic and inorganic preservatives has become fashionable in the food industry.

The most commonly used **inorganic preservatives** are **sulphur dioxide, nitrates** and **nitrites**. Sulphur dioxide is used in gaseous form, in solution as sulphurous acid, or as sulphites of sodium, potassium or calcium. It prevents the browning of foods and also inhibits the growth of moulds, and it is used extensively in the preservation of fruit juices and dried fruits. Sulphur dioxide is known to destroy vitamin B, but it helps to preserve vitamin C, however, its use is also associated with asthma.[31] Sodium and potassium nitrate and nitrite are used mainly in the curing of meats and in some cheeses, but concern about their possible carcinogenic effect has prompted stricter control over these compounds in some countries. Their use is restricted in most European countries, and because they have the potential to form **nitrosoamines** and to interfere with the metabolism of infants and young children, they may not be used in infant foods in the UK.[28]

Nitrites have a powerful antimicrobial action, but they also influence the flavour and colour of the food. The pink colour of bacon and ham is due to their action on haemoglobin which is converted to nitrosohaemoglobin. Although the use of these compounds is restricted in infant foods, this does not prevent the consumption of treated foods by young children. Indeed, cured meats are advertised as the ideal food for growing children, an issue that should be of some concern to responsible adults. Sodium nitrite can also cause headaches, skin rashes and gut disturbances.[4] Another prohibited inorganic preservative is **boric acid** which is not used because it is cumulative, however it is still used for the preservation of caviar.[28]

The most extensively used **organic preservatives** are **benzoic acid, 4-hydroxybenzoates, salicylic acid, parachlorobenzoic acid, dehidroacetic acid, propionic acid, sorbic acid** and **sodium diacetate**. Many of these products are used in the preservation of breads and flour confectionery. Benzoic acid and benzoates are used for the preservation of some jams, fruit juices, desserts, tinned fruits, salad creams, yoghurt, sauces and margarines. It is also an effective agent against the growth of yeasts and moulds. Benzoic acid is also a natural ingredient in some small berries. Benzoic acid has been implicated in urticaria and most of the symptoms associated with a sensitivity to tartrazine.[35]

Flavour enhancers

Monosodium glutamate (MSG) and the ribonucleotides **disodium inosinate** and **disodium guanylate** are commonly used as

Light petroleum	Ethyl acetate
Trichloroethylene	Butyl acetate
Dichloromethane	Amyl acetate
Dichlorodifluoro- methane	Diethyl tartrate
	Benzyl benzoate
1, 2-dichloroethane	Isopropyl myristate
Ethanol	Ethyl lactate
Methanol	Mono- and
Propan-1-ol	diglycerides
Propan-2-ol	Glycerol tributyrate
Propane-1, 2-diol	Castor oil
Glycerol	Acetone
Butan-1-ol	Butanone
Butan-2-ol	Diethyl ether
Benzyl alcohol	Carbon dioxide
Glycerol acetates	

Table 6.4. The FACC recommended list of solvents. (From reference 28)

flavour enhancers in processed foods. The use of MSG is extensive, and annual world production of this compound exceeds 300 000 tons. MSG is a neurotoxin which effects the destruction of the arcuate nucleus (AR) of the hypothalamus when administered to mice.[42,43] MSG is converted into the amino acid, **glutamic acid**, which is known to have neuroexcitory properties, and **glutamate** is also implicated in neurotransmission. Interest in MSG was stimulated after some people experienced symptoms such as tightening of the face and chest muscles and also a burning sensation in the upper body as well as headaches. This was called **Chinese restaurant syndrome**, because it was frequently experienced by patrons of Chinese restaurants and was traced to the liberal use of MSG by Chinese chefs.

Other symptoms associated with MSG are dizziness, diarrhoea, nausea and stomach cramps. Some children experience shudder attacks which may be mistaken for epilepsy, and long-term exposure in mice can lead to obesity.[42,33] The most serious side effect of MSG is, however, its neurotoxic effect which also affects the endocrine function. MSG has been reported to depress growth hormone levels, and levels of prolactin and sex hormones are also affected.[44,45,46] Such findings should make one extremely cautious of using MSG, and replacement products such as protein hydrolysates should also be avoided as they also contain large amounts of glutamate and thus have the potential to elicit similar effects.

Sweeteners

Non-carbohydrate sweeteners are divided into two classes, those with a sweetness similar to sucrose are called **bulk sweeteners** and those with a sweetness that greatly exceeds that of sucrose are known as **intense sweeteners**. Bulk sweeteners supply similar calories as sugar, but as they are not metabolized in the same way, they are used as substitutes for sugar in the preparation of diabetic foods and they are also used in foods that are stored at low temperatures such as ice-cream. Bulk sweeteners include **hydrogenated glucose syrup, sorbitol, mannitol, xylitol, lactitol** and **isomalt**. The intense sweeteners include the synthetic sweeteners (artificial sweeteners) **saccharin, cyclamate, aspartame, acesulfam-K, thaumatin, stevioside, sucralose** and **alitame**.

The most controversial sweeteners are the cyclamates and saccharin. Cyclamates are banned in many countries on the strength of laboratory experiments which indicated that they could be tetragenic and carcinogenic. The evidence for these phenomena is, however, controversial. The IARC monographs list saccharine as a chemical for which there is sufficient evidence for carcinogenicity,[37,39] but it still remains on the list of approved food additives. Aspartame is another problem sweetener because its effect is similar to that of MSG.[33]

Although the above list of food additives is by no means complete, it should be clear that the issue is indeed worthy of some concern. Legislation governing the use of food additives is not equally explicit in all countries, but most responsible bodies realize their duty in keeping the public informed. In most countries there is legislation which enforces the proper labelling of food items sold to the general public, and most nutritional organizations support the right of the public to know what is in the food they buy. In the United States new labelling guidelines are being considered with this very purpose in mind. The positions of the American Institute of Nutrition, the American Society for Clinical Nutrition and the American Dietetic Association also clearly underscore the policy that sound nutritional information should be provided to the American public. They, however, also acknowledge the fact that substantial improvement in nutrition education of the public is necessary for food labelling to serve its purpose effectively.[47] The policy of comprehensive food labelling affords each individual the opportunity to make his own choice as to what foods he wishes to buy.

Caffeine and alcohol

No discussion on healthful living would be complete without reference to caffeine and alcohol. Both these compounds play a major role in human nutrition, and the sale of commodities containing either of these substances plays a major role in the economy of many nations. Tea, coffee and cocoa are important plant exports of many nations and in some cases they are the major, or only, earners of foreign exchange. The stimulating effects of tea, coffee and cocoa are due to their **alkaloid** content. Alkaloids are complex compounds containing carbon, hydrogen, nitrogen, and usually oxygen. The nitrogen often forms part of a heterocyclic ring system and as alkaloids are usually basic compounds, they normally form salts with acids.

The alkaloids found in tea, coffee and cocoa are **caffeine, theobromine** and **theophylline**. Caffeine is found in tea and coffee, whilst theobromine is found in cocoa. Tea also contains the alkaloid theophylline, but all of these compounds have a similar structure and are derived from purines (fig. 6.1).

Tea (*Camellia sinensis*) has been used in China for thousands of years and it is cultivated extensively in Asian and African countries. Harvesting of tea takes place after flushing, which is the term used to describe the development of the new growth which occurs after pruning. For the "best" tea, only the two top leaves and the bud are used, but for coarse tea the bud and all four leaves of the flush are used. Plants protect their ephemeral (young) tissues from herbivory by concentrating secondary plant compounds, such as alkaloids, in these tissues, and it is therefore surprising that the ephemeral tissue is used to make tea. Green tea is produced by heating the harvested leaves to prevent fermentation, and black tea is produced by encouraging fermentation. After harvesting the leaves are spread out on nets to dry whilst hot air is blown over them. They are then crushed and **polyphenols** and enzymes are released and fermentation is initiated, which results in compounds that give tea its characteristic flavour. The „best" tea has high concentrations of polyphenols (called tannins, but are not the same as those used for tanning leather) which are also compounds that prevent herbivory in nature and affect the ability to digest, absorb and assimilate nutrients.

Coffee (*Coffea* spp.) is grown largely in South America, the West Indies and Africa. The harvested berries are opened and allowed to ferment in water, and are subsequently dried in the sun to produce mild coffee. Hard coffee is prepared by first drying the beans and then removing the pulp. The beans are then roasted, which changes the sugars to caramel and gives the beans their dark colour. The cocoa plant (*Theobroma cacao*) is grown for its pods, which are also fermented, and the cocoa beans subsequently dried. The beans are roasted to drive off the acetic acid, which is formed during the fermentation process, they are then ground and can then be further

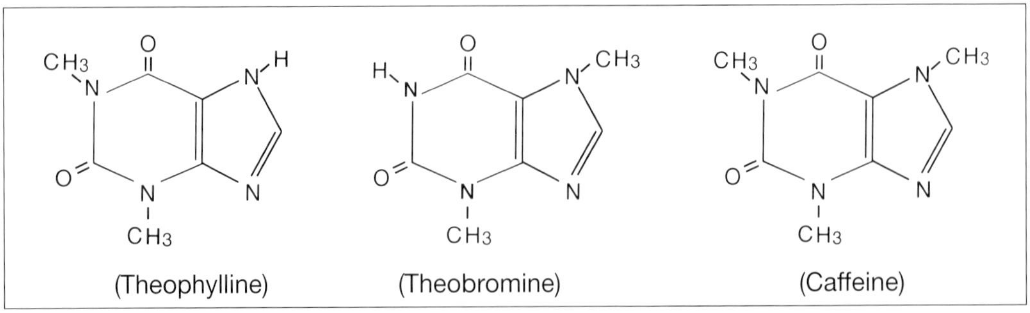

Figure 6.1 The structure of alkaloids found in tea, coffee and cocoa.

separated into cocoa butter and cocoa powder. Cocoa powder contains approximately one per cent theobromine.

Caffeine

The consumption of caffeine begins at an early age for many people. Caffeine is a natural ingredient in tea, coffee and some soft drinks, and it is used as an additive in many baked goods, frozen dairy products, sweets, gelatins, puddings and soft drinks. The quantities of caffeine in some commonly used items are summarized in table 6.5.

Based on these values the National Institute of Nutrition in Canada estimated that the average daily caffeine consumption of Canadians approximates 450 mg per day. Children also consume large quantities of caffeine in the soft drinks and sweets which they consume, and this is a matter of some concern. Adults absorb 99% of the caffeine they consume, and peak blood levels are reached within 15–45 minutes, and the half-life of the caffeine (the time it takes to eliminate 50% of the caffeine from the system) varies from 3–7.5 hours. Caffeine is found in breast milk, and can cross the placenta and thus influence the unborn child. In newborn infants the rate of elimination of caffeine is much slower than in adults, and the half-life is 82 hours. In preterm infants the half-life ranges from 62–102

Source	Caffeine (mg)
Coffee (178 ml or 6 oz)	
Approximate average	100
Average from ground beans	66–80
Automatic percolated	75–140
Filter drip	110–180
Instant regular	60–90
Instant decaffeinated	2–6
Tea (178 ml or 6 oz)	
Weak (bag)	20–45
Strong (bag)	79–110
Cola drinks (280 ml or 10 oz)	22–50
Coacoa products	
Chocolate milk (225 ml or 7.5 oz)	2–7
Hot cocoa from mix (178 ml or 6 oz)	6–30
Dark chocolate bar (56 g or 2 oz)	40–50
Milk chocolate bar (56 g or 2 oz)	3–20
Baking chocolate (28 g or 1 oz)	25–35
Medications (1 tablet or 1 capsule)	
Cold remedies	15–30
Headache relievers	30–32
Weight control aids	120–200
Some diuretics	40–100

Table 6.5. Sources of caffeine. (From reference 48)

hours.[48] Some races also experience slower clearance rates than others, and Orientals have a much slower rate of elimination than Europeans. Pregnancy and the use of oral contraceptives also substantially increase the clearance rate.

The Federation of American Societies for Experimental Biology (FASEB) reported the mean consumption of caffeine to be 0.17 mg/kg per day for babies 0–11 months old, 0.49 mg/kg/day for age group 1–5 years, 0.31 mg/kg/day in the 6–11 year age group, 0.21 mg/kg/day in the 12–17 year age group and 0.18 mg/kg/day in the 18 year and older age group. In people with high consumption levels of soft drinks, levels can be significantly higher, and for children in the 1–5 year age group levels can reach 1.8 mg/kg/day.[49] In view of concerns about the safety of caffeine, and the relatively high concentrations to which children are exposed, the FDA has reviewed the use of caffeine as additives in soft drinks.

The effects of excessive caffeine intake, which in some individuals may be manifested at levels as low as 500 mg/day, include insomnia, headache, anxiety, irritability, and depression. When consumed on an empty stomach it can produce tremors, and at consumption rates of 1g (which is not unusual for some people) can produce symptoms such as fever, agitation, trembling, rapid breathing and heart rate, cardiac palpitations, diuresis, nausea and anorexia. Still higher intakes (5–100 g or 50–100 cups of coffee) have caused tachycardia, convulsions, respiratory and heart failure and coma and death due to shock.[48] People who stop drinking beverages containing caffeine may experience equally unpleasant withdrawal symptoms, the most common of which are muscle tension, nervousness, irritability and headaches. Caffeine also effects urinary calcium excretion, particularly in postmenopausal women.[49] Rats fed instant coffee for 3 to 4 weeks also showed increased calcium loss via the urine and faeces.[50] In one study carried out on a group of women (age 50–84), it was found that the consumption of more than two units of caffeinated beverages (one unit = one cup of coffee or two cups of tea), increased the risk of hip fracture by 69%.[51] Metabolic studies have shown that the kidneys and intestinal system are directly affected by caffeine.

Of even greater concern than these immediate symptoms are the long-term dangers associated with caffeine, which can occur at lower levels and may be more subtle and difficult to detect. In studies on animals, caffeine was shown to affect the nervous system and influence such behaviours as learning, memory, motor performance, sensory function and emotional reactivity.[52,53] These findings have prompted the FASEB to voice their concerns about behavioural effects of caffeine, and effects on the development of the nervous system in children who consume large amounts of cola-type beverages.

The administration of caffeine to pregnant mice indicates that caffeine has toxic effects on the unborn offspring and can possibly produce birth defects. Some of the birth defects noted after the administration of caffeine were: cleft palate, digital defects, muscular disorders, facial deformities, anophthalmia (absence of eyes) and exencephaly (the brain lying outside the skull). In rats the situation is similar, and incomplete ossification in the offspring was also reported.

As these studies suffered from lack of certain controls and low sample numbers the FDA undertook two new studies to resolve the issue of the teratogenic effects of caffeine. These studies revealed that high doses result in death and resorption of embryos, significant reductions in foetal weight, and skeletal abnormalities such as reduced pubis size, reduced dorsal arch and missing hind digits. In fact irreversible birth defects were noted at levels as low as 80 mg/kg and other defects at levels as low as 6 mg/kg.[52] Much uncertainty still exists as to whether caffeine increases the risk of birth defects in humans, and it is premature to make such claims. Nevertheless, the studies on animals indicate that there are enough reasons for concern.

Alcohol and diet

It is an interesting phenomenon that many studies have shown that alcohol reduces the risk of coronary disease and may even have a positive influence on cholesterol levels.[54] This phenomenon has received quite some attention and has given many an excuse for not curtailing their drinking habits. The negative aspects associated with alcohol, however, far outweigh any positive effects it may have on the cardiovascular system.[55] Evidence is mounting that alcohol consumption increases the risk of cancer, particularly breast cancer, and although the relative risk is small (around 1.5), the alcohol habit is so widespread that it might account for a large proportion of breast cancers in Western countries.[56,57]

In a recent study, the effect of moderate intakes of alcohol on women 21 to 40 years old was assessed by measuring blood lipids at a time in the menstrual cycle when hormone levels were at their lowest. The subjects were given the typical US diet containing 36% fat and two 6-oz glasses of wine daily. Their total cholesterol levels remained unchanged, but there was an increase in HDL levels relative to LDL levels. This is indeed positive, but at the same time oestrogen levels rose from 7% to 37% during the menstrual cycle and this could be the reason why alcohol is associated with increased risk of breast cancer.[58] Alcohol is probably not a direct carcinogen, but **acetaldehyde**, the main metabolic product in humans is a known carcinogen. Alcohol consumption is particularly linked with high risk of rectal cancer and the relative risks in individuals consuming three or more drinks per day were 3.17 (1.05-9.57).[59] The IARC (International Agency for Research on Cancer) found that free extracts of some alcohol free beverages were also genotoxic, and the link between the consumption of alcoholic beverages, mainly beer, and rectal cancer was suggestive but not conclusive.[59]

Alcohol is known to impair the function of natural killer cells (NK) which destroy cancer cells. Even small amounts of alcohol have a significant impact, and in one study it was found that just two cans of beer (3.5% alcohol) taken over a 30 minute interval during a meal significantly impaired the activity of lymphokine-activated killer cells (LAK) thus reducing the immune system's capacity to clear virus infected cells or cells that have undergone neoplastic transformation.[60] It is sometimes claimed that alcohol contributes at least partially towards the overall nutrition, but alcoholic beverages provide little nutritive value apart from calories, and can not be equated with carbohydrates. Moreover, glucose homoeostasis is impaired by alcohol, and alcohol can affect insulin release and lead to glucose intolerance.[61] Gout is also associated with alcohol, and short-term administration to patients, who have no disorders of renal function or uric acid metabolism, show significantly increased uric acid levels which persist, in some instances, for several days. Blood lipid levels are also raised by alcohol, and triglyceride levels can increase several-fold.[62]

It has been shown that alcohol is directly injurious to the small intestine and stomach. It can cause lesions in the duodenum and may impair the absorption of many nutrients.[63] The liver is another organ that suffers from alcoholic intake and it has been shown that even daily alcohol consumption as low as 40 g (± 3 drinks) in men and 20 g (± 1½ drinks) in women resulted in a statistically significant increase in the incidence of cirrhosis in well-nourished persons.[62] Vitamin metabolism is also impaired by alcohol, and reduction of liver stores of folacin, niacin, thiamin, vitamin B6 and vitamin B12 have been described. Fat-soluble vitamins are also negatively affected, and alcoholics have been found to have very low stores of vitamin A and vitamin D. Moreover, alcohol also results in greater renal losses of minerals, particularly zinc, calcium and magnesium, and the absorption of these minerals may also be impaired.[62]

A whole-food lifestyle, together with avoidance of harmful compounds, would circumvent many of the pitfalls associated with modern living. Whole foods will supply all the vitamins and minerals that the body requires to function normally, and at the same time most whole foods come prepacked in nature's own wrappings. Many whole foods are naturally preserved, and fresh products allow one to largely avoid the many additives associated with processed foods. A diet consisting largely of fresh fruits, vegetables, grains, seeds, nuts and legumes can provide a whole new eating experience, and with a little bit of ingenuity will provide a satisfying alternative lifestyle.

References

1. Dwyer, J.T. 1988. Health aspects of vegetarian diets. *Am.J.Clin.Nutr.* 48:712–38.
2. Position paper on food nutrition misinformation on selected topics. 1975. *J.Am.Diet.Assoc.* 66:277–280.
3. Medeiros, D.M., Bock, M.A., Ortiz, M., Raab, C., Read, M. Schutz, H.G., Sheehan, E.T., Williams, D.K. 1989. Vitamin and mineral supplementation practices of adults in seven western states. *J.Am.Diet.Assoc.* 89:383–386.
4. Read, M.H., Medeiros, D. Bendel, R., Bhalla, V., Harril, I., Mitchell, M., Schutz, H.G., Sheehan, E.T., Standal, B.R. 1986. Mineral supplementation practices of adults in seven western states. *Nutr.Res.* 6:375
5. WHO. 1989. *Global Nutrition Status Update*. Geneva: WHO Publications, 1989.
6. Scrimshaw, N.S. 1996. Nutrition and Health from Womb to Tomb. *Nutrition Today,* 31 (2) March/April pp. 55–67.
7. Ross, A.C. 1991. Vitamin A: Current understanding of the mechanism of action. *Nutrition today*. Jan./Feb. 1991, pp. 6–12.
8. Jacobs, C., Dwyer, J.T. 1988. Vegetarian children: appropriate and inappropriate diets. *Am.J.Clin.Nutr.* 48:811-8.
9. Johnston, P.K. 1988. Counselling the pregnant vegetarian. *Am.J.Clin.Nutr.* 48:901–5.
10. Lindberg, A.S., Leklem, J.E., Miller, L.T. 1983. The effect of wheat bran on the bioavailability of vitamin B-6 in young men. *J.Nutr.* 113:2578–86.
11. Reynolds, R.D. 1988. Bioavailability of vitamin B-6 from plant foods. *Am.J.Clin.Nutr.* 48:863–7.
12. Callender, S.T., Spray, G.H. 1962. Latent pernicious anaemia. *Br.J.Haematol.* 8:230–40.
13. Leitzmann, C. 1993. Vitamin B_{12}. Aktueller Stand der Forschung. *Fit fürs Leben* 6/93:12-15.
14. Herbert, V. 1988. Vitamin B-12: plant sources, requirements, and assay. *Am.J.Clin.Nutr.* 48:852–8.
15. Sherman, A.R. 1992. Zinc, copper, and iron nutriture and immunity. *J.Nutr.* 122:604–609.
16. Hallberg, L., Rossander-Hulten, L. 1991. Iron requirements in menstruating women. *Am.J.Clin.Nutr.* 54:1047–58.
17. Greger, J.L. 1987. Mineral bioavailability / new concepts. *Nutrition today*. July/August 1987, pp. 4–9.
18. Kaneko, K., Masaki, U., Aikyo, M., Yabuki, K., Haga, A., Matabo, C., Sasaki, H., Koike, G. 1990. Urinary calcium and calcium balance in young women affected by high protein diet of soy protein isolate and adding sulfur-containing amino acids and/or potassium. *J.Nutr.Sci.Vitaminol.* 36:105–116.
19. Einhorn, T.A. Levine, B. Michel, P. 1990. Nutrition and bone. *The Orthopaedic Clinics of North America*. 21:43–50.
20. Howe, J. 1990. Postprandial response of calcium metabolism in postmenopausal women to meals varying in protein level/source. *Metabolism.* 39:1246–1252.
21. Blank, R.P., Diehl, H.A., Ballard, G.T., Melendwz, R.C. 1987. Calcium metabolism and osteoporotic ridge resorption: A protein connection. *J. Prosthetic Dentistry*. 58:590–595.
22. Kitano,T., Esashi, T., Azami, S. 1988. Effect of protein intake on the mineral (calcium, magnesium, and phosphorus balance in Japanese males. J.Nutr.Sci.Vitaminol. 34:387–398.
23. Greger, J.L. 1989. Effect of dietary protein and mineral on calcium and zinc utilization. *Critical Reviews in Food Science and Nutrition.* 28:249–271.
24. Godowski, P.J., Picard, D. 1989. Steroid Receptors. How to be both a receptor and a transcription factor. *Biochemical Pharmacology.* 38:3135–3143.
25. Hunt, J.R., Johnson, L.K. 1992. Dietary protein, as egg albumen: Effects on bone composition, Zinc bioavailability and zinc requirements of rats, assessed by a modified broken-line model. *Am.Inst.Nutr.*122:161–169.
26. Erdman, J.W., Garcia-Lopez, J.S., Sherman, A.R. 1987. Processing and fortification: how they

References

affect mineral interactions? in *Nutrition '87*, Levander, O.A., Ed., American Institute of Nutrition, Bethesda, MD.

27. Murphy, E.W., Willis, B.W., Watt, B.K. 1975. Provisional tables on the zinc content of foods. *J.Am.Diet.Assoc.* 66:345–355.

28. Kirk, R.S., Sawyer, R. 1991. Pearsons composition and analysis of foods. 9th. edition. Longman Scientific & Technical UK.

29. Waslien, C.I., Rehwoldt, R.E. 1990. Micronutrients and antioxidants in processed foods _ analysis of data from 1987 food additives survey. *Nutrition today* July/August 1990.

30. Graham, D.M., Filer, L.J., Bigelow, S.W. 1990. Assessing dietary exposure to food additives: A new approach. *Food Tech*. July 1990, pp. 94, 96.

31. Murdoch, R.D., Iessof, M.H., Pollock, I., Young, E. 1987. Effects of food additives on leukocyte histamine release in normal and urticaria subjects. *J. of the Royal College of Physicians of London*. 21:251–256.

32. Finegold, B.F. 1975. Why your child is hyperactive. Random House, New York.

33. Weiss, B. 1983. The behavioral toxicity of food additives. Nutrition Update. Vol.1. Ed. Weiniger, J. and Briggs, G.M. John Wiley & Sons, New York, pp. 21–38.

34. Goyette, C.H., Conners, C.K., Pettit, T.A., Curtis, L.E. 1978. Effects of artificial colors on hyperkinetic children: A double blind challenge study. *Psychopharmacol. Bull*. 14:39

35. Warrington, R.J., Sauder, P.J., McPhillips, S. 1986. Cell-mediated immune responses to artificial food additives in chronic urticaria. *Clinical Allergy*. 16:527-533.

36. Schaubschläger, W.W., Zabel, P., Schlaak, M. 1987. Tartrazine-induced histamine release from gastric mucosa. *Lancet*. 39:800–801.

37. Poulsen, E. 1991. Safety evaluation of substances consumed as technical ingredients (food additives). *Food additives and contaminants*. 8:125–134.

38. Haigh, R. 1986. Safety and necessity of antioxidants: EEC approach. *Food. Chem.Toxic*. 24:1031.

39. Tricker, A.R., Preussmann, R. 1990. Chemical food contaminants in the initiation of cancer. *Proceeding of the Nutrition Society*. 49:133-144.

40. Kagan, V., Serbinova, E., Novikov, K., Ritov, V., Kozlov, Y., Stoytchev, T. 1986. Toxic and protective effects of antioxidants in biomembranes. *Arch.Toxicol.Suppl*. 9:302–305.

41. Hemeda, H.M., Klein, B.P. 1990. Effects of naturally occurring antioxidants on peroxidase activity of vegetable extracts. *J.Food Sci*. 55:184–185,192.

42. Olney, J.W. 1969. Brain lesions, obesity and other disturbances in mice treated with monosodium glutamate. *Science*. 164:719–721.

43. Belluardo, N., Mudo, G., Bindoni, M. 1990. Effects of early destruction of the mouse arcuate nucleus by monosodium glutamate on the age-dependant natural killer activity. *Brain Research*. 534:225–233.

44. Bloch, B., Ling, N., Benoit, R., Wehrenberg, W.B., Guillemin, R. 1984. Specific depletion of immunoreactive growth hormone-releasing factor by monosodium glutamate in rat median emminence. *Nature*. 307:272–273.

45. Terry, L.C., Epelbaum, J., Martin, J.B. 1981. Monosodium glutamate: acute and chronic effects on the rhythmic growth hormone and prolactin secretion, and somatostatin in the undisturbed male rat. *Brain Research*. 217:129-142.

46. Olney, J.W. 1971. Glutamate induced neuronal necrosis in the infant mouse hypothalamus. *J.Neuropath.Exp.Neurol*. 30:75–90.

47. Position statement on food labelling. American Institute of Nutrition and the American Society for Clinical Nutrition. 1990. Nutrient labeling of food products under consideration. *Nutrition today*. May/June 1990.

48. Review from the National Institute of Nutrition in Canada. 1987. Caffeine: A perspective on current concerns. *Nutrition Today*. July/August 1987, pp. 36–38.

49. Massey, L.K., and S.J. Whiting. 1993. Caffeine, urinary calcium, calcium metabolism and bone. *J.Nutr*. 123:1611–1614.

50. Jeh, J.K. and Aloia, J.F. 1986. Differential effect of caffeine administration on calcium and vitamin D metabolism in young and adult rats. *J.Bone Minr. Res*. 1:251–258.

51. Kiel, P. et al. 1990. Caffeine and the risk of hip fracture: the Framingham study. *Am. J. Epidemol*. 132:675–684.

52. Nightingale, S.L., Flamm, W.G. 1983. Caffeine and health. Current status. Nutrition Update. Vol.1. Ed. Weiniger, J. and Briggs, G.M. John Wiley & Sons, New York, pp. 3–19.

53. Kirsh, K.R., Pinzone, M.G., Forde, J.H. 1974. Spontaneous locomotor activity changes

evoked by caffeine in mice. *Fed.Proc*. 33:466.

54. Rimm, E.B., Giovannucci, E.L., Willett, W.C., Colditz, G.A., Ascherio, A., Rosner, B., Stampfer, M.J. 1991. Prospective study of alcohol consumption and risk of coronary disease in men. *Lancet*. 338:464–68.

55. The Surgeon General's Report on Nutrition and Health. 1988. DHSS publ. no. 88-50210. Washington, DC: US Government Printing Office.

56. Editorial, Hospital Update. 1991. Breast cancer and dietary factors. *Hospital Update*. November 1991, pp. 3–4.

57. Graham, S. 1987. Alcohol and breast cancer. *N.Engl.J.Med.* 78:1211–1213.

58. Clevidence, B. 1995. Alcohol and blood cholesterol. *Nutrition Today* July/August 1995. 30 (4) p. 141.

59. Bingham, S.A. 1996. Epidemiology and mechanisms relating diet to risk of colorectal cancer. *Nutrition Research Reviews*, pp. 197–239.

60. Thylan. S. 1996. Soaking cells. *New Scientist*. 13 July 1996.

61. Phillips, C.B., Safrit, H.F. 1971. Alcoholic diabetes: induction of glucose intolerance with alcohol. *J.Am.Med.Assoc.* 217:1513.

62. Shaw, S., Lieber, C.S. 1983. Nutrition and alcohol: a clinical perspective. Nutrition Update. Vol.1. Ed. Weiniger, J. and Briggs, G.M. John Wiley & Sons, New York, pp. 79–104.

63. Gottfried, E., Korsten, M.A., Lieber, C.S. 1978. Gastritis and duodenitis induced by alcohol: an endoscopic and histologic assessment. *Am.J.Gastroenterol*. 70:586.

Part 2

An alternative Lifestyle

Chapter 7
The whole-food alternative

Faced with the overwhelming evidence that animal products, particularly in these modern times, must be regarded as a health hazard, and that diets high in fats and proteins are associated with degenerative diseases, the question may be asked: "What is there left to eat?" The problem becomes particularly pressing if one considers that modern processed and refined foods, with their high salt content, scores of additives and disproportionate relationships of nutrients are not exactly conducive to good health.

In spite of the abundance of food in industrial countries, many individuals are undernourished, not because of a lack of food, but because of poor choice of nutrients. Indeed, malnutrition often takes the form of over-nutrition.[1] Refined foods together with high fat consumption are largely to blame for the tremendous increase in obesity and associated degenerative diseases so prevalent in Western society. The most common pathophysiological conditions associated with obesity are: Sudden death, cardiomyopathy, Pickwickian/sleep apnea syndrome, pituitary/gonadal dysfunction, Acanthos nigricans, osteoarthritis, diabetes mellitus as well as various forms of cancer.[2,3]

Most people are uninformed regarding the principles of wholesome nutrition, and in a survey conducted among laity, medical practitioners and scientists, it was found that most of these people blamed genetic factors, lack of willpower, physical inactivity, carbohydrate craving, repeated dieting and depression as the most likely causes of obesity. The solution to the problem was mainly sought in restricting the intake of certain foods, particularly carbohydrates and fats, or in the use of drugs.[4] However, neither of these solutions is acceptable, as they will induce a vicious circle from which it is difficult to escape. More and more drugs will be taken, depression will increase, which in turn will lead to even more drug utilization.

In our modern society, social pressures induce many people to follow restrictive diets, in order to lose weight, and there has been a veritable explosion in the weight-loss industry. It is a fact, however, that the weight-loss programmes have very poor success records, and it has been estimated that 90% of all dieters who lose weight in a diet programme, regain that weight within two years.[5,6] The ethics of obesity treatment have also been questioned, and the scientific fraternity realizes that the methods of weight-reduction must be reevaluated.[7,8] Moreover, it has been found that these programmes often have psychological effects, and depression may indeed be more intense after a short-lived weight loss.[9] Furthermore, many studies have shown that individuals who have had a major weight loss, do not enjoy improved health.[10] This is not surprising, as many weight-loss programmes advocate a high-protein, low-carbohydrate diet which, as we have seen, is not conducive to good health. The problem is so acute that it has even been recommended that regulations governing the weight-loss industry in the USA should be strengthened, in order to protect consumers.[11]

The reasons for the poor nutritional regimes followed by people living in affluent societies are multifactorial, and Dr. Frances Berg, editor of *Healthy Weight Journal* has proposed a concept of **dysfunctional eating** to describe this phenomenon.[12] Whereas normal eating is geared to nourish the body and is regulated by hunger and satiety, dysfunctional eating is focused on eating for other reasons such as thinness, body shaping, comfort, pain or stress relief, anxiety, anger or loneliness. These factors show that there is more to eating than just the consumption of food. Social pressures and psychological condition play a vital role in the overall health of any individual. A healthy lifestyle must thus include more than just good food, it must include a physical exercise programme, periods of rest, sunshine, social interaction and trust. Important as the psychological conditions of individuals are in dictating eating habits, most people are, however, gaining weight merely because they are on high fat diets containing a large proportion of refined foods. For the majority of people the answer obviously does not lie in dieting, but what is needed is a permanent change of lifestyle that will not only address the issue of obesity, but will also lead to an improved health status.

A vegetarian whole-food nutritional programme can provide all the nutrients we need without being restrictive in terms of the quality, variety and quantity of foods consumed. The common attitude towards vegetarian nutrition, however, is one of negativism, and conjures up images of carrots and lettuce leaves. Indeed, the reverse is true. A vegetarian whole-food programme can provide a veritable taste explosion. Foods that hitherto have never been heard of or even considered for human consumption, can provide a variety of tastes and textures which will surprise even the staunchest of critics. Eating constitutes one of the great pleasures of human existence, and one should never be satisfied with second best.

With the explosion of the healthy lifestyle industry in the Western world, many conflicting and often complicated eating practices are suggested to people seeking an alternative lifestyle. A few simple rules are, however, all that is necessary to ensure adequate nutrition:

1) First and foremost, nutrient needs must be met by a **variety of foods**. A varied diet does not, however, mean eating a great variety of foods at one meal, as this would place great demands on the digestive system, but rather that a varied overall diet be followed.

2) A healthy diet should include the **right combinations** of food groups to ensure optimum protein and energy consumption.

3) It is also important to ensure that **compatible foods** be consumed at any one meal so as to avoid the excessive formation of fermentation products in the stomach and small intestine.

It should also be remembered that the digestive system is not a machine that can be worked twenty four hours a day. The stomach is a living organ and should be granted periods of rest. Two to three well-balanced meals is all that is required for an adult to obtain all the nutrients that are required. Eating between meals robs the body of its vitality, but fortunately, a whole-food nutritional programme will go a long way in reducing the constant craving for snacks between meals. It is suggested, that meals be spaced at least four to five hours apart, so that the gastric glands have time to recover and large heavy meals should be avoided just before retiring to bed. During sleep there is a decline in metabolic activities which will impact negatively on the digestive process. The result is a restless night and a greater concentration of fermentation products from poorly digested food. In this day and age, it is difficult for working people not to have the main meal in the evenings, but if this cannot be avoided, then the meal should be eaten several hours before going to bed.

What is whole food?

"Whole food is food that contains all the nutrients in the same proportions as found in nature."

Man has a propensity to interfere with the natural packaging of food, a process which is termed **"refining"**. In the process of refining, foods are separated into components, and these are then consumed independent of each other. Grain is, for example, separated into bran, germ and white flour, and one or more of these components is eliminated from refined foods. Most often it is the germ which is discarded in view of its spoiling qualities, but the germ contains the essential fatty acids which are require for the formation of healthy cell membranes and prostaglandins. The fat in the germ comes prepacked with the right quantities of vitamin E to prevent the formation of harmful free radicals through the process of autoxidation. Furthermore, the germ also contains vitamin B-5, which is needed for carbohydrate metabolism. Separating the carbohydrate-rich endosperm from the germ thus robs us of the means of optimally utilizing these carbohydrates.

The removal of the bran interferes with intestinal motility, and this in turn leads to constipation, and a host of associated diseases. Even more illogical is the modern concept of consuming the daily bran ration in one meal. A breakfast consisting largely of bran will certainly assist intestinal motility of the food ingested, but will do nothing for subsequent meals. The only way to ensure a correct relationship between nutrients and fibre, is to consume whole food. It is also of little value to add bran and other refined products in order to try and rectify imbalances in refined foods, as one can never achieve the optimal relationship with which whole food was originally endowed.

The same applies for all grains, legumes, nuts, fruits, and vegetables. Refined, separated, texturized vegetable proteins are much harder to digest than whole foods, and extracted fats and sugars are responsible for a host of physiological disorders. Though the exclusive consumption of refined foods must be considered a health hazard, this does not mean that whole foods may not be processed, which is an entirely different procedure.

The foods may be ground, liquidized, combined with other foods and cooked or baked to change their taste and texture, as this processing does not remove any of the original nutrients. Many vegetarians consume meat analogues instead of meat, but meat analogues, such as gluten and soya-protein products are, in fact, refined foods that are high in sodium and low in iron and fibre content, and their consumption should be limited. A new attitude is needed; there must be a moving away from concentrated foods such as animal products and meat analogues, to proper combinations of whole foods.

General guidelines to healthful living

As more information on nutrition-related diseases has become available, so guidelines for healthful living have changed to bring them in line with current thinking. The modern guidelines as suggested by most health bodies are summarised in table 7.1.

For vegetarians, in addition, increased consumption of cereals, nuts, and legumes is recommended, together with fortified soy milk or nut milk.[13,14,15] A whole-food programme can answer all these requirements and will provide essential nutrients in the right proportions.

High-protein diets should also be avoided, and carbohydrates rather than proteins, should enjoy pride of place. A balanced diet must, however, contain adequate quantities of all the primary nutrients, and it is suggested that carbohydrates should comprise approximately 60-70% of the diet, and proteins and fats the remaining 30-40% (fig.7.1). There is, however, no hard and fast rule concerning this relationship, and some people may require more of the oil-rich foods than others, particularly if they tend to be underweight. A whole-food programme automatically ensures an appropriate relationship between primary nutrients, and there is no need to be armed with a calculator when preparing a meal. Adjustments to suit the individual needs are all that is required, and in the case of young children who are vegetarians, it should be remembered that they also need to proportionally consume more of the energy-, protein-rich foods such as grains, legumes, and nuts, than do adults, in order to boost their energy intake as discussed in chapter 5.[16,17]

Ensuring proper food combinations

Good nutrition is not just a question of eating wholesome food. It also entails the consumption of foods in proper combinations. The subject of food combinations is one of the most confused issues in the health literature, and at times the requirements set can be so overwhelming that even the most ardent of health-conscious individuals could become discouraged. Numerous charts and tables are presented and the most exacting combinations prescribed. Common suggestions in this regard are that some foods should only be eaten by themselves, proteins and carbohydrates should not be mixed in a meal, and even that foods grown above the ground should not be combined with foods grown below the ground. If all these suggestions were to be implemented at the same time, meal planning would become very exacting. Nevertheless, certain basic rules pertaining to the subject of food combinations do exist, and can be usefully applied. Some important ones in this regard are: Ensuring a balanced proportion of acid- and alkaline-forming foods in the diet, combining foods that have roughly similar digestion times so as to prevent fermentation and the accumulation of toxins, and selecting food combinations in the overall diet that will provide balanced proportions of macro- and micro-nutrients. To achieve this the kitchen does not have to be changed into a laboratory, and in primitive societies these criteria are met naturally and without the need for advanced training on the subject of nutrition.

Combining acid- and alkaline-forming foods

Food can be either acid-forming, or alkaline-forming. The elements in the food, to a large extent, determine whether there will be **acidosis** or **alkalosis** after the digesting of the food. Minerals are the main controllers of the acid-alkaline levels once the products of digestion have either been converted to alkaline or acid ash. A list of the acid- and alkaline-forming minerals is presented in table 7.2.

Human blood is slightly alkaline at pH 7,4 and is maintained at this level by acid-base re-

---

1. **A reduction in protein intake.**
2. **A reduction in fat intake.**
3. **An increased intake of fibre.**
4. **An increased intake of complex carbohydrates.**
5. **Avoidance of obesity.**
6. **Avoidance of refined foods.**
7. **Avoidance of alcohol.**
8. **Eating a variety of fresh fruits and vegetables.**

Table 7.1. Guidelines to healthful living as recommended by most health bodies.

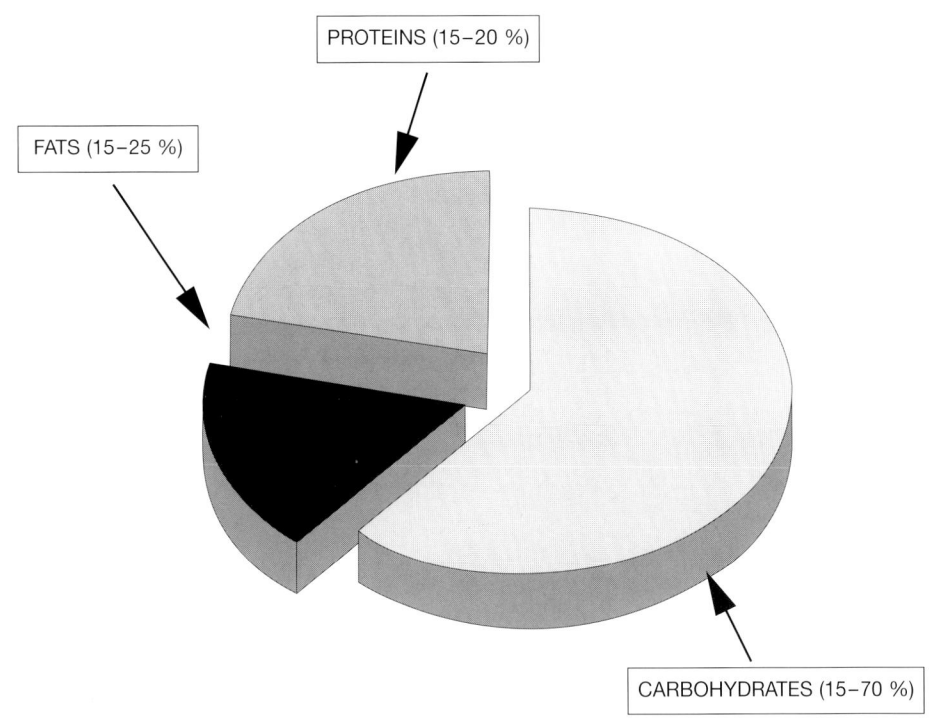

Figure 7.1. Recommended consumption of primary foods.

gulatory mechanisms. The lungs and kidneys are the two organs which regulate the acid-base balance. The lungs take care of volatile substances such as CO_2, and the kidneys eliminate nonvolatile acids, such as lactic acid, ketone bodies (derived from fatty acid metabolism), sulphuric acid (produced in the metabolism of protein) and phosphoric acid produced in the metabolism of phospholipids. Even slight variations in the blood pH will have a profound effect on the regulation of the acid-base balance. For example, during metabolic acidosis, bone mineral is decomposed in order to contribute to the buffering of the

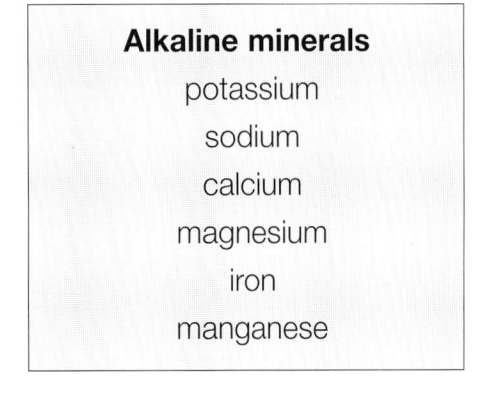

Acid minerals	Alkaline minerals
phosphorus	potassium
sulphur	sodium
silicon	calcium
chlorine	magnesium
fluorine	iron
iodine	manganese

Table 7.2. The main acid- and alkaline-forming minerals.

acid load. In one study carried out on mice, it was found that when pH fell below 7.4, then calcium efflux of bone took place, when the pH was above 7.4, then calcium influx into the bone took place whilst at pH 7.4 there was no net flux.[18] A diet which is acid-forming is thus a diet which will place excessive demands on the system, and can lead to increased susceptibility to disease. Besides contributing to calcium loss from bone, high-acid diets will lead to impaired immune responses, early aging and eventual renal impairment. In cases of renal impairment there is excessive retention of acidic catabolites such as phosphates and sulphates and in addition ammonia exchange is poor, which leads to further acidosis. In the overall diet it is, therefore, important to choose more alkaline-forming foods than acid-forming foods as presented in figure 7.2.

In table 7.3 the main categories of alkaline and acid-forming foods are presented. It is important to note that both alkaline- and acid-forming foods are required in the diet, but the balance should always favour alkalinity as shown in figure 7.2. Moreover, it should be noted that animal products are generally highly acid forming, which is another reason why they should be avoided. Meals that contain large proportions of acid-forming food groups should be balanced with meals containing mainly alkaline-forming foods, particularly fruits.

From table 7.3 it is evident that animal products are highly acid-forming, and the invertebrate foods, such as the crabs, lobsters and oysters are the most acid-forming in this category. Diets high in animal products are also rich in purines which lead to uric acid formation and enhance kidney stone formation.[21]

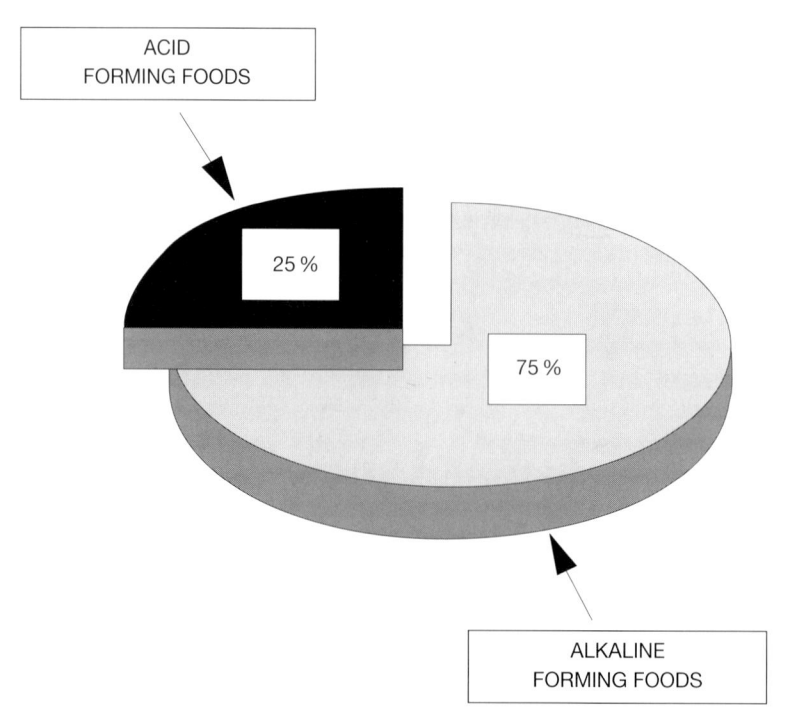

Figure 7.2. The suggested ratio of alkaline- to acid-forming foods.

High acid (15–40)	High alkaline (16–37)
Meats bacon, beef, chicken, crabs, eggs, fish, ham, lamb, liver, lobster, mutton, oyster, pork, turkey, veal.	**Dried fruits** apricots, figs, raisins **Fruits** olives **Sweetener** molasses **Vegetables** beet greens, Swiss chard, dandelion greens.
Medium acid (2.0–11) **Grains and legumes** barley, corn, lentils, oats, peanuts, rice, rye, wheat. **Nuts** Brazil nuts, walnuts. **Dairy products** cheese (hard and soft)	**Medium alkalinity (5–15)** **Fresh fruits** Most fruits including: apricots, bananas, blackberries, cantaloupe, cherries, currants, dates (dried), lemons, limes, loganberries, mango, nectarines, oranges, peach, persimmons pineapple, raspberry, tangerine. **Vegetables** Most vegetables including: beets, carrots, celery, cucumber, kale, kohlrabi, lettuce, parsnips, potato, pumpkin, sauerkraut, sweet potato, tomatoes, watercress. **Legumes** lima beans, navy beans, peas. **Nuts** almonds, chestnuts, coconuts.
Low acid (1–2) **Fruits** cranberries, plums. **Fats** butter, cream, oils.	**Low alkalinity (0.1–5)** **Fresh fruits** apple, blueberries, gooseberries, pear, strawberries, watermelon. **Grains** millet, sorghum. **Legumes** kidney beans, snap beans, soya beans. **Vegetables** asparagus, broccoli, cabbage, cauliflower, eggplant, okra, onions, peppers, radish, squash, turnip.

Table 7.3. Acid and alkaline ash food groups. The figures in brackets represent the percentage alkalinity or acidity. The grouping of fruits and vegetables is listed according to common usage and not biological classification. (From references 19 and 20)

Grains are mildly acid-forming, but when eaten together with the neutral or alkaline-forming legumes, fruits or vegetables, will not only supply an excellent protein with a well balanced mix of amino acids, but the combination will also be overall alkaline-forming.

Of the alkaline-forming foods, the dried fruits are most alkaline-forming, and all vegetables and fruits in general, with the exception of plums and cranberries, are alkaline-forming. Strange as this may seem, this means that even the lemon with its high organic acid content is overall alkaline-forming, because the acids are weak and once metabolized, the lemon has more alkaline than acidic components. The same holds true for all the other acid-tasting fruits in the list. Fruits or vegetables, in addition to a grain-legume combination, will thus ensure an overall shift towards alkalinity.

Animal products are particularly acid-forming, in view of their high sulphur, and phosphorus content. Purines that are present in animal foods are degraded in the course of their metabolism to uric acid, and the greater the consumption of these foods the greater the uric acid load becomes. People living in Western countries, particularly the affluent classes, are also at greater risk of forming kidney and gallstones.[22,23] Both these stone types consist of calcium-oxalate, whereas gallstones, in addition contain cholesterol.

Meat in the diet results in acid urine, which results in negative calcium balance as a result of increased calcium loss in the urine.[24] In addition, meat has a significant effect on the acid-base balance of the body, which in turn could lead to substantial bone loss.[18,25] The reason for this is probably the high sulphur content of meat, as calcium loss has been attributed to the excretion of sulphate which is derived from amino acid metabolism.[26] Combining animal foods such as cheese, eggs and meats with plant foods will lead to fermentation and toxin accumulation, as the digestion of these foods takes much longer than that of the plant foods.

Another source of acidity in the body is oxalic acid in food. Oxalic acid is not metabolized by the body, and combines with calcium to be eliminated as calcium-oxalate. Certain foods and beverages, including tea, cocoa products such as chocolates, peanuts, beets, spinach, rhubarb, Swiss chard, and black pepper, are high in oxalates and can thus also place an acid load on the system.[27] As oxalic acid is excreted in the form of calcium oxalate, its elimination entails calcium loss, and there is a tendency to form crystals if consumption of these foods is high.[28] It has, however, been found that if vegetarians consume foods high in oxalates, the urine composition of vegetarians is such that the formation of calcium oxalate crystals is inhibited. The relative risk of gallstone formation is 1,9fold greater in non-vegetarians than in vegetarians, and the risk of kidney stone formation is also less in vegetarians than in non-vegetarians.[27] It has also been shown that the problem for non-vegetarians seems to lie in the nature of the animal proteins which they consume,[29,30] a vegetarian diet with emphasis on variety, would substantially reduce the acid load on the system.

Combining fruits and vegetables

Fruits and vegetables are both essential components of a healthy diet. Fruits are rich in vitamins and minerals and they require a shorter digestion time than do vegetables, as the principle sugar in fruit is fructose which requires no further digestion. Vegetables, on the other hand consist mainly of complex carbohydrates, and also have a different ratio of soluble to non-soluble fibres.

Because of the differences in composition, fruits and vegetables have different digestion and stomach retention times and the eating of fruits and vegetables at the same meal can lead to fermentation in the stomach. Symptoms produced by incorrect combinations include flatulence, halitosis and all the conditions associated with an acid system. Vegetables take on average two hours longer to digest than fruits, and it has been suggested that fruits be only eaten by themselves, however, the consensus of opinion is that fruits and vegetables combine well with grains, nuts and legumes but do not combine well with each other. The digestion of the protein component in grains, nuts and legumes in the stomach takes place rapidly and provided that the system is not subjected to free fats, animal proteins, or excessive quantities of high-protein foods, this digestion takes place rapidly enough to prevent fermentation. It is therefore not necessary to eat fruits only by themselves, and a breakfast consisting of grains and fruits is therefore not only compatible, but advisable, particularly for young children who need high energy foods to start the day.

Another issue that can be confusing is the question as to what should be regarded as a fruit and what should be regarded as a vegetable. Biologically the products of a blossom containing seed must be considered fruits, however, in terms of their composition and also their common usage, some biological fruits are more like vegetables in that their principle carbohydrate is not fructose but complex carbohydrates. To confuse the issue even further, some fruits and vegetables are neutral and produce no adverse effects when combined with either fruits or vegetables at the same meal. The neutral vegetables are mainly the high-water content vegetables with very low starch content and the neutral fruits are largely the high fat content fruits such as avocados and olives. In table 7.4 a list of likely compatible and non-compatible combinations is presented. It must be noted, however, that this list is not iron clad as no hard and fast rule exists in this regard, and what works well for one individual may cause discomfort for another. Nevertheless, it is intended to provide a starting point for the selection of compatible combinations.

It is important to vary the diet. **Variation** must be the watchword for healthful living. Some foods contain components which will suppress the uptake of vitamins and minerals in other foods, so that even if all the elements required by the system should be present in one meal, not all of them may be maximally utilized in that particular combination. By varying the combinations, however, we not only make life more interesting, but we also ensure a balanced uptake of essential nutrients.

Combining grains and legumes

If a vegan vegetarian diet is followed, protein needs must be met by combining plant protein sources, as plants generally do not contain complete proteins. All plant foods contain some protein, and the digestion of these proteins will contribute to the amino acid pool from which the body will construct its own proteins. The body does not store proteins as such, but the amino acid pool is maintained for a sufficient period of time to augment amino acid requirements from one meal to the next and it is therefore not necessary to obtain all the required amino acids during any one meal. Nevertheless, it is important to ensure that foods containing balanced proportions of all the essential amino acids be consumed over a 24-hour period, even if they are not consumed at the same meal.

Some vegetarians follow very restrictive diets where nutritional needs are supplied by only one, or a few plant food sources such as rice, but such diets will be totally inadequate. Although, the quantities of essential amino acids in plant foods are not the same as those in animal foods, proper combinations will supply all the body's needs.[13,31] One such combination is the combination of grains and legumes, which supplies a protein of exceptional quality. The amino acid profiles of individual grains and legumes do not always supply adequate quantities of the essential amino acids if eaten by themselves, but if eaten together, or separately over a 24-hour period, the amino acid pool will be supplied with all the essential amino acids the body requires.

Grains are relatively low in the amino acid lysine, and supplementation with legumes or nuts will provide excellent protein. Legumes and grains go well together as the simple peanut butter sandwich will demonstrate, and preparing meals that contain both of these

```
┌─────────────────── INCOMPATIBLE ───────────────────┐
│                                                    │
│   ┌── COMPATIBLE ──┐    ┌── COMPATIBLE ──┐         │
```

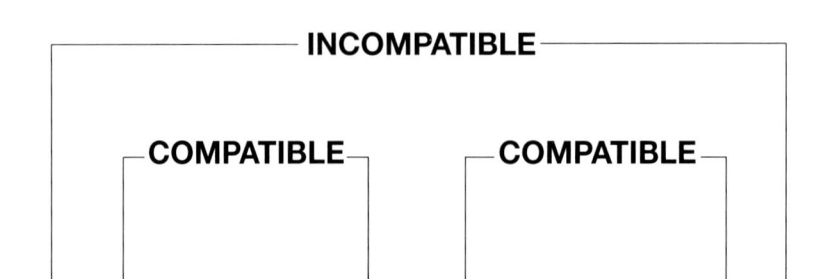

Fruit	Neutral	Vegetables
Most fruits: Apples Apricots Bananas Blackberries Blueberries Cantaloupe Cherries Cranberries Currants Dates Gooseberries Lemons Limes Loganberries Mango Nectarines Oranges Peach Pear Persimmons Pineapple Plums Raspberries Strawberries Tangerines Watermelons etc.	**All grains:** Barley, Buckwheat, Bulgur, Corn, Millet, Oats, Rice, Rye, Sorghum, Wheat etc. **All legumes:** Carob, Chick peas, Kidney beans, Lentils, Lima beans, Mung beans, Peanuts, Soya beans etc. **All nuts:** Almonds, Brazil, Cashews, Chestnuts, Coconuts, Hazelnuts, Macadamias, Pecans, Walnuts etc. **All seeds:** Linseed, Poppy seed, Pumpkin seed, Sesame, Sunflower etc. **Some vegetables:** Cucumber, Herbs, Lettuce, Sprouts, Tomatoes (?), Watercress **Some fruits:** Avocados, Olives	**Most vegetables:** Artichokes Asparagus Broccoli Beets Brussels sprouts Cabbage Carrots Cauliflower Celery Eggplant (Brinjal) Green beans Green peppers Kale Kohlrabi Leeks Okra Onions Parsnips Potato Pumpkin Radish Spinach Squash Sweet potato Turnip etc.

Table 7.4. Compatible combinations of plant foods.

plant protein sources will not only provide nourishing meals, but will also give peace of mind. Adequate nutrition for young children is always a matter of concern, and whilst legumes or grains might be adequate for adults, the combination is more than adequate, even for young children. Studies in rats[31] and humans confirm that suitably combined vegetarian foods supply up to many times the minimum essential amino acid requirements.[32]

The concern for adequate proteins often leads to an overemphasis of legumes and nuts in the vegetarian diet, and the proportions in which these foods are consumed are mostly incorrect. Heavy protein dishes consisting largely of legumes, will not only produce flatulence, but will also lead to excessive protein katabolism with its associated problems. When combining grains and legumes, the quantity of grains should exceed that of the legumes or other high protein source. Legume dishes can be made very tasty by incorporating vegetables into the recipe as in the case of casseroles, and this will naturally make the legume dish less concentrated.

Much can be learnt from Eastern, Middle Eastern and Mediterranean cultures regarding the use of whole foods such as whole grains, legumes, seeds and nuts in the preparation of tasty dishes. A whole new range of tastes and textures is available from these foods that will more than compensate for any foods given up in the interest of health. These foods can be purchased from health shops, but as these are often quite expensive it may be wise (and fun) to scout around farming co-operatives and Eastern markets, particularly Indian, Malaysian and Chinese markets, to obtain the best buys. Furthermore, a few modern kitchen appliances such as a strong blender and mixer will greatly increase the range of dishes that can be prepared, and will also be a time saver. Expensive kitchen appliances are not essential to adopting this lifestyle, as has been proved by the many tribes that have not had the advantages of modern technology at their disposal but enjoy a healthy lifestyle based on whole foods.

Grains

Grains have formed the mainstay of human nutrition for thousands of years, and it is indeed a pity that modern man has so restricted the use of this primary food source in his diet. The few grains that are still consumed are robbed of most of their nutrient value through the process of refining, and it is therefore not surprising that this generation is characterized by disease and obesity. Refined foods supply largely empty calories, and they not only rob the body of essential nutrients, but they also take away one's appetite for wholesome foods. Eating whole grains will certainly lead to improved health and they can provide a whole new eating experience. The grains can be prepared in many ways as long as the components are not removed by refining.

Grains are classed as carbohydrate foods, as they contain on average 75% starch, and in addition to starch, whole grains contain some 10–15% protein, 2% fat and are also rich in fibre, vitamins and minerals. Grains contain important quantities of the B-group vitamins, and if incorporated regularly in the diet they can contribute substantially to the daily requirements for this group. Ascorbic acid (vit.C) is lacking in grains, but if sprouted, this vitamin is also produced. Vitamin A and D are also absent in grains, but yellow maize contains the carotenoids cryptoxanthin and small amounts of α- and β-carotene, which are vitamin A precursors. Grains also contain anticarcinogenic compounds such as **inositol hexaphosphate** and other compounds with suspected anticancer activity (see table 7.18).

The germ of grains contain tocopherols (vitamin E) which are natural antioxidants and protect the body against the formation of free radicals. The germ also contains some complete protein, and the vitamins in the germ are essential to carbohydrate and fat metabolism, but because it is the component of wheat that spoils first, it is mostly removed in the refining process. Thiamin, riboflavin, niacin and vitamin B-6 are all present in grains, but the quantities can vary depending on the kind of grain and on the soil and climatic conditions. The bran is rich in the B-complex vitamins and fibre, but it is also removed in the refining process.

Refined grains rob the body of essential dietary components and will lead to decreased vigour and gastrointestinal disturbances, particularly constipation. In modern societies it has become customary to offset this imbalance by adding wheat-germ or bran to the diet. Indeed, some modern breakfasts can consist almost entirely of bran under the assumption that one is getting a good, healthy start for the day. Eating a daily ration of fibre in one meal, does nothing for subsequent meals and contributes little to solving the problems associated with a low fibre diet. The nutrients in a high bran and wheat germ diet are in the form of proteins, fats and minerals. However, the protein and mineral composition of bran and germ are totally disproportionate to the overall needs of the body as the ratio of protein to utilizable carbohydrate is such that energy requirements must be met by metabolizing proteins or fats. Unrefined grains will supply primary nutrients, vitamins and minerals in well-proportioned quantities. They will ensure gastric regularity, and lead to better overall health.

Whole grains can be used in a variety of ways: The grains can be soaked and cooked whole like rice, they can be sprouted and eaten raw or cooked in stir fries etc., porridges can be prepared from cooked rolled grains or liquidized soaked whole grains, grains can be used in baked dishes or in patties or they can be roasted and used in muesli and granola. Sprouted grains, or grains soaked to the point of sprouting, can be eaten raw but most grains should be well cooked before eating because they contain protein inhibitors which inhibit the activity of digestive enzymes.[33,34] These inhibitors are, however, inactivated by heat or sprouting. Grains (dry or soaked) can be readily frozen for storage if they are to be kept for long periods of time. Again, it can be emphasised, that it is important to concentrate on variety, as different grains have different attributes as the following discussion will show.

Barley (*Hordeum vulgare* or *H. sativum*)

The composition of barley is presented in table 7.5.

There are many varieties of barley, and it has been cultivated for centuries, particularly for the preparation of beer which was already drunk by the ancient Egyptians.[38] Besides being one of the major raw materials of beer, it was used as a food source by the ancient civilizations of China, Egypt, Greece and Rome, and in countries with cold climates it is still used extensively today. Barley is known for its heat-producing qualities and should become a regular component of soups, stew and breakfast cereals, particularly in winter. Barley can also be used in baking where it

	Energy (cal)	Carb. (g)	Prot. (g)	Fat (g)	Fibre (g)	Ca (mg)	P (mg)	Fe (mg)	K (mg)
Dry	350	79.0	8.0	1.0	–	16	189	2.1	160
Cooked	120	27.6	2.7	0.6	2.2	3	70	0.2	40
	Mg (mg)	Zn (mg)	Vit. A (IU)	Vit. B1 (mg)	Vit. B2 (mg)	Vit. B3 (mg)	Vit. B5 (mg)	Vit. B6 (mg)	Vit. E (mg)
Dry	35	–	0	0.1	0.05	3.1	1	0.22	–
Cooked	7	0.7	0	0	0	0.9	0	–	–

Table 7.5. The composition of barley. The figures are for 100 g portions. (From ref. 35,36,37)

will add flavour and retain moisture, and if sprouted, it will add even greater nutritive value to the diet. Barley is easy to digest and is rich in pantothenic acid (vitamin B-5) which is essential for the intermediary metabolism of carbohydrates, fat and protein. Because vitamin B-6 is incorporated into co-enzyme A, it is involved in the release of energy from carbohydrates and in the metabolism of fatty acids which probably accounts for barley's heat-producing qualities.

Corn (maize, mealie) (*Zea mays*)

The composition of corn or maize is presented in table 7.6.

Corn often means different things to different nations, but most often it refers to the grain which grows on the cob. It is also known as maize and it forms the staple diet of many nations. Corn was cultivated in South America where the American Indians referred to it as "the daughter of life". Maize meal is used extensively by African nations but unfortunately here too the refined product is nowadays preferred.

Yellow maize and sweet corn contain carotene, and thus contribute to vitamin A requirements, but overall maize is lower in nutritive value than most other grains. Furthermore, as maize meal has a large capacity for water absorption, it is not advisable to rely extensively on cooked maize meal porridges to supply one's energy needs, as a look at the composition table will show. It should be noted that cooked maize meal porridge will absorb up to six times its mass in water, and if eaten as the sole energy supplier will thus fill the stomach largely with water without providing sufficient energy. This is particularly important in the case of young children, as they have a limited stomach capacity.[39,40]

African people prepare maize meal in such a way that far less moisture is retained and the cooked product then has a dry, crumbly texture. This is known as **"putu"**, and prepared in this way the energy per volume is greatly increased. Putu can then be eaten as one would eat rice together with stews and vegetables, or it could be combined with stewed fruit to make a very palatable breakfast. Combining corn with legumes will improve the protein and mineral quality, and the quality of corn bread will thus be enhanced by adding a little soy flower to the mixture. If these points are borne in mind, corn can form a versatile, nutritious part of the diet.

Millet (*Panicum miliaceum*)

The composition of millet is presented in table 7.7.

There are many kinds of millet, but the common millet is known as Proso millet (*Panicum miliaceum*) which originated in Egypt or

	Energy (cal)	Carb. (g)	Prot. (g)	Fat (g)	Fibre (g)	Ca (mg)	P (mg)	Fe (mg)	K (mg)
Meal (yellow)	320.0	56.8	9.2	4.3	8.1	3	195	2.8	293
Porridge (white)	66.0	13.6	1.6	0.5	1.0	0	32	0.5	46
On cob	108.0	21.0	3.3	1.3	4.1	2	103	0.6	249
	Mg (mg)	Zn (mg)	Vit.A (IU)	Vit.B1 (mg)	Vit.B2 (mg)	Vit.B3 (mg)	Vit.B5 (mg)	Vit.B6 (mg)	Vit.E (mg)
Meal (yellow)	87	1.74	476	0.44	0.17	1.7	–	–	1.75
Porridge (white)	14	0.29	0	0.07	0.02	0.2	–	–	0.23
On cob	32	–	217	0.22	0.07	1.6	0.88	–	0.44

Table 7.6. The composition of corn. The figures are for 100 g portions. (From ref. 35,36,37)

Arabia. The name Proso is the Russian name for millet. Millet is used extensively in Eastern countries, particularly India and China, and it is a must for the health conscious as it is not only highly nutritious, but is also one of the few alkaline grains. Millet belongs to the sorghum family of grains and is rich in magnesium and iron, the latter being one of the minerals that vegetarian diets can be low on. The mineral composition of millet is beneficial to the nervous system, and for arthritis sufferers this grain is highly recommended in view of its alkaline-forming properties.

Millet has a very hard outer casing and must be dehulled before it can be eaten. Many people are disappointed with millet because they buy the intact seed, which is suitable for birds, but provides quite a chewing experience for humans. Dehusking is normally done mechanically, and the dehusked product can be bought from health outlets. If millet is not available in the area in which one lives, then it is worthwhile ordering it by post. Millet is also a very versatile grain, and it can be prepared in a variety of ways. Prepare a millet porridge for breakfast or liquidize the cooked grain and use it to form the basis of delicious puddings. Millet flour can be used in conjunction with other flours in baking, and the high soluble fibre content gives the flour excellent binding qualities so that it can be used for binding patties, nut and legume roasts and can substitute for eggs in recipes that require eggs for binding.

Oats (*Avena sativa*)

The composition of oats is presented in table 7.8.

Whole oats is the best grain source of calcium, and together with its other minerals contributes to healthy bones and teeth. Moreover, oats has the highest fat content of all the grains and is second in terms of protein quality. The fat in oats is rich in oleic acid and the essential fatty acid, linoleic acid, and oats thus has an excellent fatty-acid composition. Another endearing quality of oats is its natural fibre composition which, in view of its unique blend of soluble fibres, assists the body in keeping cholesterol levels down and also ensures that the products of carbohydrate digestion are released slowly into the bloodstream. This ensures a constant supply of energy to the body rather than the glucose surge associated with refined foods. All these qualities combined, make oats, together with fruit, the ideal breakfast food.

It has long been known that the fibre in grains has an effect on cholesterol and triglyceride levels, and tends to reduce the levels of both.[41] It has now been clearly established that oat bran is not only the most efficient in achieving this objective,[42] but that the LDL cholesterol level, associated with arterial disease, is furthermore lowered by oat bran.[43] Sustained slow release of glucose during starch digestion is highly desirable to prevent hypoglycaemia and to ensure a constant supply of energy to the system. Here again it is oats fibre which outperforms all other grains in

	Energy (cal)	Carb. (g)	Prot. (g)	Fat (g)	Fibre (g)	Ca (mg)	P (mg)	Fe (mg)	K (mg)
Raw	331.0	75	10	2.8	–	22	325	7	475
	Mg (mg)	Zn (mg)	Vit.A (IU)	Vit.B1 (mg)	Vit.B2 (mg)	Vit.B3 (mg)	Vit.B5 (mg)	Vit.B6 (mg)	Vit.E (mg)
Raw	180	–	0	0.75	0.38	2.3	–	–	2

Table 7.7. The composition of millet. The figures are for 100 g portions.(From ref. 35,36,37)

The whole-food alternative

preventing glucose surges by slowing down the rate of glucose release.[44]

Oats is one of the few grains which requires very little to no cooking and is, therefore, ideally suited for raw consumption in the form of muesli. Consumption of uncooked oats will also supply more energy per spoonful, as the stomach will not be filled with the water that the grains so readily absorb. This is why a muesli or granola breakfast is ideally suited for young children with their limited stomach capacity. Together with nuts and dried fruits, oats will provide a champion breakfast.

The best oats to purchase is either coarsely rolled oats, or groats which is the dehusked whole grain of oats. The latter can be obtained from health stores and some seed outlets and is highly recommended. If a grain mill is available, or even a coffee grinder, the groats can be freshly ground and used in many dishes to add flavour or to thicken and to bind. Groats can also be cooked whole like rice and can be eaten as such or it can be eaten as a breakfast grain together with fruit. Another advantage of eating muesli, granola or the whole oat berries, is that it will compel one to properly chew one's food, and as starch digestion commences in the mouth, this is particularly important. Finally, oats is the ideal food for convalescing or sick people as it is easily digested and serves to improve the electrolyte balance.

Rice (*Oryza sativa*)

The composition of rice is presented in table 7.9.

The commonest rice species is *Oryza sativa*, and the different varieties of this rice can be divided into two main groups, the **japonica** and the **indica** types. The japonica types are the short-grained varieties, whereas the indica types are the long-grained varieties. Besides these, there are also many other varieties of rice, of which some grow on unflooded plains. Rice was first cultivated in India and today it is one of the most extensively used grains in the world, with China and India producing most of the world's crop. Modern transport has, however, made rice available to virtually every country in the world. Like millet, rice belongs to that elite group of alkaline grains and should thus play an important part in our diet, as alkaline-forming foods should form the bulk of our daily nutrient intake.

Even a cursory glance at the composition-table of rice, will show that brown rice is far superior to white refined rice in terms of its nutrient content. It almost seems that, whenever nature provides something exceptionally good, then man must rob the product of its exceptional components. Refined rice should not form a regular component of the diet, as it will lead to all the pitfalls associated with a highly refined diet. Some complain, that brown rice is to chewy compared to refined

	Energy (cal)	Carb. (g)	Prot. (g)	Fat (g)	Fibre (g)	Ca (mg)	P (mg)	Fe (mg)	K (mg)
Raw	384.0	67.0	16.0	6.3	5.6	52	474	4.2	350
Cooked	62.0	10.8	2.6	1.0	0.9	8	76	0.7	56
Muesli	368.0	66.2	12.9	7.5	7.4	200	380	4.6	600
	Mg (mg)	Zn (mg)	Vit.A (IU)	Vit.B1 (mg)	Vit.B2 (mg)	Vit.B3 (mg)	Vit.B5 (mg)	Vit.B6 (mg)	Vit.E (mg)
Raw	148	3.07	101	0.73	0.14	0.8	1.25	0.01	0.80
Cooked	24	0.49	16	0.11	0.00	0.1	0.20	–	–
Muesli	100	2.20	–	0.33	0.27	2.7	–	0.14	3.20

Table 7.8. The composition of oats. The figures are for 100 g portions. (From ref. 35,36,37)

rice. This problem can be lagely resolved by soaking the rice before cooking it, but it should also be remembered chewing is beneficial in terms of the digestive process.

The protein in rice is the perfect partner to the proteins in legumes and the combination of these two will provide a complete protein. Moreover, of all the grains, rice has the best percentage available protein. There are many varieties of rice on the market, so there is room for experimentation. Moreover, rice flour can be used for creating a variety of exciting dishes as well as cakes and puddings.

Rye (Secale cereale)

The composition of rye is presented in table 7.10.

Rye probably originated in Afghanistan and Turkistan, where the wild species still grows today. Rye has only been in circulation since the bronze era,[45] and since that time it has become firmly established as one of the major grains of Europe. Rye is well adapted to colder climates and gives yields over shorter periods of time than do other grains. In the past, rye was considered a weed and in America it is still sometimes referred to as "black wheat" and even in Europe it was still designated as cattle fodder in the 1980 European Community listings.[45] The Germans are particularly fond of rye, and they would certainly balk at the idea that rye could be termed cattle fodder.

Rye is rich in minerals, particularly potassium, and also contains substantial amounts of the B-group vitamins, however, it is relatively gluten-free and thus will produce very firm, dense bread, such as pumpernickel, if baked by itself. The best way to achieve the best baking results with rye flour, is to combine it with wheat flour or to use the grain **Triticale**, which is a hybrid of wheat and rye, and can be used to bake delicious ready-made rye bread. The combination of rye and wheat flour will produce a lighter bread and improve the protein quality, and do wonders to the flavour.

Sorghum (Sorghum vulgare)

The composition of sorghum is given in table 7.11.

Sorghum is native to Africa and Asia, and

	Energy (cal)	Carb. (g)	Prot. (g)	Fat (g)	Fibre (g)	Ca (mg)	P (mg)	Fe (mg)	K (mg)
Brown (R)	354	76.0	7.4	1.80	–	32	216	1.6	210
White (R)	354	78.0	6.5	0.75	–	23	91	0.9	89
Brown (C)	119	23.9	2.5	0.60	1.3	12	73	0.5	70
White (C)	109	23.5	2.0	0.10	0.7	10	28	0.2	28
Flour	371	79.1	7.2	0.70	0.2	7	90	0.4	104
	Mg (mg)	Zn (mg)	Vit. A (IU)	Vit. B1 (mg)	Vit. B2 (mg)	Vit. B3 (mg)	Vit. B5 (mg)	Vit. B6 (mg)	Vit. E (mg)
Brown (R)	86	–	0	0.43	–	4.60	1.00	0.05	1.50
White (R)	6	–	0	0.01	–	–	–	–	0.02
Brown (C)	54	–	0	0.09	0.02	1.40	0.35	–	1.54
White (C)	4	0.36	0	0.02	0.01	0.04	0.20	–	0.10
Flour	–	–	0	0.06	0.03	1.40	–	–	–

R = Raw, C = Cooked.

Table 7.9. The composition of rice. Figures are for 100 g portions. (From ref. 35,36,37)

it is an alkaline grain which is available in both a red and a white variety. This grain is widely used as cattle fodder, but man can certainly benefit from its consumption. Sorghum flour can be combined with wheat in bread, added to other grains and cooked as a porridge or it can be cooked as a porridge by itself. The whole grain is available from seed shops, farming co-operatives or from health outlets. In order to make one's own flour from sorghum or to make porridge, a wheat mill can be used or, the grain can be blended together with water in a high-speed blender until smooth and creamy. Home-prepared sorghum has a rich flavour, probably because more of the volatile components are retained compared to bought sorghum products.

Wheat (*Triticum*)

The composition of wheat and wheat products is presented in table 7.12.

Different varieties of wheat are grouped according to the number of chromosomes which their somatic cells contain. After rice, wheat is the most-used grain crop in the world. The world's annual harvest of wheat exceeds 95 million metric tons per year (that of rice is 186 million tons) and for billions of people it is the staple grain. Wheat has been grown for thousands of years, and the rise and fall of nations has been determined by the success or failure of the wheat crop. Many strains of wheat have been developed, but the development of short-stemmed varieties, that are less prone to wind damage, has revolutionized the wheat industry. However, traditional wheat varieties still have their place in many areas of the world, because they are adapted to particular areas and are resistant to local diseases.

Whole-grain wheat is one of the best sources of primary protein, and also supplies essential minerals and vitamins in appreciable amounts. The components of wheat all have their own unique properties. The bran is very different from the rest of the seed in that it has a high-fibre content and also contains a fair amount of lipids. The germ, on the other hand has a high-lipid content, and although wheat contains only about 2% lipid in total, the separated germ contains approximately 12% lipid and is also rich in vitamin E. Finally, the endosperm consists of cells containing starch granules and protein, and the composition of these proteins is most important in determining the baking quality of the flour.

Another important product of wheat is **Bulgur wheat**, also known as lapsi or cracked wheat. Bulgur is one of the staple grains of Middle Eastern countries, particularly Turkey. Traditionally, wheat is cooked in large tin-lined copper pots on an open wood fire, and then it is laid out on clean sheets to dry in the sun. Subsequently it is sent to the mills where it is cracked, and the recipes for its use depend on the final size of the cracked grains. Bulgur wheat is a very consumer-friendly wheat, as it is pre-cooked and thus takes very little preparation time. It also has a unique flavour and is very palatable. Bulgur is normally prepared like rice, and sautéed together with onions and green peppers it is

	Energy (cal)	Carb. (g)	Prot. (g)	Fat (g)	Fibre (g)	Ca (mg)	P (mg)	Fe (mg)	K (mg)
Raw	334	73	12	1.7	–	38	376	3.7	467
	Mg (mg)	Zn (mg)	Vit. A (IU)	Vit. B1 (mg)	Vit. B2 (mg)	Vit. B3 (mg)	Vit. B5 (mg)	Vit. B6 (mg)	Vit. E (mg)
Raw	115	–	–	0.43	0.22	1.6	–	–	–

Table 7.10. The composition of rye. The figures are for 100 g portions. (From ref. 35,36,37)

particularly tasty. In some countries it is not readily available, but most health outlets should stock it.

Bread

The protein composition of wheat gives it its unique character, and also makes it possible to bake a leavened bread. Bread is the staff of life and should form an essential component of a healthy lifestyle. Even a cursory glance at the composition tables will show that bread provides vastly more energy and nutrients per unit mass than does any other cooked grain. The reason for this lies in the fact that a large proportion of the water, added in the preparation, which to begin with is only a one to one ratio, is evaporated during the baking process, thus providing a high-energy food which should take pride of place in our diets. Furthermore, bread prepared from whole-grain flour will not be fattening and will contribute substantially to one's overall health and well-being. There is nothing as pleasant as the aroma and taste of a good home-baked bread, and no home should have to forgo the pleasure of enjoying this commodity. In today's society the art of bread baking has to a large extent been lost, and modern milling techniques have so changed the composition of wheat flour, that it has, indeed, become difficult to produce a product which will impart all the goodness of whole wheat.

In the past, wheat was milled by stone mills, and all the components of the wheat would be finely ground. Modern mills no longer use stones, and they automatically separate the components of the wheat. Milling involves successive stages during which the bran, the germ and the endosperm are gradually separated from each other. Most mills today use rollers to crush the wheat, and in the first crushing, the rollers are set relatively far apart, thus merely cracking the wheat kernels. Separation of the components is achieved by sieving or bolting, and successive rollers produce finer and finer products. The first process removes most of the bran, and during the crushing action of the rollers, some of the fat in the germ is squeezed out, thus allowing the germ particles to stick together. The high lipid content of the germ causes this component to be lighter than the rest, and it is therefore also readily separated by shaking and bolting. At each stage the fine flour consisting mainly of the endosperm accumulates, and eventually forms the bulk of the milling process. By combining and blending the different components of the milling process, many different flour varieties are produced, but the germ is seldom used in these combinations, in view of its spoiling qualities.

A good wholesome bread should contain all the components of wheat, and it is advisable to scout around for a supplier of whole flour. Some mills will still produce a whole flour, or they will be willing to produce such a

	Energy (cal)	Carb. (g)	Prot. (g)	Fat (g)	Fibre (g)	Ca (mg)	P (mg)	Fe (mg)	K (mg)
Raw	355	61.5	8.8	2.9	2.0	18	192	3.9	317
Cooked	43	7.5	1.1	0.4	0.2	2	23	0.5	39
	Mg (mg)	Zn (mg)	Vit.A (IU)	Vit.B1 (mg)	Vit.B2 (mg)	Vit.B3 (mg)	Vit.B5 (mg)	Vit.B6 (mg)	Vit.E (mg)
Raw	102	2.30	0	0.40	0.13	3.4	–	–	–
Cooked	12	0.28	0	0.05	0.00	0.4	–	–	–

Table 7.11. The composition of sorghum. The figures are for 100 g portions. (From ref. 35,36,37)

product upon request. Failing this, flour can be obtained from stone mills which are still operative, or the grain can be milled in household mills which are becoming more and more popular. Bread baked from stone, or home-ground flour, is a feast and will be difficult to give up once one has developed a palate for it. Bread is so versatile. By the addition of different ingredients it is possible to change the whole character of a loaf of bread. Adding herbs, onions or garlic will produce a delicious savoury loaf, whereas the addition of sweet ingredients or fruits, will produce a totally different culinary experience. The art of bread baking should be regained.

The art of bread baking

Sadly, many people have given up baking home baked bread, particularly whole-wheat bread, because they have obtained such poor results from their attempts. Often the bread produced is good for building houses, but totally unsuited for human consumption, and so the prospective bread baker has given up in despair and reverted to buying light and fluffy commercial products. This need, however,

	Energy (cal)	Carb. (g)	Prot. (g)	Fat (g)	Fibre (g)	Ca (mg)	P (mg)	Fe (mg)	K (mg)
Dry	330	69.0	14.0	2.2	–	36	383	23.1	370
Cooked	79	16.2	2.4	0.6	0.6	14	49	0.9	–
Germ	363	46.0	26.0	10.0	20.3	72	1118	9.4	827
Bran	240	70.0	16.0	5.0	–	130	1400	16.0	1200
Flour (ww)	318	65.8	13.2	2.0	9.6	35	340	4.0	360
Flour (cake)	350	80.0	9.8	1.2	3.4	15	110	1.5	140
Bread (ww)	268	40.3	3.5	3.4	8.9	64	211	3.5	322
Bread (Rye)	243	51.7	9.1	1.1	–	75	147	1.6	145
Pumpernickel	207	43.7	8.4	2.0	3.2	58	154	2.2	193
Bulgar	353	76.0	11.2	1.8	–	29	338	5.6	229
Bulgar (canned)	181	32.6	5.9	–	–	20	195	1.4	112
	Mg (mg)	Zn (mg)	Vit.A (IU)	Vit.B1 (mg)	Vit.B2 (mg)	Vit.B3 (mg)	Vit.B5 (mg)	Vit.B6 (mg)	Vit.E (mg)
Dry	160	–	0	0.57	0.12	4.3	–	–	–
Cooked	27	–	0	0.03	0.03	0.8	–	–	–
Germ	336	12.50	0	2.00	0.68	4.2	2.20	0.92	15
Bran	450	16.20	0	0.80	0.40	20.0	3.00	0.90	0
Flour (ww)	140	3.00	0	0.46	0.08	5.6	0.80	–	1
Flour (cake)	20	0.70	0	0.10	0.02	0.7	0.30	–	0
Bread (ww)	88	2.32	0	0.35	0.12	4.0	0.63	–	0
Bread (Rye)	–	–	0	0.18	0.07	1.4	–	–	–
Pumpernickel	49	1.38	0	0.27	0.20	2.3	–	–	–
Bulgar	–	–	0	0.28	0.14	4.5	–	0.22	–
Bulgar (canned)	–	–	0	0.06	0.04	3.0	–	–	–

Table 7.12. The composition of wheat and wheat products. The figures are for 100 g portions. (From ref. 35,36,37)

not be the lot of anyone if a few elementary procedures were rigorously adhered to. As with any other subject, it is always better to adhere to procedures if the principles involved are first understood, so before addressing the subject of bread baking, a brief discussion of the chemical process seems appropriate.

The chief proteins found in all cereals are **prolamines** and **glutelins**, and the relationship between these proteins varies from grain to grain. Wheat is unique, in that it contains a prolamine called **gliadin**, and a glutelin called **glutenin** in approximately equal proportions. The presence of gliadin and glutelin in the endosperm of wheat, gives wheat flour its unique baking qualities, because in the presence of water and mechanical agitation, these two protein fractions will form a tough, elastic complex known as **gluten**.[46] Gluten does not occur as such in wheat, but it is formed when the dough is kneaded and it will form an elastic, gummy product as the gluten will absorb water and swell up to 200%. The properties of the gluten, that is formed in the kneading process, will depend on the quality of the flour but in general, hard wheats will form a gluten of good strength.

The gluten that develops in the kneading process, acts as a trap for the gases produced by the yeast, which is added to the dough mixture to make the bread rise. The mixed dough must have the texture of chewing gum, which should not break when attempting to spoon out a portion, but should be elastic with good stretching ability. The yeast produces carbon dioxide as an excretory product during the fermentation period, and because it also produces new offspring, which also produce carbon dioxide, the dough will rise as the gas becomes trapped in the gummy gluten mixture. Some strains of yeast produce more gas than others and a number of other components of the dough also influence the rate of gas formation. As yeast is a living organism, it is obvious that it will only grow vigorously if its nutritional needs are met.

Yeast cells utilize sugars to provide for their metabolic needs, and as these are broken down, carbon dioxide is produced as a by-product. The sugars present in flour are mostly glucose, fructose and sucrose, with the first two being present mainly in the germ which is mostly removed in commercial flours. To speed up the rate of fermentation, sugar is normally added to the mixture, but as too much sucrose in dough will slow down the rate of fermentation, it is advisable to bear this in mind when adding sugars to the mixture. The bread recipes given in this book thus use monosaccharide sugar sources to circumvent this problem.

The quality of bread thus depends on a few fundamental principles, which if adhered to should greatly improve the product which is produced. The lightness, texture and taste of the loaf will be determined by the quality of the grains used, by the combination of grains used, by what is added to the dough and by the mechanical preparation of the dough.

Mechanical preparation

The gluten can be developed either by mixing or kneading, but it is essential that it is developed sufficiently to trap the carbon dioxide produced by the yeast. Undermixing will produce a heavy, dense bread which is difficult to digest, and will also discourage the baker. Overmixing will produce a sticky, less rubbery mixture which can also decrease the volume of the loaf.

Other ingredients

The ingredients added to a dough mixture are very important and will influence the quality of the end-product. A few factors to consider are:

a) **Grains**: In general the addition of flours, other than wheat, will produce denser loaves of bread, but the flavour and nutritional value can be improved. It is advisable to experiment until a happy compromise is reached which suits one's individual taste.

b) **Sugar**: Sugar can be added as yeast nutrient, but a fructose or glucose source would produce faster and tastier results. It is suggested that fruit or dried fruit such as raisins be added in liquidized form to provide a monosaccharide sugar form.

c) **Malt**: It is often customary to use malt extract, and malted barley in bread recipes, but this practice should be limited, as the malt contains proteolytic enzymes which break down the gluten in the dough, making it sticky, difficult to handle and producing a tacky bread of poor volume. Proteolytic enzymes also occur in the wheat flour itself, and this is desirable as it improves the gluten, however, too much will produce adverse results and that is why an addition of enzymes in malt and malted products can cause a problem.

d) **Salt**: Sodium chloride (table salt) improves the quality of the gluten that is developed, and can thus be added to the bread mixture. Salt will also improve the taste.

e) **Milk**: Milk contains factors which increase proteolytic enzyme activity, and raw or pasteurized milk should not be added to the dough.

f) **Heat**: Finally it should be remembered that grains contain factors which will limit their digestibility, but as these factors are normally neutralized by exposure to heat, it is advisable not to bake very large loaves of bread, so that the heat can penetrate deep into the loaves during baking. This will also ensure that the yeast cells are all killed during the baking process, as it is not advisable to ingest live yeast cells, as these will rob the body of essential nutrients. Live yeast cells, like all living organisms, require nutrients in order to continue their life processes and will thus absorb vitamins and nutrients from the system. If the loaves are, however, small and well-baked, the yeast cells will be killed and will themselves be digested thus adding to the nutrient supply.

The production of a quality bread is thus influenced by many factors, but adherence to the few principles outlined above, will produce an acceptable product. With a little practice and experimentation, it should, however, soon be possible to produce bread of the highest quality.

Legumes

As mentioned previously, legumes form the perfect companions to grains in terms of providing balanced proteins. Moreover, they supply an abundance of essential fatty acids, complex carbohydrates, vitamins and minerals, and most of them are alkaline-forming. Like the grains, legumes supply far more nutrients on a weight basis than do foods with a high water content, making them the ideal energy food particularly for young children.[47] Legumes generally have a low-fat content, but some varieties have considerable concentrations of fat, thus greatly boosting the energy content of these varieties. Underweight people could benefit from a higher consumption of the fat- and energy-rich varieties such as chick peas and soya beans in particular. Peanuts also have a very high energy content and they also have the highest fat content (49.2 g/100 g), but in view of their acid-forming character and oxalic acid content their use is often discouraged. It is encouraging to know that vegetarians cope well with the oxalic acid in foods, a fact which has been coupled to the absence of animal proteins.[29,30] Legumes with a high-fat content can also be used to make milk substitutes, and in this regard, the soya bean must rate supreme, however, most of the high-protein/high-fat varieties can be used to make highly nutritious milk substitutes.

Legumes have received some bad press, because their consumption is associated with flatulence and intestinal discomfort. If a few basic principles about their physiology and composition were understood, and the preparation adjusted accordingly, these side-effects could all be avoided. Dried legumes are dormant seeds that will only germinate under the right conditions. The nutrients and enzymes required during germination and early growth of the plant are thus inactive, and will only become active once the conditions are right for germination. The activated enzymes will then liberate nutrients from the stored foods in the legume as required by the developing plant. The enzymes present in the seeds include lipases, proteases and carbohydrate-digesting enzymes such as amylase which are similar to the enzymes found in the digestive tracts of humans. These enzymes are dormant in the dry seeds, because specific enzyme suppressants present in the seeds inhibit their activity. These enzyme suppressants will also inhibit the activity of human digestive enzymes and reduce the availability of nutrients from legumes.

Salivary and pancreatic **amylase inhibitors** have been found in grains and legumes, a trypsin inhibitor is present in black-eyed peas, kidney beans, lima beans, navy beans and soya beans,[48] and **lipase inhibitors** have also been isolated from soya beans.[49] Moreover, legumes contain **tannin** and **phytic acid** which render minerals unavailable for absorption, and in addition they contain carbohydrates such as **raffinose** and **stachyose** which are not broken down by human amylase. Raffinose is a trisaccharide consisting of glucose, fructose and galactose, and stachyose is a tetrasaccharide consisting of glucose, fructose and two molecules of galactose. These two oligosaccharides form additional storage carbohydrates, besides starch, and are only converted to a usable form when the seeds germinate. The list seems daunting indeed, and is enough to discourage anyone from eating legumes. If, however, we realize that these substances are rendered inactive during germination, then we merely have to simulate this process in order to eliminate the problem of suppressants.

Soaking, germination, fermentation, and cooking all reduce the effect of phytate and tannin in legumes,[50] and germination and cooking will also destroy the enzyme inhibitors.[34] Enzymes within the legume will then be activated, and raffinose and stachyose will be broken down, and the longer the germination process is allowed to continue, the lower the concentrations of the oligosaccharides will become. Sprouting legumes is thus the ideal way of improving their digestibility, and even if the sprouts are blanched before eating, it will not reduce the quality or the content of the proteins within the legume.[51] The quality of the proteins in beans, will also be improved by cooking, particularly if moist, rather than dry heat is used to prepare the legume.[52] Roasted legumes such as roasted peanuts or soya beans will, therefore, have poorer protein quality than the cooked product. The digestibility of legume proteins can also be increased by changing the method of processing. The proteins in legumes are only partially digested in the small intestine if they are eaten whole, but if they are liquidized before eating, then the protein can be 90% digested.[53]

It is essential to soak beans in plenty of water before using them (soak overnight or preferably longer) and discard the excess water as this will remove some of the tannin and will also activate the enzymes in the legume. It is not sufficient to soak the beans in just enough water so that all the water is soaked up into the beans, as this will not remove the suppressants. Soaking overnight in plenty of water is normally sufficient, but longer soaking periods are even more beneficial. Regular rinsing and discarding of the water will remove most of the suppressants and will eventually lead to sprouting, and once they have reached this stage they can be eaten raw without ill effect. Soaked beans can be placed in freezer bags and frozen for later use, thus eliminating the waiting period. If desirable, the husks of the beans can also be removed, and this will increase the protein content and lower the fibre content. Soaked legumes can then be cooked as is, or liquidized and used in a variety of recipes. Sprouting is one of the best ways of consuming legumes, but soaked and cooked legumes, particularly if properly prepared, are very nutritious, wholesome foods that can form a regular component of the diet.

Gas production will also be reduced if smaller portions of legumes are consumed during mealtimes as soaked, and even cooked legumes, will still contain some carbohydrates which cannot be broken down by human amylase and these resistant starches will pass through to the colon where bacteria will break them down anaerobically. The products of this fermentation process will be short-chain fatty acids and gas, and the fatty acids will be absorbed by the mucosa of the colon, and form the nutrients of choice for these cells.[54] The digestion-resistant carbohydrates are not digested in the small intestine, but they are fermented by the colonic bacteria and contribute to the increase in the number and bulk of the bacterial population. They also aid in the absorption of water, thus increasing the faecal bulk, they contribute to the production of anticarcinogenic compounds (see chapter 3), and thus offer protection against large bowel cancer.[53,55,56] It has been argued, the presence of phytic acid residues in legumes can adversely affect the bio-availability of iron in legumes, but it is ironic that the ability of phytic acid to chelate iron is also responsible for its antioxidant and anticarcinogenic properties.[57,58]

As stated earlier, variety in the diet is what is required in order to gain the most benefit out of all types of foods, and fear of shortages of nutrients need not exist if this principle is

Legume	Energy (kcal)	Carb. (g)	Prot. (g)	Fat (g)	Fibre (g)	Ca (mg)	P (mg)	Fe (mg)	K (mg)
Baked beans	64.0	10.3	5.1	0.5	7.3	45	91	1.4	300
Broad beans (r)	338.0	58.0	25.0	1.7	–	27	157	2.2	471
Carob (flour)	182.0	90.0	4.3	–	–	279	73	4.0	911
Chick pea (r)	320.0	50.0	20.2	5.7	15.0	140	300	6.4	800
Chick pea (c)	107.0	16.7	6.7	1.9	5.0	47	100	2.1	266
Haricot (r)	271.0	45.5	21.4	1.6	25.4	180	310	6.7	1160
Haricot (c)	93.0	16.6	6.6	0.5	7.4	65	120	2.5	320
Kidney beans (r)	273.0	49.8	5.9	1.1	21.6	85	320	5.9	1700
Kidney beans (c)	95.0	17.1	7.1	0.3	5.1	19	87	1.7	400
Lentil (r)	340.0	48.3	24.7	1.1	11.8	79	377	6.8	790
Lentil (c)	106.0	15.6	7.8	0.0	3.7	25	119	2.1	249
Lentil sprouts (r)	106.0	19.0	9.0	0.6	3.1	25	173	3.2	322
Lima bean (r)	345.0	64.0	20.0	1.6	–	72	385	7.8	1529
Lima bean (c)	137.0	25.8	8.4	0.5	–	29	154	3.1	612
Mung beans (r)	340.0	60.0	24.0	1.3	–	118	340	7.7	1028
Mung bean sprout (r)	30.0	4.8	3.0	0.2	1.1	13	54	0.9	149
Mung bean sprout (c)	21.0	3.4	2.0	0.1	0.8	12	28	0.7	101
Peanuts	580.0	10.2	26.8	49.2	8.3	86	506	1.9	703
Peanut butter	591.0	8.2	28.5	51.1	7.6	33	374	1.8	685
Peas, split (r)	310.0	56.6	22.1	0.4	11.9	33	270	5.4	910
Peas, split (c)	118.0	21.9	8.3	0.3	5.1	11	120	1.7	270
Pinto bean (c)	147.0	27.0	8.3	0.6	–	48	164	3.0	490
Soya (r)	403.0	28.6	34.1	17.7	4.9	226	554	8.4	1677
Soya (c)	130.0	9.2	11.0	5.7	1.6	73	179	2.7	540
Soya flour	352.0	28.2	45.3	7.2	14.3	240	640	9.1	2030
Soya (tofu)	85.0	2.5	7.5	4.2	–	90	126	1.9	42

Table 7.13 (Part 1). The composition of selected legumes. The figures are for 100 g portions (r = raw, c = cooked). (From ref. 35,36,37)

Legume	Mg (mg)	Zn (mg)	Vit.A (IU)	Vit.B1 (mg)	Vit.B2 (mg)	Vit.B3 (mg)	Vit.B5 (mg)	Vit.B6 (mg)	Vit.E (mg)
Baked beans	31.0	0.70	0	0.07	0.05	0.50	–	0.12	0.06
Broad beans (r)	–	–	220	0.28	0.17	1.60	–	–	–
Carob (flour)	–	–	Tr	0.05	0.05	1.60	–	–	–
Chick pea (r)	6.4	–	317	0.50	0.15	1.50	–	–	–
Chick pea (c)	2.1	–	106	0.17	0.05	0.50	–	–	–
Haricot (r)	180.0	2.80	0	0.45	0.13	2.50	0.70	0.56	–
Haricot (c)	45.0	1.00	0	0.11	0.06	0.70	–	–	–
Kidney beans (r)	164.0	2.80	0	0.45	0.13	2.50	1.00	0.58	–
Kidney beans (c)	33.0	1.00	0	0.14	0.07	0.70	–	–	–
Lentil (r)	77.0	3.13	60	0.37	0.22	2.00	1.38	0.61	1.27
Lentil (c)	25.0	1.00	20	0.07	0.06	0.60	0.31	0.11	–
Lentil sprouts (r)	37.0	–	45	0.23	0.13	1.10	0.58	0.19	–
Lima bean (r)	180.0	–	–	0.48	0.17	1.90	–	–	–
Lima bean (c)	–	–	0	0.13	0.06	0.70	–	–	–
Mung beans (r)	–	–	80	0.38	0.21	2.60	–	–	–
Mung bean sprout (r)	21.0	0.41	21	0.08	0.12	0.70	0.38	0.09	–
Mung bean sprout (c)	14.0	0.47	14	0.05	0.10	0.08	0.24	–	–
Peanuts	88.0	6.62	0	0.29	0.10	14.80	2.09	0.40	8.31
Peanut butter	175.0	2.92	0	0.15	0.11	13.40	0.92	0.39	4.70
Peas, split (r)	130.0	4.00	250	0.70	0.20	3.20	2.00	0.13	0.00
Peas, split (c)	30.0	1.20	83	0.11	0.06	1.00	–	–	0.00
Pinto bean (c)	–	–	Tr	0.18	0.09	0.39	–	–	–
Soya (r)	–	3.52	80	1.10	0.31	2.20	1.70	0.81	20.43
Soya (c)	–	1.20	30	0.21	0.09	0.60	–	–	20.43
Soya flour	290.0	4.87	–	0.90	0.36	2.40	2.10	0.68	–
Soya (tofu)	–	–	0	0.06	0.03	0.08	–	–	–

Table 7.13 (Part 2). The composition of selected legumes. The figures are for 100 g portions (r = raw, c = cooked). (From ref. 35,36,37)

followed. Fear of dietary protein shortages often prompts people to consume large quantities of legumes in a highly concentrated form, and the legume is then blamed for intestinal discomfort. Highly concentrated protein dishes of any kind, including high protein legumes, will increase the proportion of undigested protein entering the large intestine, which in turn will increase the concentration of potentially harmful substances derived from nitrogen.

If the above criteria are followed, legumes can form a trouble free component of the diet that provides numerous benefits including protection against degenerative diseases. Use raw sprouted legumes in salads, or enjoy them together with bread and fruits. Use soaked or sprouted beans in stews, roasts or patties and eat them in combination with grains to provide high quality protein and variety on the table. There are so many different kinds of legumes with so many different tastes and textures, that it will take a lifetime to sample them all. Some of the more common varieties include pea varieties such as **chick peas** and **split peas** and then there are the **lentil varieties** and **kidney beans, lima beans, mung beans, soya beans, broad** beans, **carob beans** and even the humble **peanut**. In this section only a few of the stalwarts will be discussed with which one can stock the kitchen, but by scouting around the markets many more varieties can be discovered which can provide a variety of tastes and textures to liven up ones diet. Table 7.13 gives the composition of some of the most commonly used legumes.

Carob (*Ceratonia siliqua*)

The carob tree is native to Mediterranean countries and its seeds are borne in large, long pods. The tree is a member of the locust family of plants and it is probable that this is the food source used by John the Baptist in Biblical times. It is from this background that the fruit of the carob tree is also known as 'St. John's bread'. The carob bean has a singular composition, as much of its carbohydrate source is in the form of fructose rather than complex carbohydrate. Carob is also rich in vitamins and minerals, particularly calcium, has a low-fat content and contains 8% protein. Furthermore, it contains pectin which ensures that the fruit sugar that is present is released gradually into the bloodstream. The natural sweet taste of carob, makes it the ideal substitute for cocoa and cocoa products such as chocolate.

In the Middle East, carob is very popular and is used extensively for making sweets and drinks. Indeed, the carob tea vendor is a marvellous sight in the streets of the ancient cities of Palestine.

Carob powder is a must in the kitchen and can be used to make hot 'chocolate' drinks as well as to give a chocolate flavour to puddings, fruit and 'milk' shakes and cakes. Carob chocolate can also be purchased from health shops and some enlightened supermarkets, and as carob is caffeine free, it can be used with a clear conscience and is safer for children. There are different varieties of carob powder available, ranging in taste from sweet to bitter, and it is advisable to purchase the sweet varieties if they are to be used for sweetening purposes.

Chick peas (Garbanzo) (*Cicer arietinum*)

Chick peas are native to western Asia and are very popular in Mediterranean countries, and many traditional dishes are prepared from this versatile legume. In Middle Eastern countries **hummous**, which is a mixture of chick peas, sesame seeds, oil, spices and lemon juice, is prepared from chick peas, and **falafel**, which is the filling for Arab bread, also has a chick-pea base. Chick peas can be used in stews, roasts, patties and a variety of spreads including an excellent substitute for butter. Sprouting greatly improves the protein, vitamin and mineral availability and also reduces the concentration of indigestible carbohydrates present in the pea.

Chick peas are a very rich source of iron, and even cooked chick peas will supply almost double the amount of iron of an equivalent portion of steak. Calcium levels are also high in chick peas, exceeding those of steak by many times, and in view of the protein composition of the peas, more of this calcium can be retained than if the protein were of animal origin. Furthermore, a meal combining grains, particularly rice, with chick peas, will supply a complete protein meal superior to that of meat.

Kidney beans (*Phaseolus vulgaris*)

The genus *Phaseolus* includes a great variety of beans including the variety used for making baked beans, and more and more strains of this genus are being developed and cultivated worldwide. The beans were originally cultivated by American Indians and were also used extensively on the islands of the West Indies. After the discovery of the New World, they were introduced into Europe in the 16th century and since then have also been known as 'French beans', a name that has become associated with the green varieties that are served in the pod as a vegetable.

Kidney beans can be prepared in many ways, and it is always useful to consult the merchants in oriental markets as to the traditional ways of preparation. Some varieties of kidney beans are very large and soft so that they can be fried and served as a substitute for meat products. Some of the more common varieties of dried beans that can be tried, include the common **haricot beans, navy beans, calico beans, snap beans, Mexican black beans** and **pinto beans**. Pinto beans are an excellent source of protein, and are also very tasty.

Bean diets are known to lower cholesterol levels and improve the HDL:LDL ratio by as much as 17%.[59] In a study done on canned beans, it was found that serum cholesterol levels were lowered by 13% and triglyceride levels by 12% after just 3 weeks of use, when compared to controls.[60,61] This is good news for people suffering from cardiovascular diseases, and beans are thus highly recommended for keeping cholesterol and blood-fat levels in check and improving the overall health status of the cardiovascular system. Canned beans (depending on brand) can cause flatulence, as the beans are either not soaked for sufficient time periods, or in a large enough volume of water to eliminate the enzyme suppressants. Nevertheless, canned beans are healthy and convenient, but nothing beats home prepared beans in tomato or other sauce. Normally the small white varieties of kidney beans are used to prepare beans in tomato sauce, but another bean which can be used to create tasty dishes is the **adzuki bean** (*Phaseolus angularis*) which also contains some 20% protein.

Lentils (*Lens esculenta*)

Lentils are native to western Asia, from where they were introduced to the Mediterranean region. Lentils are a must for every household. They require very little preparation time if properly prepared, and supply a superb package of nutrients. Because of the small size of some lentils varieties, lentils are often cooked like rice without pre-soaking. This is not a harmful procedure in itself, but because the lentil also contains the enzyme suppressants and digestion resistant storage carbohydrates common to legumes, it is advisable to soak them like any other legume before cooking. Lentils have always formed an important component of the human diet, and indeed, birthrights have been sold for them. They have also been found in Egyptian tombs, presumably because pharaohs believed that lentils would sustain them even after death.

Lentils are known to be an energy food, and this is probably due to the high concentration of B-group vitamins in combination with the carbohydrates present in this legume. This combination makes them the ideal food for active people like hikers and sportsmen. The carbohydrates in legumes are released slowly into the bloodstream after digestion, thus ensuring a steady, sustained supply of sugar to the system. The slow release of glucose into the bloodstream provided by legumes can be very beneficial to people suffering from hypoglycaemia, and it also ensures that the active person will be able to produce a sustained energy output over a long period of time. Lentils are rich in minerals, particularly iron and contain substantial amounts of proteins. Of all the legumes, however, lentil proteins have one of the lowest amino acid scores,[62] which means that the combination of amino acids present in this legume are of such a nature, that they will not supply adequate quantities of essential amino acids if eaten by themselves. The answer again lies in combining lentils with grains, particularly rice, for a balanced supply of essential amino acids. Lentils are ideal for sprouting, and the nutrient value is improved by this process. Sprouts provide a good source of vitamin C, and the vitamin B content is also improved by sprouting. Lentils sprout very readily and are versatile in their use. Try lentil sprouts in soups and stews, or eat them raw in salads or on sandwiches.

Lima and Sieva beans (*Phaseolus lunatus*)

Lima beans are indigenous to tropical America, and in Britain they are known as **butter beans**. They are also known as **sieva beans**, **pole beans** or **curry beans**. Lima beans are a high-energy food with a high carbohydrate content, and they are easy to prepare as they require less cooking time than most beans. The protein content of lima beans is high and they have a high amino acid score which once again will be much improved by combination with grains. One of the endearing qualities of lima beans is that they have a soft, creamy texture and are 13,1% alkaline-forming. Furthermore, they have a high concentration of potassium, magnesium, iron and calcium. Lima beans can be used like peas, and they can be incorporated into many different dishes and make excellent bean loaves.

Mung beans (*Vignia aureus*)

Mung beans are native to India and they form an important component of the human diet in Asia, where the whole or split seeds are used. Mung beans can be sprouted, cooked or ground into a flour. Mung beans provide an important protein source, and together with cereals, provide complete proteins. In the East, the beans are either sprouted, or used to make **Dhal**, soups and curries, and in India, foods such as **Idli** and **Dosa** consist of mixtures of rice and mung beans.[50] The popularity of mung beans has also increased in Western cultures and mung beans, particularly sprouts, are being used more and more extensively. The beans can be ground into a flour, which can be used to make noodles, breads and biscuits.

Mung beans belong to the genus *Vignia* comprising a number of related species, of which the **cow pea** (*Vignia unguiculata*) and the **mung bean** (*Vignia radiata*), have all been cultivated for human consumption for centuries. Cow peas are extensively cultivated in African countries and are relatively cheap. This factor, and the fact that they have a very high-protein concentration (ranging from 22.8–26.8 g/100 g dry matter) make them ideally suited to the extraction of bean milk to be used as infant formulas in poorer countries. Such milk-extracts contribute more protein to the RDA of both infants and children up to three years of age, than does human milk.[63]

Mung beans are deficient in sulphur amino acids such as methionine, but they are rich in lysine, so it is important to include grains in the diet to gain the maximum benefit from the high protein concentrations that are present. It is also important to remember that the processing techniques discussed earlier be applied when preparing mung beans, as they also contain enzyme suppressants, indigestible carbohydrate varieties and substances which interfere with ion absorption. Soaking, cooking and sprouting, all reduce the concentrations of these metabolic suppressants and the sprouted mung bean in particular is highly nutritious. Sprouting mung beans, reduces the quantities of raffinose, phytic acid and tannin, and it increases the quantities of glucose, galactose, sucrose, folic acid, vitamin C and inorganic phosphorus. Furthermore, the bioavailability of iron is increased by sprouting, fat metabolism is stimulated, and the digestibility of protein is enhanced.[50] Sprouts should be allowed to grow for at least 3 to 4 days, as the nutrient availability increases with time, and after 72 hours of sprouting, the true digestibility of the proteins will be improved by as much as 12.8% over that of the ungerminated bean. Raw sprouts will provide a high-vitamin content, and whilst stir frying or blanching of mung bean sprouts will have little effect on the protein and fat availability, it will reduce the vitamin C content by as much as 50%. As a whole food diet, which includes plenty of fruits and vegetables, supplies ample vitamin C, there is certainly nothing wrong in using sprouts in stir fries occasionally.

Soya beans (*Glycine max*)

Soya beans have been a staple food throughout Asia for thousands of years, and according to tradition was one of five sacred crops named by Chinese emperor Shengnung. It is only recently that the soya bean has been introduced into Western society, and apparently it was first brought to the United States in 1804 as ballast on board a ship.[64] It was not until 1890 that soya bean crops were being considered, and by 1917 only 50 000 acres were under cultivation in the United States. From this humble beginning, soya bean production in the United States has steadily increased, and today it is the second most important cash crop in that country, and produces about half of the total world crop. Sadly most of this is used for animal fodder, but the potential for human nutrition is being recognized more and more. Indeed, the consumption of whole and processed soya products has increased dramatically, though not always for the correct reasons.

Whole soya beans are an excellent source of protein, and after peanuts, is the legume which contains the most oil. In addition, soya beans are a good source of fibre, calcium, iron, zinc, phosphorus, magnesium, thiamin, riboflavin, niacin, and folacin. It is, therefore, not surprising that the greater stamina of northern Chinese over their rice-eating southern counterparts is associated with the consumption of soya beans. Today, whole soya beans and traditional soy products such as **tofu, soy milk, miso,** and **tempeh** are being consumed more frequently in the Western world, and in addition a new generation of soy products has been developed which tends to substitute for meat and dairy products. These second generation soy products tend to be low fibre, and are high-protein foods, which in the interest of healthful living should not form a regular component of the human diet. In the United States, 90% of soya beans consumed by humans is in the form of soy-protein products.[64]

The proteins in soya beans are of a very high quality, but as is the case with most legumes, the levels of sulphur amino acids can be limiting. Soy-protein isolates, however, contain sufficient quantities of all the essential amino acids, including the sulphur amino acids, to meet the needs of adults, and probably infants as well. In fact, isolated soy protein is the sole protein source for some infant formulas.[65] Combinations of soya with grains will, however, definitely supply adequate quantities of essential amino acids for all age groups. The fibre found in soya beans is also very beneficial as it not only facilitates the movement of food through the intestines, but also has a considerable cholesterol-lowering effect.[65]

Whole soya, and products made from whole soya, will certainly benefit the consumer, and can more than adequately replace animal products. It is important, however, to follow the general procedures of preparation for legumes, as soya beans also contain the enzyme suppressants and indigestible carbohydrate components common to the legume family. The concentrations of these compounds are considerably reduced through soaking and heat treatment, thus largely eliminating their adverse effect on digestion and bio-availability of nutrients. The small concentrations of suppressants which remain, are insufficient to hamper nutrient availability, and can play an important role in disease prevention, as many of these compounds have been recognized as anticarcinogens.

Compounds in soya beans which act as anticarcinogens are the **isoflavins, protease inhibitors, phytic acid, saponins, phytosterols (e.g. phytoestrogen)** and **phenolic acid.**[64] Isoflavins in soya beans are present in fairly high concentrations and seem to offer protection against mammary cancer, and may even protect against endometrial and ovarian cancer.[64] It has been suggested that the low incidence of breast and colon cancer in countries such as Japan and China is diet-related, and may be linked to the high consumption of soya beans in these countries. In 1990 the National Cancer Institute held a workshop to examine this relationship.[66]

The protease inhibitors in soya beans are largely destroyed by heating, but not all activity is destroyed.[64] Raw soya beans do have high concentrations of these protease inhibitors and these could adversely affect protein utilization and have been known to cause pancreatic hypertrophy in rats. However, in populations that consume cooked soya bean products no such adverse effects have been noted. The principle protease inhibitors in soya beans are the **Kunitz trypsin inhibitor** and the **Bowman-Birk trypsin** and **chymotrypsin inhibitor**, but these compounds also inhibit colon, lung and oral cancer. In addition, the protease inhibitors also suppress the transformation of cells into malignant cells, and they suppress the production of other carcinogenic compounds such as hydrogen peroxide.[64] The small quantities of inhibitors consumed will thus, on balance, be beneficial to the consumer.

Cooked whole beans and soya products such as tempeh, natto and miso still contain most of the nutrients present in the unprocessed beans, but in the case of soy milk and products prepared from this milk, some of these nutrients are lost. Soy milk and soy milk products such as tofu and soy cheeses will be low in calcium, and this should be borne in mind when planning to substitute soy milk for cow's milk in the diet of children. Table 7.14 gives the nutrient composition of some common soy foods.

Soy milk

Soy milk is an excellent substitute for cow's milk and is far more digestible and compatible with human nutritional requirements than is cow's milk. The amount of fat in soy milk is less than that of cow's milk, but the oil in soy beans consists mainly of mono- and polyunsaturated fats and is cholesterol free, in contrast with the fat in cow's milk which consists of saturated fats and is not cholesterol free. The oil in the soya bean and soya bean milk also contains a considerable quantity of essential fatty acids, particularly α-linolenic acid, and thus provides a convenient source, together with whole grains, for meeting the body's requirements for these essential fatty acids. In addition, soya beans are also rich in vitamin E, thus preventing harmful oxidation of these polyunsaturated fatty acids.

In contrast to cow's milk, the proteins in soy milk are readily digestible and do not produce the adverse side-effects associated with casein, the principle protein of cow's milk. Ca-

Component	beef steak	cow's milk	raw, dry soybean	cooked soybean	roasted soybean	sprouted soybean	miso
Water (g)	61.10	87.90	10.00	71.00	2.00	69.10	41.00
kcal	190.00	61.00	403.00	130.00	471.00	128.00	206.00
Protein (g)	30.80	3.30	34.10	11.00	35.20	13.10	11.80
Lipid (g)	7.40	3.30	17.70	5.70	25.40	6.70	6.10
Carbohydrate (g)	0.00	4.70	28.60	9.20	33.60	8.90	28.00
Fibre (g)	0.00	0.00	4.90	1.60	4.60	2.30	2.50
Calcium (mg)	6.00	119.00	226.00	73.00	138.00	67.00	66.00
Iron (mg)	3.40	0.10	8.40	2.70	3.90	2.10	2.70
Zinc (mg)	5.90	0.40	3.52	1.20	3.10	1.17	3.30
Thiamin (mg)	0.09	0.00	1.10	0.21	0.10	0.34	0.10
Riboflavin (mg)	0.40	0.2	0.31	0.09	0.15	0.12	0.25
Niacin (mg)	6.30	0.1	2.20	0.60	1.40	1.10	0.86
Vitamin B–6 (mg)	0.33	0.00	0.81	–	0.21	0.18	0.22
Vitamin E (mg)	0.29	0.10	20.43	20.43	–	–	–
Folacin (µg)	17.00	5.00	171.00	171.00	211.00	172.00	33.00

Table 7.14 (Part 1). Composition of selected soyfoods per 100 g portions. Values for steak and cow's milk are given for comparison. (Adapted from ref. 37, 64)

Component	natto	okara	soymilk	soy sauce (tamari)	tempeh	firm, raw tofu	regular, raw tofu
Water (g)	55.00	82.00	93.00	66.00	55.00	70.00	85.00
kcal	212.00	77.00	33.00	60.00	199.00	145.00	76.00
Protein (g)	17.70	3.20	2.80	10.50	19.00	15.80	8.10
Lipid (g)	11.00	1.70	1.90	0.10	7.70	8.70	4.80
Carbohydrate (g)	14.40	12.50	1.80	5.60	17.00	4.30	1.90
Fibre (g)	1.60	4.10	1.10	0.00	3.00	0.15	0.08
Calcium (mg)	217.00	80.00	4.00	20.00	93.00	205.00	105.00
Iron (mg)	8.60	1.30	0.60	2.38	2.30	10.50	5.40
Zinc (mg)	3.00	–	0.23	0.43	1.80	1.57	0.80
Thiamin (mg)	0.16	0.02	0.16	0.06	0.13	0.16	0.01
Riboflavin (mg)	0.19	–	0.70	0.15	0.11	0.90	0.05
Niacin (mg)	0.00	–	0.15	3.95	4.60	0.38	0.20
Vitamin B-6 (mg)	–	–	0.40	0.20	0.30	0.09	0.05
Vitamin E (mg)	–	–	–	–	–	–	–
Folacin (µg)	–	–	1.50	18.20	52.00	29.30	15.00

Table 7.14 (Part 2). Composition of selected soyfoods per 100 g portions. Values for steak and cow's milk are given for comparison. (Adapted from ref. 37, 64)

Miso = Cooked soybeans inoculated with *Aspergillus oryzae*, fermented and pressed into a paste.
Natto = Cooked soybeans inoculated with the bacterium *Bacillo natto*, fermented, and commonly wrapped in straw.
Okara = The pulp remaining after the extraction of soymilk from the beans.
Roasted soybeans = Whole soybeans that are dry or oil roasted until crunchy.
Soymilk = Soaked soybeans are heated in hot water, liquidised, squeezed through a cheesecloth to obtain the soymilk.
Soy sauce = Cooked soybeans inoculated with *Aspergillus oryzae*, shaped into nuggets, incubated, mixed with salt and the mash (called moromi) aged. It is then pressed to yield Soy sauce (tamari).
Tempeh = Cooked soybeans inoculated with *Rhizopus oligosporus*, producing a chunky cake.
Tofu = Soymilk is coagulated with either calcium or magnesium salt (**nigari**), and the curd pressed. The degree of pressing produces hard or soft tofu.

sein is known to elicit a hypercholesterolaemic effect when fed to a variety of animals, and will even result in the animals developing arteriosclerosis.[67] These effects were diminished in rabbits if casein was replaced with soy protein.[67] With the exception of vitamin B-12, soy milk also contains substantially higher concentrations of the B-group vitamins than does cow's milk. Vitamin B-12 can, however, be added to home-made soy milk, as is currently being done in the case of commercial soy milks and infant formulas. Contrary to popular belief, fermented soy products also do not contain vitamin B-12, except if it was added or is present as a contaminant. The vitamin B-12 that is presumed to be present in these foods is in the form of analogues, and not as cobalamine, which is the active vitamin.[68]

In the past, soy milks were rather unpalatable as a result of a strong beany flavour, however, this drawback has to a large extent been eliminated and sales of soy milk have rocketed in countries where the new generation of milks is readily available. The beany flavour of soy milk is caused by the action of enzymes such as **lipoxygenase** during the preparation process. Modern processing thus inactivates lipoxygenase through heat treatment whilst at the same time ensuring that the solubility of the other soya proteins is not too greatly affected, as this would reduce the amount of soluble protein that can be extracted from the milk. Heating soaked, dehulled beans to 80–85 °C for not more than 2 minutes will inactivate the lipoxygenase whilst still allowing 80% of the protein to be extracted from the beans.[69] It was also found that soaking dehulled beans at 70 °C for 5 minutes prior to liquidizing and extracting of the milk would reduce the **n-hexanal** content of the soy milk and improve the flavour.[70]

Commercial soy milk and soy products are a great time saver, but for the industrious or for those living in areas where these products are not available or too expensive, soy milks can be prepared at home, which will rival any of the modern commercial products. Moreover, the concentrated soy bean extract can be used to make a variety of sauces and soy cheeses such as tofu, which is obtained by precipitating the protein from the milk. These products can be incorporated into many dishes to improve their nutritional value, texture and taste. Try some of the recipes given in the last chapter.

Nuts and oilseeds

Nuts provide numerous health benefits and are one of the best sources of primary proteins, essential unsaturated fats, minerals and vitamins. The combination of nutrients in nuts is superior to that found in any animal product, and nuts should, if possible, become a regular component of the diet. Nuts have a high-fat content, but in view of their exceptional nutrient density, they offer concentrated nutrition with a relatively low-calorie content. In spite of their high-fat content, nuts will not be fattening if consumed in moderation. Unfortunately, nuts are quite expensive, although this depends on the grade of nuts and the place of purchase, and the inclination is to forgo the pleasure of making regular use of this commodity. Most nut recipes will require that the nuts be liquidised or processed in some way, and one can purchase broken nuts which are cheaper, for this purpose. On a weight-for-weight basis nuts are very good value for money and, in addition, the versatility of nuts makes them a culinary delight. Nuts can be eaten raw, they can be used to prepare delicious nut milks, creams and sauces, and they can be used in a variety of other ways in cooked meals. It only takes a small quantity of nuts to achieve great results, and even expensive nuts can be used for making creams and milks that will compare favourably in price with dairy products. Where economic considerations are paramount, however, oilseeds can be used to substitute for many of the qualities of nuts, and they can replace nuts in most recipes which require them.

The protein composition of nuts and oilseeds is of exceptional quality, and the essential amino acids are well supplied. The proteins are also readily digestible, and do not require the excessive stomach acid secretion necessary for the digestion of animal proteins, thus making them totally compatible with other plant foods. Moreover, just 150 g of nuts will supply all the protein needs of the average adult and it should thus be self-evident why the addition of even small quantities of nuts to meals will ensure that the amino acid requirements are met.

Nuts and oilseeds have a high fat content, but the fat is present as unsaturated fats, and the accessory nutrients required for metabolizing these fats are also present, thus ensuring maximum utilization of these nutrients without the detrimental effects associated with the use of animal fats. The fatty acids, **palmitic acid**, **oleic acid** and **linoleic acid** form the largest portion of the fatty acid composition of nuts[71] and seeds, but the relative amounts of these vary in the different products. In nuts, the monounsaturated fats, rich in oleic acid, are the most abundant, and nuts thus provide a healthy source of energy whilst at the same time being friendly to the cardiovascular system. Almonds, for example, contain 52% fat but 67% of this is in the form of monounsaturated fat and this, together with the proteins and fibre in whole almonds, contributes to a lowering of blood cholesterol levels.[72] The high-oil content of nuts can thus be of particular benefit to people living in cold environments to provide additional heat energy.

The oils in whole nuts and seeds also come prepacked with antioxidants which prevent the formation of free radicals which are associated with tumour development. Antioxidant substances have been found in sesame seeds,[73] and vitamin E, a natural antioxidant, is present in high concentrations in whole nuts and seeds. Other compounds in seeds and nuts also contribute to a lowering of cholesterol levels, thus making these high-fat foods extremely user friendly. In this regard, it can be mentioned that sesame seeds contain the compound **sesamin**, a lignin from sesame oil, which lowers cholesterol levels by decreasing the rate of absorption from the intestine, increasing the rate of faecal excretion and inhibiting its formation in the liver.[74] For vegan vegetarians, nuts and seeds together with oil rich legumes form the most important source of fats, and it is essential that these be used to effectively to maintain adequate body weights. It is important to note here again that growing children need higher proportions of fat than adults, and nuts and seeds can be used to augment their fat supplies.[17] Even adults that struggle to maintain adequate BMI's, can increase their fat consumption by adding more of these oil rich foods to their diets.

The nutrient and amino acid composition of some of the more common nuts and seeds is given in tables 7.15 and 7.16.

Almonds (*Prunus amygdalus* var. *dulcis*)

The almond tree, *Prunus dulcis*, is closely related to the peach, plum and apricot tree, but the seed rather than the fleshy fruit, is the edible portion. The seeds of apricots have many things in common with almonds, and they, like almonds, are also utilized in the manufacture of traditional almond products such as marzipan. Almonds constitute the world's largest nut crop with California producing some 70% of the total world crop annually. Almonds are available in a number of varieties, the most common of which is the **Nonpareil** variety which is a flat nut and has a mild, sweet flavour. Other common varieties include the **Mission** variety which is a round nut with a rough dark skin particularly suited to roasting, the **Carmel** variety which is similar to the Nonpareil variety and the **California** variety which is a blend of several related varieties. Another type of almond is the bitter almond which contains high concentrations of benzaldehyde, which give it a pungent flavour, and for this reason it is not widely cultivated.

Almonds are the most alkaline of all nuts and this, together with their balanced composition of nutrients, makes them one of the most beneficial foods. Almonds have a 52% fat content, and 67% of this is in the form of unsaturated fat, consisting mainly of palmitic, oleic and linoleic acids.[71,72] The combination of essential oils, proteins and fibre in almonds have been found to lower cholesterol levels, and almonds are also one of the richest sources of vitamin E, which is a natural antioxidant, preventing the formation of free radicals. Moreover, almonds supply appreciable quantities of the B-group vitamins, particularly niacin, and are also rich in calcium, and magnesium which promotes healthy nerve function. Almonds consist of 18,6% protein, and if combined with other nuts, particularly cashews and Brazil nuts, the protein availability improves. Almonds are ideal companions of cereals,[75] and should, therefore, be one of the nuts of choice for muesli and other breakfast foods. Another way to enjoy almonds, is to convert them into almond butter or nut milk, the latter being particularly tasty and value for money. If almonds are blanched, then the brown skin is easily removed, and they have a milder flavour and a softer texture and nut butters made from blanched nuts may thus have greater eye appeal and a milder taste.

Brazil nuts (*Bertholletia excelsa*)

As the name suggests, Brazil nuts are native to Brazil. They consist of 14,4% protein and are the richest natural source of the

The whole-food alternative

Nuts/Seeds	Energy (kcal)	Carb. (g)	Prot. (g)	Fat (g)	Fibre (g)	Ca (mg)	P (mg)	Fe (mg)	K (mg)
Almonds (toasted)	586	16.7	20.4	50.8	6.2	283	550	4.9	773
Brazil nuts	656	3.3	14.3	66.2	9.5	176	600	3.4	600
Cashew nuts	574	32.0	15.3	46.4	0.7	45	490	6.0	565
Chestnuts (roasted)	245	40.1	3.2	2.2	12.9	29	107	0.9	592
Coconut (dried)	660	0.2	6.9	64.5	23.5	26	3	3.3	543
Coconut (raw)	345	2.8	3.3	33.5	12.4	14	113	2.4	356
Hazelnuts	632	5.5	13.0	62.6	9.8	188	321	3.3	445
Hickory nuts	700	13.0	14.0	70.0	–	–	–	2.8	–
Macadamia nuts	702	8.4	8.3	73.7	5.3	70	136	2.4	368
Pecan nuts	667	16.6	7.8	67.6	1.6	36	291	2.1	392
Pinenuts	515	13.4	24.0	50.7	0.8	26	508	9.2	599
Pistachio nuts	577	22.9	20.6	48.4	1.9	135	503	6.8	1093
Walnuts	642	11.8	14.3	61.9	6.5	94	317	2.4	502
Pumpkin seeds	553	15.0	29.3	46.4	–	51	1144	11.2	990
Safflower seeds	615	12.0	19.0	59.0	–	–	620	–	–
Sesame seeds	588	6.4	26.4	54.8	3.0	131	776	7.8	407
Sunflower seeds	570	14.6	22.8	49.6	4.2	116	705	6.8	689

Nuts/Seeds	Mg (mg)	Zn (mg)	Vit. A (IU)	Vit. B1 (mg)	Vit. B2 (mg)	Vit. B3 (mg)	Vit. B5 (mg)	Vit. B6 (mg)	Vit. E (mg)
Almonds (toasted)	305	4.92	0	0.13	0.60	2.86	0.26	0.074	50.27
Brazil nuts	225	4.59	0	1.00	0.12	1.60	0.24	0.251	7.60
Cashew nuts	260	5.60	0	0.20	0.20	1.40	1.22	0.256	0.57
Chestnuts (roasted)	33	0.57	24	0.24	0.18	1.30	0.55	0.497	–
Coconut (dried)	90	2.01	0	0.06	0.10	0.60	0.80	0.300	–
Coconut (raw)	32	1.10	0	0.07	0.02	0.50	0.30	0.054	0.73
Hazelnuts	285	2.40	67	0.50	0.11	1.10	1.15	0.612	33.73
Hickory nuts	160	–	–	0.55	–	–	–	–	–
Macadamia nuts	116	1.71	0	0.35	0.11	2.10	–	–	–
Pecan nuts	128	5.47	128	0.85	0.13	0.90	1.71	0.188	3.10
Pinenuts	–	4.25	0	0.81	0.19	3.60	–	–	–
Pistachio nuts	158	1.34	233	0.82	0.17	1.10	–	–	5.20
Walnuts	169	2.37	124	0.38	0.15	1.00	0.63	0.558	2.62
Pumpkin seeds	–	–	71	0.24	0.19	2.40	–	–	–
Safflower seeds	–	–	–	1.10	0.40	2.20	–	–	–
Sesame seeds	347	10.25	66	0.72	0.09	4.70	0.68	–	–
Sunflower seeds	354	5.06	50	2.29	0.25	4.50	1.40	1.250	52.18

Table 7.15. The composition of selected nuts and seeds. The figures are for 100 g portions. (Adapted from ref. 37)

amino acid methionine. Combining Brazil nuts with other nuts, particularly cashews and pistachios, or with grains and legumes, will thus greatly enhance the overall protein availability from these food combinations. Legumes are generally poor in methionine and rich in lysine, and the two thus form the perfect partners. With a little bit of imagination, meals can be prepared that are not only nutritious, but are also tasty. Use the nuts to create delicious nut butters, sauces or creams and milks, and in this way create meals which taste rich and creamy whilst at the same time being free from the unhealthy side effects normally associated with such meals.

Cashew nuts (*Anacardium occidentale*)

Cashew nuts are also native to Brazil and they were introduced to India by the Portuguese. Today India is the greatest producer of cashew nuts. Cashew nuts are the actual fruits of the Cashew tree, but the tree also produces a false fruit known as a **cashew apple**, which is very popular in the regions where the trees grow. Cashew nuts have high concentrations of essential amino acids, but the methionine concentration is limiting. To obtain maximum benefit from the proteins, cashew nuts should be combined with Brazil nuts or other foods to augment the supply of methionine. Moreover, cashews are a good source of zinc and other minerals and vitamins. Cashew nuts can be expensive and it is advisable to find a supplier of broken nuts, as these are less expensive. If the nuts are to be used in cooking, it makes little difference if they are broken or whole. Nuts are easily stored, and broken cashew nuts can be bought in bulk when the price is right, and kept in the freezer.

The beauty of cashew nuts is their versatility. The low-fibre content makes it possible to create the smoothest creams which are truly delicious and unique in taste. Moreover,

Nuts/Seeds	TRY (mg)	THR (mg)	ISO (mg)	LEU (mg)	LYS (mg)	MET (mg)	PHE (mg)	VAL (mg)	ARG (mg)	HIS (mg)
Rump steak	189	715	848	1327	1415	402	666	899	1045	562
Chicken	250	877	1088	1490	1810	537	811	1012	1302	593
Almonds	176	610	873	1454	582	259	1146	1124	2729	517
Brazil nuts	187	422	593	1129	443	941	617	823	2247	367
Cashew nuts	471	737	1222	1522	792	353	946	1592	2098	415
Coconut (meal)	199	770	1076	1605	908	421	1038	1268	2899	414
Hazelnuts	211	415	853	939	417	139	537	934	2171	288
Pecan nuts	138	389	553	773	435	153	564	525	1185	273
Pistachio nuts	–	610	880	1520	1080	370	1090	1340	–	–
Walnuts	175	589	767	1228	441	306	767	974	2287	405
Pumpkin seeds	560	933	1737	2437	1411	577	1749	1679	4810	711
Safflower meal	675	1462	1914	2740	1525	731	2605	2446	4623	985
Sesame seeds	331	707	951	1679	583	637	1457	885	1992	441
Sunflower seeds	343	911	1276	1736	868	443	1220	1354	2370	586

Table 7.16. The essential amino acid composition of selected nuts and seeds, with values for rump steak and chicken given for comparison. The figures are for 100 g portions. Values for arginine and histidine are given because they too can be limiting. (From ref. 17)

TRY = Tryptophan, THR = Threonine, ISO = Isoleucine, LEU = Leucine, LYS = Lysine, MET = Methionine, PHE = Phenylalanine, VAL = Valine, ARG = Argenine, HIS = Histidine

cashews make a superb milk and the best sauces. If blended in water, the resultant milk will naturally thicken to a creamy sauce if brought to the boil, and other ingredients can then be added to create the sauce of choice. In this way white sauces, garlic sauces, sour creams or sweet creams can be created which will be a delight, and they will be economical too. A little nut cream can also be added to stews as a finishing touch to create a stroganoff type of taste.

Chestnuts (*Castanea sativa*)

The sweet chestnut is a true nut, and like the oak and the beech it belongs to the family *Fagaceae*. Chestnuts are native to the Mediterranean region, and the Romans were responsible for their distribution in Europe. In France and in Italy, some 200 varieties of chestnuts are cultured. Chestnuts can be eaten raw, but they are normally cooked or roasted and are often used as a stuffing. One of the most delicious ways of eating chestnuts is, however with sugar, and glazed chestnuts are a popular delicacy in Europe and the Far East. In regions where chestnuts are common, they are also ground into flour and used for making porridge and even bread, or they are eaten as a vegetable. Chestnuts have a lower protein- and fat-content than most other nuts but they are nevertheless a nutritious food, rich in carbohydrates and are very adequately supplied with vitamins and minerals. In view of their composition, one can partake more liberally of chestnuts than of the other nut varieties.

Coconut (*Cocos nucifera*)

Coconuts probably originated on the islands of the Malayan Archipelago but today they are distributed throughout the tropical regions of the world. The coconuts are the stones of the drupes borne by the coconut palm, and the endosperm of these stones is the edible portion. The endosperm can be eaten raw, or it is dried and used in confectionery or for the extraction of oil. The oil of the coconut is unusual, in that it is rich in saturated fats (86%) and contains only small amounts of mono- and polyunsaturated fats. The oil in coconuts is best consumed in the coconut as it then comes prepacked with all the necessary ingredients for metabolizing it.

Hazel nuts (*Corylus avellana*)

Hazel nuts are also known as **Filberts** or **Cob nuts** depending on their country of origin. They contain a high proportion of essential oils and supply a well-balanced mixture of vitamins and minerals. Hazel nuts contain a high concentration of vitamin E which prevents oxidation of the polyunsaturated fats, and it is also one of the few nuts which contains vitamin A, which is a natural antioxidant and has cancer-preventing properties. The B-group vitamins are also well represented in hazel nuts, particularly vitamin B-5 and B-6. Moreover, hazel nuts are an excellent source of minerals, particularly the minerals manganese, selenium and zinc, but the protein composition is such that combinations with other nuts, grains or legumes are required in order to obtain the maximum benefit. Hazelnut butters make a pleasant spread and will add variety to the table.

Macadamia nuts (*Macadamia ternifolia*)

Australia is the home of the macadamia nut, but today it is cultivated in many countries, particularly Hawaii and African countries. The macadamia is a member of the protea family *(Proteaceae)* and the stones it produces are known for their very hard shells. Macadamias have a very high oil content (73,7%) and they make a superb, snow-white cream or milk if blended in water. The high-fat content also makes macadamia nuts ideally suited for making nut butters. Moreover, macadamia nuts are rich in calcium, magnesium, phosphorus and vitamins.

Pecan nuts (*Carya illinoensis*)

Pecan nuts belong to the family *Juglandaceae*, to which also the walnut belongs. Pecans are native to the southern states of the USA and to Mexico. Like hazel nuts, pecan nuts do not contain high concentrations of essential amino acids, and their total protein content is also quite low. Their fat content is, however, high and they contain a good balance of minerals and vitamins, including vitamin A. The oil in pecan nuts is also rich in essential oils.[71] Pecan nuts make great snacks, they can also be used in breakfast foods and be used in baking.

Pistachio nuts (*Pistacia vera*)

Pistachio nuts grow in very dry areas in poor soil, and they have been grown for centuries in the Mediterranean region, and are the nuts of choice in the Middle Eastern countries. Pistachio nuts are delicious, and they are excellent food value, being a good source of fibre, proteins with a good blend of essential amino acids, vitamins and minerals.[76] The amino acid tryptophan is, however, in short supply, and in order to obtain maximum protein value it would be good to combine pistachios with other sources of this amino acid, such as seeds, some legumes, particularly soya beans, or cashew nuts. Pistachios are a good source of the minerals calcium, potassium and iron and they have a high vitamin A content. Moreover, they are nutrient-dense and offer an excellent balance of calories for concentrated nutrition. Pistachios can be milled, used in desserts, breads or savoury products and will be an asset in any kitchen.

Walnuts (*Juglans regia*)

Walnuts come in two varieties, the **European walnut** and the **black walnut** which originates from America. These nuts provide a balanced all-round nutritional package, with all the main nutritional components being present in useful amounts.[77] The protein content of the black walnut is higher than that of the European walnut, but both provide excellent protein value because of their balanced composition of essential amino acids. Combinations with other protein sources would, once again, improve protein availability. Add walnuts to muesli or enjoy them just as they are.

Seeds

Seeds provide balanced nutrient packages comparable to those of nuts, and the oil-rich seeds can substitute for nuts in many of the recipes that require nuts as an ingredient. Seeds can be used in a variety of ways to add versatility to the diet, and their health-providing properties will certainly benefit the consumer. The oil in oilseeds consists largely of polyunsaturated fats, monounsaturated fats and small quantities of saturated fats which come prepacked in the whole seeds with the necessary antioxidants to prevent autoxidation. The problems associated with extracted oils, as discussed in the chapter on oils and fats, do not apply to whole seeds and processed whole seeds, and whole seeds can thus be used to supply the essential fatty acids which our bodies require, and in addition they will also supply a balanced variety of vitamins, minerals and proteins of exceptional quality.

Pumpkin seeds

Pumpkin seeds are one of the best sources of primary proteins and they are packed with vitamins and minerals. The protein content of pumpkin seeds is high, and in some varieties can reach up to 31%. Moreover, it is a complete protein with all the essential amino acids being well supplied. A handful of pumpkin seeds will supply approximately half the daily protein needs of the average person, and a comparison with steak will show that the relative quantities of the essential amino acids in pumpkin seeds exceed those of steak. Pumpkin seeds are a good source of vitamins and minerals, particularly zinc and iron, the latter occurring in more than three times the concentration found in steak.

Pumpkin seeds are relatively inexpensive, and they can be incorporated into many dishes to improve the protein quality and to enhance the flavour. To prepare one's own pumpkin seeds, simply remove the seeds from the pumpkin, and spread them out to dry. The seeds can also be dried in the oven, and a light roasting will make them extremely palatable. Hulled seeds are easier to buy than to prepare oneself, but the unhulled seeds can be eaten as a snack, or they can be ground fine in a coffee grinder to be used in bread or protein dishes. Used in this way they add spice to the food which compares favourably to commercial stocks and food flavourants, and they improve the nutritional value of the meal.

Sesame seeds (*Sesanum indicum*)

Sesame seeds are a superb food originating from the Middle East, where this versatile seed has found a variety of uses. Many traditional dishes, cookies and cakes, sweets and spreads include sesame seeds as one of the prime ingredients. The most common form in which sesame seeds are available is in the hulled form, which is the form of choice for spreads and sweets, as the unhulled form is slightly bitter. Sesame seeds should be crushed or ground into a paste before consumption, as the small seeds will pass through the intestine without being digested. If sesame seeds are ground until the oil is released, a paste is formed that is called **Tahini**. Tahini originated in Turkey and is a nutrient-rich spread that can substitute for butter. Other Middle Eastern delicacies include **Halva**, a sweet that is sesame-based. Moreover, sesame seeds can be used to make a wholesome milk which can be used as a substitute for cow's milk, and can also be used in cooking or for making home-made ice-cream.

Sesame seeds contain almost 30% complete protein of good quality, with all the essential amino acids, particularly methionine, being present in substantial amounts. The oil in sesame seeds is a mixture of the glycerol esters of oleic and linoleic acids, and it also has some unique features. It contains the compound **sesamin**, a lignin from sesame oil, which lowers cholesterol levels by decreasing the rate of absorption from the intestine, increasing the rate of faecal excretion and inhibiting its formation in the liver.[74] Moreover, sesame seeds contain antioxidant substances[73] which act as preservatives and give the ground seeds and sesame oil a long shelf life. Sesame seeds are a good source of the minerals magnesium, zinc, calcium and iron, and the calcium levels are in fact, more than twenty times higher than in steak, and the iron concentration is more than three times as high as in steak. Of course, people would consume more steak than sesame seeds and, therefore, obtain more iron from this source than from the seeds, but if sesame seeds were regularly incorporated into foods such as bread or spreads, they could make a significant contribution to dietary mineral requirements.

Sunflower seeds (*Helianthus annuus*)

Sunflower seeds are native to America, and contain almost 23% primary protein, and all the essential amino acids are well supplied. The 50% fat content of sunflower seeds consists mainly of polyunsaturated fats of which the essential fatty acid, linoleic acid, comprises some 30% of the total fat content, and the mono-unsaturated fatty acid, oleic acid, accounts for some 10% of the total fat content. The vitamin E content of sunflower seeds is very high, and this is vital in view of the high levels of polyunsaturated fats. The relationship between the polyunsaturated fats and vitamin E prevents autoxidation of the fatty acids and production of free radicals. For this reason it is safe to use whole and freshly ground or liquidised sunflower seeds on a regular basis in contrast to the consumption of large amounts of extracted oils, such as sunflower-seed oil, which have been associated with an increased incidence of cancer (see chapter on fats).

Sunflower seeds are a good source of the minerals calcium, phosphorus, magnesium and iron and are one of the prime suppliers of B-group vitamins. This together with their high vitamin E and balanced primary nutrient content, makes them an energy food that we would do well to exploit. Use sunflower seeds in baking and incorporate them into breakfast foods such as muesli and granola. Furthermore, they can be used to prepare nutritious sauces and mock cheeses, or they can be added to nut or other milks to improve their nutritional value.

Fruits and vegetables

Numerous studies have shown that the daily consumption of fruits and vegetables is associated with decreased risk of a host of diseases, including many forms of cancer.[14] Fruits and vegetables are rich in substances which offer protection against this disease which has become such a major killer in our century. The substances most associated with protection against cancer include: **fibre**, vitamins (particularly **vitamins A, C** and **E**), **carotenoids**, some minerals and some organic compounds known as secondary plant compounds (**phytochemicals**). Pytochemicals that play a protective role against cancer include substances such as **phenols, polyphenols, β-sitosterol, isothiocyanates, thiocyanates, dithiolthiones, flavones** and **indoles** which occur in many plant foods, but are particularly abundant in cruciferous vegetables such as cabbage, broccoli, cauliflower and brussels sprouts.

Vitamin A or its precursor ß-carotene, found in dark-green or yellow fruits and vegetables, has been found to be particularly effective in preventing epithelial, lung and oesophageal cancer,[78,79] and has also been correlated with decreased incidence of bladder cancer. Vitamin C lowers the risk of stomach and oesophagus cancer, and probably affords this protection by acting as an antioxidant in much the same manner as would vitamins A and E. The flavonoids are plant pigments which are very common in plants, and also act as powerful antioxidants,[80] and probably afford their protection against cancer in this way. It has also been found, that the consumption of vegetables in general, and cruciferous vegetables in particular, induces enzymes which rid the body of harmful metabolites, thus acting as powerful cleansers and reducing the risk of cancer.[81]

Approximately 14 classes of phytochemicals, which can block cancer development, have been identified, and it is even envisaged that these compounds could be routinely added to commercial foods to act as cancer preventers. The concentration of these phytochemicals is, however, relatively low in natural foods, and excessive intake in this way would probably do more harm than good. The best way to obtain maximum protection against disease, is to consume the foods as nature intended, by following a whole-food programme. In table 7.17 a list of foods with cancer-preventative properties is presented in the order of importance as currently understood, and in table 7.18 the distribution of the major phytochemicals in food plants, associated with cancer prevention, is presented. The precise mechanism of action of these phytochemicals is not yet fully understood, but current understanding of their impact on cancer initiation and promotion is summarised in figure 3.5.

Fruits

The benefits of fruit in the diet cannot be overemphasized, but the very wholesomeness of fruit has, unfortunately, led to many misconceptions and inappropriate diets. Just because something is good, does not mean that it is necessarily complete in all its attributes, or should be regarded as a sole source of nutrients. Man's diet should be based on a variety of foods, of which fruit should be an important component. Moreover, it should be remembered that fruits contain a high percentage of water, and would not provide sufficient energy if this were the sole source of nutrients. This is particularly important in the case of young children who still have a limited stomach capacity, and the use of dried fruit can augment their energy intake. Even a cursory look at the composition tables will show that energy content of dried fruit is approximately four times as high as that of fresh fruit. The composition of fresh and dried fruit is presented in tables 7.19 and 7.20.

The whole-food alternative

HIGH	Garlic, Cabbage, Licorice, Soybeans, Ginger *Umbelliferae* (carrots, celery, parsnips)
MEDIUM	Onions, Tea, Tumeric Citrus (orange, lemon, grapefruit) Wholewheat, Flax, Brown rice, *Solanaceae* (tomato, eggplant, peppers) *Cruciferae* (broccoli, cauliflower, brussels sprouts)
MODERATE	Oats, Mints, Oregano, Cucumber, Rosemary, Sage, Potato, Thyme, Chives, Cantaloupe, Basil, Tarragon, Barley, Berries

Table 7.17. *Possible cancer-preventive foods and ingredients arranged in order of effectiveness. (Adapted from ref. 82)*

	Garlic	Green tea	Soybeans	Grains	Cruciferous	Umbelliferous	Citrus	Solanaceous	Cucurbitaceous	Licorice	Flax seed
Sulfides	×				×						
Phytates			×	×							
Flavonoids		×	×	×	×	×	×	×	×	×	×
Glucarates		×		×	×		×	×			
Carotenoids			×	×	×	×	×	×			
Coumarins		×	×	×	×	×	×	×	×	×	×
Mono-terpenes	×				×	×	×	×	×		
Tri-terpenes	×		×	×	×	×	×	×	×	×	
Lignans			×								×
Phenolic acids	×	×	×	×	×	×	×	×	×	×	×
Indoles					×						
Isothiocyanates					×						
Phthalides						×					
Polyacetylenes						×					

Table 7.18. *Distribution of some of the major cancer-preventing phytochemicals in food plants. (Adapted from ref. 82)*

Fruit	Energy (kcal)	Carb. (g)	Prot. (g)	Fat (g)	Fibre (g)	Ca (mg)	P (mg)	Fe (mg)	K (mg)
Apples	59	12.2	0.2	0.4	3.1	7	7	0.2	115
Apricots	48	9.0	1.4	0.4	2.1	14	19	0.5	296
Avocados	161	5.3	2.0	15.3	2.1	11	41	1.0	599
Bananas	92	20.4	1.0	0.5	3.0	6	20	0.3	396
Berries*	52	8.7	0.8	0.4	4.1	20	14	0.4	146
Cantaloupe	35	6.8	0.9	0.3	1.6	11	17	0.2	309
Cherries	72	21.8	1.2	1.0	1.5	15	19	0.4	224
Custard-Apple	101	21.8	1.7	0.6	3.4	30	21	0.7	382
Figs	74	15.8	0.8	0.3	3.4	35	14	0.4	232
Gooseberries	44	7.6	0.9	0.6	2.6	25	27	0.3	198
Granadilla	97	7.5	2.2	0.7	15.9	12	68	1.6	348
Grapefruit	32	7.5	0.6	0.1	0.6	12	8	0.1	139
Grapes	71	16.1	0.7	0.6	1.7	11	13	0.3	185
Guava	51	6.3	0.8	0.6	5.6	20	25	0.3	284
Kiwi fruit	67	14.2	1.0	0.6	2.8	29	34	0.4	370
Kumquat	63	12.7	0.9	0.1	3.7	44	19	0.4	195
Lemons (peeled)	29	8.9	1.1	0.3	0.4	26	16	0.6	138
Loquats	47	11.6	0.4	0.2	0.5	16	27	0.3	266
Lychees	66	16.0	0.8	0.4	0.5	5	31	0.3	171
Mangos	65	15.4	0.5	0.3	1.6	10	11	0.1	156
Melons (white)	35	7.6	0.5	0.1	1.6	6	10	0.1	271
Mullberries	43	8.4	1.4	0.4	1.4	39	38	1.9	194
Olives (green)	422	-	0.9	11.0	4.4	61	17	1.0	91
Oranges	47	9.8	0.9	0.1	2.0	40	14	0.1	181
Papaya	39	8.9	0.6	0.1	0.9	24	5	0.1	257
Peaches	43	9.9	0.7	0.1	1.2	5	12	0.1	197
Pears	59	12.6	0.4	0.4	2.5	11	11	0.3	125
Persimmons	70	17.1	0.6	0.2	1.5	8	17	0.2	161
Pineapple	49	10.9	0.4	0.4	1.5	7	7	0.4	113
Plums	55	11.0	0.8	0.6	2.0	4	10	0.1	172
Pomegranate	68	17.0	1.0	0.3	0.2	3	8	0.3	259
Prickly pears	41	7.8	0.7	0.6	1.8	56	24	0.3	220
Quince	57	8.9	0.4	0.1	6.4	11	17	0.7	197
Strawberries	30	5.1	0.6	0.4	1.9	14	19	0.4	166
Tangerines	44	9.3	0.6	0.2	1.9	14	10	0.1	157
Watermelon	32	6.9	0.6	0.4	0.3	8	9	0.2	116

*Represents the average for Blue-/Black- and Raspberries.

Table 7.19 (Part 1). The composition of selected fresh fruits. The figures are for 100 g portions. (Adapted from ref. 37)

Fruit	Mg (mg)	Zn (mg)	Vit. A (IU)	Vit. B1 (mg)	Vit. B2 (mg)	Vit. B3 (mg)	Vit. B5 (mg)	Vit. B6 (mg)	Fol. (µg)	Vit.C (mg)
Apples	5	0.04	53	0.01	0.01	0.1	0.06	0.048	3	6
Apricots	8	0.26	2612	0.03	0.04	0.6	0.24	0.054	9	10
Avocados	39	0.42	612	0.11	0.12	1.9	0.97	0.280	62	8
Bananas	29	0.16	81	0.05	0.10	0.5	0.26	0.578	19	9
Berries*	14	0.28	132	0.04	0.06	0.6	0.19	0.050	6	20
Cantaloupe	11	0.16	3224	0.04	0.02	0.6	0.13	0.115	17	43
Cherries	11	0.06	214	0.05	0.06	0.4	0.13	0.036	4	7
Custard-Apple	18	–	–	0.08	0.10	0.5	0.14	0.221	–	19
Figs	17	0.15	142	0.06	0.05	0.4	0.30	0.113	–	2
Gooseberries	10	0.12	290	0.04	0.03	0.3	0.29	0.080	–	28
Granadilla	29	–	700	0.00	0.13	1.5	–	–	–	30
Grapefruit	8	0.07	124	0.04	0.02	0.3	0.28	0.042	10	34
Grapes	6	0.05	73	0.09	0.06	0.3	0.02	0.110	4	11
Guava	10	0.23	792	0.05	0.05	1.2	0.15	0.143	–	184
Kiwi fruit	19	0.17	–	0.02	0.01	0.2	–	–	–	118
Kumquat	13	0.08	302	0.08	0.10	–	–	–	–	37
Lemons (peeled)	9	0.06	29	0.04	0.02	0.1	0.19	0.080	11	53
Loquats	13	0.05	1528	0.02	0.02	0.2	–	–	–	1
Lychees	10	0.07	0	0.01	0.07	0.6	–	–	–	72
Mangos	9	0.04	3894	0.06	0.06	0.6	0.16	0.134	–	28
Melons (white)	11	0.18	40	0.08	0.02	0.6	0.21	0.059	53	25
Mullberries	18	–	25	0.03	0.10	0.6	0.21	0.041	–	36
Olives (green)	22	–	300	0.00	0.00	0.0	0.02	0.020	–	0
Oranges	10	0.07	205	0.09	0.04	0.3	0.25	0.060	30	53
Papaya	10	0.07	2014	0.03	0.03	0.3	0.22	0.019	–	62
Peaches	7	0.14	535	0.02	0.04	1.0	0.17	0.018	3	7
Pears	6	0.12	20	0.02	0.04	0.1	0.07	0.018	7	4
Persimmons	9	0.11	2167	0.03	0.02	0.1	–	–	–	8
Pineapple	14	0.08	23	0.09	0.04	0.4	0.16	0.087	11	15
Plums	7	0.10	323	0.04	0.10	0.5	0.18	0.081	2	10
Pomegranate	–	–	–	0.03	0.03	0.3	0.60	0.105	–	6
Prickly pears	85	–	51	0.01	0.06	0.5	–	–	–	14
Quince	8	–	40	0.02	0.03	0.2	0.08	0.040	–	4
Strawberries	10	0.13	27	0.02	0.07	0.2	0.34	0.059	18	57
Tangerines	12	0.10	920	0.11	0.02	0.2	0.20	0.067	20	31
Watermelon	11	0.07	366	0.08	0.02	0.2	0.21	0.144	2	10

*Represents the average for Blue-/Black- and Raspberries.

Table 7.19 (Part 2). The composition of selected fresh fruits. The figures are for 100 g portions. (Adapted from ref. 37)

Fruit	Energy (kcal)	Carb. (g)	Prot. (g)	Fat (g)	Fibre (g)	Ca (mg)	P (mg)	Fe (mg)	K (mg)
Apples	243	61.2	0.9	0.3	4.7	14	38	1.4	450
Apricots	238	42.4	3.7	0.5	19.4	45	117	4.7	1378
Currants	283	67.4	4.1	0.3	6.7	86	125	3.3	892
Dates	275	65.6	2.0	0.5	7.9	32	40	1.2	652
Figs	255	49.5	3.1	1.2	15.9	144	68	2.2	712
Peaches	239	49.8	3.6	0.8	11.5	28	119	4.1	996
Pears	262	64.0	1.9	0.6	5.7	34	59	2.1	533
Prunes	239	48.5	2.6	0.5	14.2	51	79	2.5	745
Raisins	300	71.8	3.2	0.5	7.3	49	97	2.1	751

Fruit	Mg (mg)	Zn (mg)	Vit.A (IU)	Vit.B1 (mg)	Vit.B2 (mg)	Vit.B3 (mg)	Vit.B5 (mg)	Vit.B6 (mg)	Fol. (µg)	Vit.C (mg)
Apples	16	0.20	0	0.00	0.16	0.9	–	0.125	–	4
Apricots	47	0.74	7240	0.01	0.15	3.0	0.75	0.156	10	3
Currants	41	0.66	73	0.16	0.14	1.6	0.05	0.296	10	5
Dates	35	0.29	50	0.09	0.10	2.2	0.78	0.192	13	0
Figs	59	0.51	133	0.07	0.09	0.7	0.44	0.224	8	1
Peaches	42	0.57	2163	0.00	0.21	4.4	0.24	0.067	11	5
Pears	33	0.39	3	0.01	0.15	1.4	–	–	–	7
Prunes	45	0.53	1987	0.08	0.16	2.0	0.46	0.260	4	3
Raisins	33	0.27	8	0.16	0.09	0.8	0.05	0.249	3	3

Table 7.20. The composition of selected dried fruits. The figures are for 100 g portions. (Adapted from ref. 37)

Fruit contains one of the most readily utilizable forms of energy available to man, namely the simple carbohydrate **fructose**, or fruit sugar, which needs no digestion and is readily absorbed by the body. Fruit contains soluble fibres (such as **pectin**), which retard the uptake of fructose, so that the sugar enters the bloodstream at a controlled rate. This unique relationship between fructose and fibre is extremely important in preventing post-prandial (after meal) glucose surges which are associated with hypoglycaemia. This is significant, in view of the modern trend to substitute sugar (sucrose) with refined fructose. The ingestion of substantial amounts of fructose, also leads to hypoglycaemia, as it facilitates the conversion of glucose to glycogen,[83] and can also lead to increased cholesterol levels.[84] The best way to consume fructose is thus in the fruit, which once again underlines the fact that a whole-food programme should be the programme of choice. The isolation and regular consumption of refined foods in whatever form, will always prove to be detrimental to health in some form or other. The use of whole fruits such as dates and currants, which are high in natural sugars, will satisfy the sweet tooth without overburdening the system.

Because fruit is so readily digestible, some people are of the opinion that fruit should only be consumed by itself and never in combination with other foods, but the very composition of fruit belies this theory. Fruits contain components which assist in the absorption and utilization of nutrients found in other foods such as grains and legumes, and the simultaneous ingestion of fruits, grains, legumes or other compatible foods can thus only be advantageous. Moreover, the soluble-fibre composition of fruit prevents over-rapid absorption of the natural fruit sugar found in fruit and the digestive products of the complex carbohydrates found in grains and legumes, thus ensuring a gradual, constant supply of these nutrients. Fruit can certainly be eaten on its own, but for a more sustained energy supply, combination with grains, nuts and legumes would be advantageous. Fruits combine well with any of the compatible neutral foods listed in table 7.4, but it should be remembered, that fruit should not be eaten together with vegetables, as discussed in the section on food compatibility.

Fruit is an excellent cleanser, and the rich supply of vitamins and minerals makes it an ideal food that should not only be regarded as a dessert or a snack, but together with grains, nuts and legumes it can provide nutritious main meals. For example, hamburgers made with whole-grain bread, a legume/nut based patty served with sprouts and a delicious nut or tomato sauce together with a variety of fruit will satisfy even the most discerning of culinary experts. Fruit should be made a part of the everyday lifestyle, and the blessings that would flow from this habit would be too numerous to mention.

Each fruit is unique and supplies its own particular blend of vitamins, minerals and primary nutrients. In order to obtain the maximum benefit from the bounty of fruit, it is essential to concentrate on variety and to look beyond the handful of fruits that have become common household foods. There is a fruit for all occasions and a fruit for each season. Winter fruits such as citrus and guava have an exceptional vitamin C content, as if they were designed to meet the increased demands for this vitamin during the winter months, and the lipid content of winter varieties of avocados is also higher than that of summer varieties so as to supply extra energy during the cold months. It is as if a fruit in season is there to supply some or other specific need of the body essential for that time of year, and by including a variety of fruits and enjoying fruit in season, the attributes of each kind can be maximally exploited. With so many different fruits available, particularly in this age of transportation and international export, it is possible to enjoy a variety of fruits.

Fruits can be arbitrarily divided into categories according to their distinguishing characteristics or according to the regions in which they are most successful. There are stone fruits, pip fruits, grapes, berry fruits, citrus fruits, tropical and subtropical fruits. The families of plants from which we derive our fruits, have been exploited by man for thousands of years both for their fruits and for medicinal purposes, and many different cultivars with different tastes and characteristics have been developed. The following discussion of some of the more common fruits will hopefully encourage the reader to look beyond just apples and bananas to satisfy the fruit tooth.

Stone Fruits

The stone fruits belong to the genus *Prunus* of the family *Rosaceae* which includes a wide variety of other fruits. The genus *Prunus* contains such varied forms as **almonds, apricots, cherries, plums, peaches** and **nectarines**, of which only a few will be discussed here.

Apricots *(Prunus armeniaca)*

Apricots are native to China and Siberia and they were introduced into the Mediterranean region about 100 BC. Apricots are an early summer fruit and they contain substantial quantities of vitamin A (over 2 600 IU per 100 g) the anti-cancer, antioxidant vitamin. Vitamin C and the B-group vitamins are well supplied in apricots as are the minerals calcium and phosphorus. Each of these attributes are of course enhanced in dried apricots, so that a mere 100 g of dried apricots will contain in excess of 7 000 IU of Vitamin A. Include dried apricots in muesli and other dishes or by soaking and blending they can be converted into spreads which can be enriched by mixing in some nut butter.

Cherries (*Prunus avium*)

Cherries are one of the earliest stone fruits to mature in the summer, but they are difficult to culture in home gardens, because of the climatic restrictions and the fact that birds love them. There are a number of varieties of sweet cherries, and then there is the sour cherry (*Prunus cerasus*) which is less restricted in its climatic requirements. Cherries contain fair amounts of vitamin A and C, and the minerals calcium, phosphorus and magnesium are also well supplied. Cherries are delightful as is, or in cakes, pastries and puddings. Cherry preserves are also a delight.

Peaches and nectarines (*Prunus persica*)

The peach originated from China, and not Persia as its scientific name suggests. Peaches and nectarines are plentiful in mid-summer and there are many varieties to choose from. In mid-season it is time to take advantage of the lower prices and to purchase them in bulk as this is the most economical way. Peaches are a good source of vitamin A, but the other vitamins and minerals are also well supplied. Dried peaches contain over 2 000 IU of vitamin A per 100 g and are thus an excellent fruit to include in muesli, convert into spreads or preserves or to be eaten as is.

Plums and prunes

Plums and prunes comprise several species of the genus *Prunus*. The common plum (*Prunus domestica*), also called the European plum, probably originated from southwestern Asia and includes the blue plums and prunes. The red plums (*Prunus salicina*), or Japanese plums, are not as commercially significant as the European plum, and require warmer summers than the European plums. Plums are one of the few acid-forming fruits, and in view of the body's need for a greater proportion of alkaline foods than acid foods, some have advocated abstinence from plums. There is no reason whatsoever to abstain from plums. Plums are low acid-forming, and a varied lifestyle should include sufficient alkaline foods to counteract the low acidity of plums. Of course, plums should not form the only item of diet over protracted periods, but they are certainly healthy and are a good source of vitamins and minerals, particularly vitamins A and C. People suffering from arthritis, gout or other ailments aggravated by an acid condition can be advised to restrict the consumption of plums.

Contrary to plums, prunes are an alkaline fruit rich in vitamins and minerals. Dried prunes contain substantial quantities of vitamin A, and the minerals calcium and magnesium are also well supplied. Prunes also have medicinal value, and have a mild, natural laxative effect which can be used to advantage particularly in the case of older people or young children.

Pip Fruits

The common pip fruits are **apples** and **pears** which are also part of the family *Rosaceae*, which also comprises a number of fruits of lesser economic significance.

Apples (*Malus domestica*)

Apples are of ancient and complex hybrid origin. They are the most important world fruit crop, and cultivars can be numbered in their thousands. Apples have long formed part of the Western diet, and they were probably cultivated in Greece as early as 600 BC, although their origin dates from the earliest of times. Apples are rich in minerals and vitamins, and contain fructose and soluble fibre in balanced proportions. Apples have a bit of everything, and the old maxim of the doctor and the apple contains more than a grain of truth. Apples, contain remedial phytochemicals and fair amounts of biotin and vitamin C. This balanced blend of nutrients is precisely what gives the apple its everyday appeal. Apples are versatile and can be prepared in a variety of ways so that one need not tire of apples.

Pears (*Pyrus communis*)

The European pear (*Pyrus communis*) is the most common pear in the Western world, and there are numerous varieties characterized by their juicy flesh and distinctive pear flavour. The Asian pears are derived from a different species, possibly *Pyrus pyrifolia*, they are more apple shaped and have a less distinct pear flavour. They tend to be crisp, but some varieties have a very juicy flesh. Like apples, pears contain a bit of everything, and dried pears in particular are an energy food which will supply useful quantities of vitamins and minerals.

Grapes

Grapes belong to the genus *Vitis*, which falls under the family *Vitaceae*. The genus includes many varieties of grapes from table grapes to wine grapes. The European grape (*Vitis vinifera*) probably originated in the region of the Caucasus mountains between the Caspian sea and the Black sea, and it is still widely cultivated as are many other species of grapes. Grapes have a higher carbohydrate content than most fruits, and thus supply fair amounts of energy. Moreover, they are a good source of the minerals manganese and silicon, and other vitamins and minerals are well supplied.

Some members of the genus are medicinal, especially those with a high quinine content, some are eaten fresh or used in juice and wine-making, whilst some are suitable for drying. The dried varieties are the **sultanas** and **raisins**. These dried varieties are excellent sources of vitamins and minerals, particularly calcium, phosphorus, iron, and the vitamins A, B-group and C. All the varieties have a high carbohydrate content and are exceptionally sweet, particularly if dried, and can thus be used as a substitute for sugar. Liquidized raisins in bread provide an excellent medium for yeast activity, and add a superb flavour to the bread whilst increasing the mineral and overall nutrient content.

Quinces (*Cydonia oblonga*)

The quince is another member of the *Rosaceae* family, and in antiquity the fruit was used as a love token associated with Venus. Quinces are cultivated mainly for their high pectin content which makes them ideally suited for the production of jellies. Because of this property they are often added to other fruits when preparing preserves or fruit jellies. Because the fruit is unpalatable raw in view of its astringency, it is usually eaten cooked.

Berry Fruit

Particularly noteworthy berries are the **blueberries** and **cranberries** (*Vaccinium*), **black, red** and **white currants** as well as **gooseberries** (*Ribes*), **raspberries** and **brambles** (*Rubus*) and **strawberries** (*Fragaria*). A number of plant families contribute to the berry fruits of the world. Strawberries, **boysenberries, blackberries, youngberries** and raspberries belong to the family *Rosaceae*, blueberries are members of the *Ericaceae*, **mulberries** fall under the *Moraceae* and gooseberries and black and red currants belong to the *Grossulariaceae*. Currants and gooseberries are hardy plants and cultured nearly up to the Arctic circle, though they fare best in cool humid climates.

Berries are a good source of minerals, particularly calcium, phosphorus, iron and silicon whilst they are rich in vitamins with the vitamin C-concentrations being particularly noteworthy. In this regard it can be mentioned that black currants are the richest fruit source of this vitamin. Moreover, berries contain fair amounts of sulphur, the element that participates in several important detoxification reactions. Toxic materials in the body are conjugated with sulphate and converted to non-toxic forms which are excreted in the urine. Sulfur is more common in vegetables than in fruits, and that is why vegetables are good cleansers. Berries thus fall into the category of foods with excellent cleansing properties.

Citrus Fruits

Citrus fruits belong to the family *Rutaceae*, and the fruits belonging to the genera *Citrus, Fortunella, Poncirus* and their intergeneric hybrids are collectively known as citrus. The fruit of citrus is a type of berry, and the ripe skin contains two pigments, **xanthophyll** and **carotene**, which are responsible for their characteristic colour. The skins also contain oils which are often used in perfumes. The white pith of citrus fruits, known as **albedo**, is also a rich source of pectin, and that is why the skins readily form jams. Citrus comes from South East Asia, and has been cultivated in China for thousands of years. It is thought that Arab traders brought the fruit to the Middle East and Palestine and it reached Europe by the year 1480. Through colonization citrus spread to North America, the Caribbean and to Southern Africa. Citrus species hybridize easily, and some popular varieties such as grapefruit have only appeared in relatively recent times. The bitter taste of the grapefruit is due to the compound **naringin**, a flavone glycoside. Some common varieties of citrus include **grapefruit, lemon, lime, orange, kumquat** and **mandarin**, including **tangerines**.

Citrus fruit is known for its high vitamin C-content, but citrus also contains substantial amounts of vitamin A, and they are an excellent source of the mineral calcium. Most of the genera yield essential oils, and citrus has medicinal properties. Citrus is one of the few groups of fruits with established cancer-preventive properties, and the compounds associated with this phenomenon are the **flavonoids, glucarates, carotenoids, coumarins, limolene, mono-** and **tri-terpenes** and **phenolic acids**.[82,85]

Oranges (*Citrus sinensis*)

The sweet orange is native to China, and important cultivars include **navels, blood oranges** and **valencias**. The sweet orange is used mainly for its juice, but it is delicious on its own.

Lemons (*Citrus limon*)

Lemons are used particularly for their juice and in food preparation. It is important to note that lemons and limes are alkaline-forming fruits in spite of their acid taste, as citric acid is a weak organic acid that is readily broken down in the body. Lemons can be used in cooking and to replace vinegar in salad dressings and spicy preserves.

Mandarins and Tangerines

Mandarins probably originate from India, and are appealing because of their loose skin. Hybridization with pomelo has produced **tangelos** which are very aromatic and have a rich fruity taste.

Subtropical and tropical fruits

The range of fruits grown in tropical and subtropical areas is far greater than that found in the colder latitudes, but modern marketing strategies have made much of the tropical bounty available to all the regions of the world. The range of fruits found in the marketplaces of tropical areas, however, still exceeds that found in temperate areas in view of the logistical problems of transporting some of the delicate fruits, and the fact that some of the minor fruits are not produced in sufficient quantities to warrant export. Those fortunate enough to travel to the far-flung regions of the world should make a point of sampling exotic fruits of the area in order to fully appreciate nature's bounty.

Avocado (*Persia americana*)

Avocados belong to the family *Lauraceae*, which is a family of aromatic evergreen trees to which cinnamon and camphor belong. Early Spanish explorers recorded the cultivation of avocado in Mexico and Peru, but today avocados are commercially significant crops throughout the tropics and subtropics. The main producing countries are Brazil, Mexico, The Dominican Republic and the USA. South Africa and Israel have also become major producers and they export large quantities to Europe. There are three distinct races of avocado, namely the **Mexican, Guatemalan** and **West Indian** races, and many different cultivars. The Mexican race is the least attractive, being small with a large pip, whereas fruits of the West Indian race are large and restricted in their distribution, as they are suited to low-altitude tropical areas. The Guatamalan race is the most common commercial race. There are many cultivars of avocado, and there is virtually a cultivar for each season, each producing fruit with distinctive flavours, ranging from a mild sweetish taste to a nutty rich flavour. The most common varieties are **Hass, Zutano, Fuerto, Hayes, Hopkins** and **Reed**.

Avocados are one of the few high-energy fruits, and they can be a meal unto themselves. Unlike most other fruits, most of the energy in avocados is in the form of fat rather than carbohydrates, although they do also contain some carbohydrates. This has led to some misconceptions, as it is sometimes assumed that avocados will induce a cholesterol problem, and its use is, therefore, often discouraged in people suffering from hypercholesterolaemia. Avocados do not contain cholesterol, and 80% of the oil in avocados consists of mono-unsaturated fats, with the remaining 20% consisting of polyunsaturated and saturated fats. This combination of oils has been shown to decrease cholesterol levels, to benefit the cardiovascular system and to lead to a lower incidence of cancer.[86] Avocados also contain a fair amount of vitamins A and E which act as natural antioxidants.

Avocados are an excellent source of the minerals magnesium, phosphorus and zinc, and the B-group vitamins. The concentrations of thiamin, Vitamin B-6 and folic acid are particularly high, with folic acid reaching concentrations in excess of 60 mg per 100 g. Folic acid requirements are particularly high during pregnancy, and avocados can contribute substantially to this need. The high concentration of these B-group vitamins enables the body to maximally metabolize the fats in the avocados, making them an ideal substitute for butter or margarines. The high fat content of avocados makes them an ideal food for growing children and vegan vegetarians to ensure adequate fat intakes. Enjoy avocado as is, or eat them with a little salt and lemon juice, or use them as a natural butter substitute on fresh home-baked bread. Avocados can also produce exciting salad dressings that will prove to be a taste sensation.

Bananas (*Musa*)

Plantains and **bananas** belong to the family *Musaceae*, and they have a complicated ancestry. The family *Musaceae* is not only useful for its fruits, but also produces fibre for textiles. Some varieties are ornamental. Bananas seldom produce seeds, and reproduction is by vegetative means. Plantains are typically thought of as cooking bananas, whilst the banana is the fruit that is eaten raw.

Bananas are nature's convenience food. Vitamins and minerals are well supplied with phosphorus, magnesium, manganese and vitamins A, B-6, folic acid and vitamin C deserving special mention. The energy content of bananas is also higher than that of most other fruits, thus making it the ideal lunch-box fruit. Bananas should be eaten ripe, as unripe bananas, like unripe mangoes, contain a protein inhibitor of salivary and pancreatic α-amylase, the enzyme that digests starch.[34] The inhibitor is destroyed during the ripening process (a ripe banana is yellow and is covered by brown spots), and heating will also destroy most protein inhibitors. The African custom of cooking green bananas between leaves will thus render the inhibitor inactive. Bananas that are still slightly green contain higher concentrations of resistant starch which contributes to the maintenance of colonic bacteria, but this in itself is not a reason for eating green bananas, as the consumption of whole foods will supply more than enough resistant starch from grains and legumes to meet the demands of the colonic bacteria. Bananas can thus be eaten as is, or they can be fried for a special treat. The texture of bananas also makes them ideally suitable for making homemade ice-cream, free of the additives of commercial varieties.

Dates (*Phoenix dactylifera*)

Date palms have been cultivated since ancient times in the arid regions of the Old World, principally northern Africa. Dates are one of the wonder foods of the Mediterranean region. They supply an abundance of vitamins and minerals, with the levels of calcium, magnesium, vitamin B-1, B-5 and folic acid being particularly noteworthy. Dates are exceptionally sweet, and can be used to substitute for sugar in many dishes. Liquidized dates are an excellent natural sweetener for porridges and breakfast foods such as granola. The sugar in dates comes pre-packed with soluble fibre, which prevents the rapid uptake of the sugar so that it will not lead to hypoglycaemia. Dates are thus a good source of natural energy which will provide maximum lift without subsequent let-down.

Figs (*Ficus carica*)

The common cultivated fig originated from western Asia and today most of the world's production occurs in the Mediterranean region, with Greece, Italy, Portugal, Spain and Turkey being the main producers. There are two main types, namely the **Adriatic** type, which is the most abundant type, and the **Smyrna** type. Figs are an excellent food known also for their remedial qualities. Dried figs supply in excess of 140 mg of calcium per 100 g and the minerals magnesium, manganese, copper and iron are also well supplied. Figs also contain a balanced vitamin composition, and the ratio of primary nutrients makes them one of the top energy fruits. It is no wonder that the rations of armies in ancient times consisted largely of dried figs. Dried figs are thus a priority fruit for people who enjoy hiking.

Guava (*Psidium guajava*)

Guavas belong to the family *Myrtaceae*, and they are the fruits of evergreen shrubs and trees. They grow in tropical and subtropical regions where two species in particular are cultivated. These are the common guava *Psidium guajava* and the strawberry guava *Psidium littorale*. Guavas come in many shapes and sizes, ranging from very small to fruits weighing in excess of 200 g. The number of seeds per fruit also varies, and the flesh colour ranges from white to yellow and salmon red. Guavas are one of the richest sources of vitamin C, supplying 184 mg per 100 g of this vital vitamin. Vitamin A and calcium are also well supplied, and the guava is thus an excellent fruit for the winter to help prevent winter ailments. Guavas can be processed into juice, jam, chutney and jelly and will thus add variety on the table.

Kiwifruit (*Actinidia deliciosa*)

There are some 36 species of kiwifruit native to Asia, and Chinese records refer to their use as far back as AD 770. It is, however, only in the twentieth century that kiwifruit has become a significant commercial crop. The main commercial cultivar to date is the **Hayward** cultivar, and New Zealand is the main producing country, although other countries are quickly following suit. As the scientific name indicates, kiwifruit is a delicious fruit, and it is also rich in nutrients. Kiwifruit is rich in calcium, phosphorus and magnesium, and it is a rich source of vitamin C, containing some 118 mg of this vitamin per 100 g.

Litchi (*Litchi*)

The genus *Litchi* is native to China, the Philippines and India, and it is particularly prized in China for its fruit. Litchis are a delicious fruit which will add flavour to fruit salads. Litchis are eaten fresh or dried, but canned litchis have become very popular. Vitamin C is present in high concentrations, the amount being approximately double that found in citrus.

Loquats (*Eriobotrya japonica*)

Loquats also belong to the family *Rosaceae* and are native to China and Japan. In Japan loquats are used to manufacture jellies, pies, jams and preserves, or they are eaten as is. Loquats are now cultivated in many regions of the world, including the Mediterranean regions, and they are easy to cultivate in the home garden. Loquats supply very useful quantities of vitamin A, the concentration being in excess of 1500 IU per 100 g.

Mangoes (*Mangifera indica*)

Mangoes are extensively used in India and Asia, and they belong to the family *Anacardiaceae*, to which also the cashew nuts belong. Two races in particular are produced worldwide, the **Indian** and **Philippine** races, and some varieties have an exquisite taste and texture. It is not for nothing that mangoes are known as the peach of the tropics. Many cultivars are free of the annoying fibre and turpentiny flavour often found in seedling mangoes, and some varieties can be peeled like a banana. The fibreless varieties can be kept in the refrigerator, and then scooped out with a spoon on a hot summer day for a really refreshing treat. Mangoes are one of the richest fruit sources of vitamin A, and the vitamin C content is also very high. A mere 100 g of mangoes contain 3 894 IU of vitamin A. It is, however, important to eat mangoes when they are ripe, because, like bananas, they contain amylase-inhibitors when they are green.

Melons and watermelons

Melons belong to the family *Cucurbitaceae* and they have been cultivated since ancient times. This family includes kinds, such as the cucumbers, which are more commonly used as vegetables. The **dessert melons** belong to the species *Cucumis melo* and include the netted summer melons and smooth-skinned winter melons. The netted variety is commonly (though incorrectly) referred to as **cantaloupes**. Watermelons belong to a different genus, and the typical watermelon (*Citrullus lanatus*) is native to tropical Africa. Watermelon cultivars vary in size, shape, colour and seed content, and it takes an expert to say when they are ripe, although a change in the ground spot colour, a slight bumpiness and a hollow sound when tapped, are good indications of ripeness.

Both winter and summer melons supply a superb array of vitamins and minerals, but the summer varieties have an exceptional vitamin A content. Over 3200 IU of vitamin A is present per 100 g in cantaloupes and the vitamin C content is also very high. Watermelons, on the other hand, are virtually pure fruit juice with good quantities of mineral and vitamins and are a treat for the whole family.

Olives (*Olea europaea*)

Olives have always occupied an important position in the diet and life of the Mediterranean and Middle Eastern cultures. In ancient times olive oil was much prized, and was used for lighting, and it also formed an important part of the rituals in the Hebrew sanctuary and temple service. The olive is one of the most nutritious fruits, and has the highest energy content of all fruits. Olives contain high concentrations of the minerals calcium, copper, magnesium, and zinc. Olives are an excellent source of essential oils, and the oil is rich in monounsaturated fats, with more than 70% of the natural oils consisting of this variety of fats. The remaining fats consist of a mixture of saturated and unsaturated fats. This combination of oil is known to lower cholesterol levels and to promote cardiovascular health,[86] and has also been associated with a reduced incidence of cancer as discussed in the chapter on fats. Of all the fats, the monounsaturated fats are least subject to autoxidation, but as all extracted oils are subject to this process, the best way to eat olive oil is in the olive.

The fruit of olives is bitter, because of the presence of certain glucosides, and olives thus have to go through an extensive preparation before they can be eaten. Olives are normally preserved in vinegar or brine, but they are best preserved in brine, as vinegar has detrimental effects. Olives can be eaten as is, or they can be used in cooking to add spice and nourishment to stews and pastas. Children (and adults) have to develop a palate for olives, but when they are used in cooking, their taste is not overwhelming. Olives can be eaten with every meal, as they are a neutral fruit, and once one has learnt the art of olive eating, they tend to become an indispensable component of the diet.

Papayas (*Carica papaya*)

The papaya tree is a giant herb rather than a tree, because it lacks woody tissue. It is also known as a pawpaw or melon tree. Papayas are native to tropical America, but they are extensively cultivated worldwide. The fruit is large, weighing from 500 g to 2 kilograms, and it may be round, cylindrical or pear-shaped, depending on the variety. The ripe fruit is normally eaten fresh, and latex is obtained from the unripe fruit from which the enzyme **papain** is extracted. Papain assists in protein digestion, and is also a stimulator of the appetite and has antibacterial properties. Papayas are a rich source of vitamins and minerals, with the levels of calcium and vitamins A and C being particularly noteworthy.

Passionfruit or Granadilla *(Passiflora)*

Passionfruit originated in the tropical highlands of South America, and a number of varieties with different tastes and colours are available. There are purple varieties (*P. edulis*), yellow varieties (*P. laurifolia*), sweet varieties (*P. ligularis*) as well as others such as the giant granadilla and the banana granadilla, and they are grown mainly for their pulp which is used as a flavourant, or for fruit juices.

Granadillas are a good source of magnesium and iron and they contain a high concentration of vitamin A and C. No fruit salad should be without some granadilla pulp to add that extra flavour.

Persimmons (*Diospyros khaki*)

Persimmons belong to the family *Ebenaceae*, of which the Ebony tree is also a member. The fruits are also known as date plums or velvet apples, and they are widely grown in Japan for the fruit and as a sugar source. Some varieties can be eaten firm like an apple (**Fuya**), whilst others are astringent and must be eaten when extremely ripe and soft (**Hachiya**). The trees are very attractive and are ideal for home cultivation. Persimmons contain large quantities of vitamin A (2 167 IU per 100 g), and will add a healthy variety to fruit meals.

Pineapples (*Ananas comosus*)

The pineapple is a member of the family *Bromeliaceae*, native to tropical South America, and is cultivated extensively in Hawaii, Brazil, Thailand, the Philippines, Malaysia and Kenya. Some varieties are used for the production of fibres for fine embroidery, whilst others are cultivated for their fruit. The fruit is used for juice production, canning and as fresh fruits. The most common cultivars are the **Cayenne, Queen** and **Spanish** groups. Pineapples were first known to Europeans from Guadeloupe when Columbus landed in 1493, and they were introduced in St. Helena in 1505. In Britain they are sometimes cultivated under glass in view of the climate. Pineapples contain average levels of nutrients, and they are a good source of the mineral manganese.

Pomegranates (*Punica granatum*)

Pomegranates belong to the family *Punicaceae*, and they are native to South West Asia. They have long been cultivated in the Mediterranean region, they grew in the hanging gardens of Babylon, and served as the inspiration for king Solomon's crown. The fruit contains seeds covered in a juicy pink pulp, which is the edible portion. The pomegranate can add to that much sought after variety in the diet.

Prickly pears (*Opuntia*)

Prickly pears are members of the cactus family *Cactaceae*, and are grown in tropical and subtropical countries. They are also known as Indian figs and they are a very rich source of minerals. They have one of the highest fruit levels of the minerals calcium and magnesium, and can contribute substantially to the requirements for these minerals.

There are many more varieties of fruits that are not dealt with in this section because they are not readily available in most areas. The list should be comprehensive enough to provide ample variation in the diet, and it is hoped that aspirant fruit eaters will be inspired to go hunting for more varieties of fruit. Remember that the Roman armies were often more hailed for the new varieties of fruits which they brought back from their conquests than for their conquests themselves.

Vegetables

The vegetable kingdom supplies an abundance of vital nutrients, and is an essential contributor to human health. Vegetables do not only provide primary nutrients, but they contain an abundance of vitamins and minerals. Moreover, vegetables help to rid the body of toxins, and they contain disease-preventive components, which include anti-cancer phytochemicals. In the United States, cancer is the second leading cause of mortality, and it has been estimated that 35% of cancer deaths are diet related. Estimates for diet related diseases range from 10–70%.[87] Statistics like these, and the fact that the consumption of fruits and vegetables has been linked to a reduced cancer risk, has led the National Cancer Institute (NCI) to recommend increased consumption of fruits and vegetables.[14] Not only are vegetables good for the prevention of cancer, but they are also beneficial for the cardiovascular system, and it has been shown that leafy green vegetables and root vegetables reduce cholesterol levels.[88,89]

Vegetables are living food packed with enzymes, vitamins and minerals, and the consumption of raw vegetables or vegetable juices would ensure an abundant supply of these essential nutrients. The introduction of raw vegetables into the diet would thus be most beneficial, and if prepared as crisp salads together with a tasty sauce, they can be very palatable. Another way to ensure a healthy intake of raw food, is by developing a taste for fresh sprouts which are easy to prepare and also supply an abundance of nutrients and enzymes. Raw vegetables also contain greater concentrations of cancer-preventing phytochemicals than cooked vegetables, as many of these compounds are destroyed by heat. The fact that raw vegetables should form a healthy component of the diet, does not, however, mean that one should go overboard and exclude all cooked vegetables from the diet. Neither should one assume that cooked vegetables are unhealthy and unfit for human consumption. The watchword is variety, and cooked vegetables certainly have their place, particularly in winter, when a plate of warm food is positively essential.

When preparing cooked vegetables, care should be taken not to overcook them, as this would lead to a loss of nutrients. Vegetables should still be crisp when cooked, and cooking them in large quantities of water is also not a good idea, as the vitamins and minerals will merely leach into the water and be discarded. A look at the composition tables will show that cooked vegetables contain lower concentrations of nutrients than do raw vegetables, and this is due to leaching. Baked vegetables, on the other hand, contain higher concentrations of nutrients, because baking is a dry process, and the evaporation of water from the vegetables will concentrate the nutrients. Preparing vegetables in waterless cookware, or through steaming will ensure minimal loss of nutrients.

Vegetables are easy to cultivate, and a home vegetable patch should be a priority for all who are in a position to possess one. Organically-grown vegetables will provide a better mix of essential nutrients than conventional vegetables that are cultivated with inorganic fertilizers. It is not always possible to obtain organically-grown vegetables, and they can also cost more than conventional ones. In a recent study it was found that organically-grown fruits and vegetables differ significantly from conventionally grown ones.[90] The nutrient levels were also affected differently in different fruits and vegetables. In potatoes it was found, for example, that the vitamin C content and that of various other nutrients was higher in conventional than in organically grown potatoes, whereas the reverse was true in the case of tomatoes, where the levels of vitamin C and that of other vitamins and minerals were higher in the organically grown varieties than conventional ones.[90] The levels of trace minerals, particularly zinc, would be higher in organically grown vegetables than in conventional kinds, but if a varied diet is followed, sufficient nutrients can be obtained from either conventional or organically grown vegetables, and there is therefore no need for advocating extreme viewpoints on the issue. The composition of some of the more common vegetables is presented in table 7.21.

Types of vegetables

Vegetables are derived from most of the families of flowering plants and also from some algae and fungi. Many different parts of the plants are used as vegetables, and these include the roots, stems, leaves, buds, flowers, fruits, and in the case of sprouts, the whole plant. As definitions for vegetables are mostly based on usage and not scientific principles, it is very difficult to define a vegetable, particularly where vegetable fruits are concerned and there is no hard and fast rule for placing some of the seed-bearing fruits in either the fruit or vegetable category. In the case of the family *Cucurbitaceae*, for example, melons are considered to be fruits because they are sweet and similar in composition to fruits, whereas cucumbers, pumpkins and squashes are considered to be vegetables, but the final placing in one category or another remains arbitrary.

As the various plant families which contribute to the vegetable kingdom often share common features, the vegetables will be discussed by family, and as the listing could constitute a book of its own, only some of the more common vegetables will be discussed in order to highlight the diversity of qualities inherent in these foods. Hopefully the list will encourage variety on the table.

Chenopodiaceae (Goosefoot family)

The goosefoot family comprises numerous genera of herbs, shrubs and vegetables, of which some are medicinal. The main vegetables in this family are: **beetroot, sugarbeet, Swiss chard** and **spinach**. These vegetables supply an abundance of vitamins and minerals, but they also contain oxalic acid, and much of the calcium is bound in the form of calcium oxalate, which is associated with the formation of kidney stones. It has, however, been found that a vegetarian diet enables the body to cope with this situation,[27] and it is not necessary for the vegetarian to eliminate these vegetables from the diet. Should there, however, be a record of kidney stones, then it would be wise to limit the use of vegetables belonging to this family.

Beetroot and Swiss chard
(Beta vulgaris)

Beetroot is native to Europe, Africa and Asia and was used as a vegetable from as early as 300 BC. The crimson root of the beetroot owes its colour to the presence of a glucoside called **betanin**, which belongs to a group of chemicals known as betacyanins. Because of its red colour, many people are mistakenly under the impression that beetroot is a cure for iron deficiency, but beetroot contains only an average amount of iron. Beetroot contains large amounts of sugar, and some varieties are cultivated solely for sugar production. The high sugar content (up to 8%) accounts for the high energy content of beetroot, but beetroot is also a rich source of the

The whole-food alternative

Vegetables	Energy (kcal)	Carb. (g)	Prot. (g)	Fat (g)	Fibre (g)	Ca (mg)	P (mg)	Fe (mg)	K (mg)	Mg (mg)
Alfalfa sprouts	29	1.6	4.0	0.7	2.2	32	70	1.0	79	27
Artichokes (c)	44	9.4	2.3	0.2	0.9	39	60	1.4	263	39
Asparagus (c)	25	2.9	2.6	0.3	1.5	24	61	0.7	310	19
Beans green (c)	35	3.9	1.9	0.3	3.9	46	39	1.3	299	25
Beetroot (c)	131	5.4	1.1	0.1	1.3	11	31	0.6	312	37
Brinjal (c)	28	3.5	0.8	0.2	3.1	6	22	0.4	248	13
Broccoli (c)	29	1.5	3.0	0.3	4.1	114	48	1.2	163	60
Brussels sprouts (c)	39	4.4	2.6	0.5	4.3	36	56	1.2	317	20
Cabbage (c)	21	2.0	1.0	0.3	2.8	33	25	0.4	205	15
Cabbage (r)	24	3.2	1.2	0.2	2.2	47	23	0.6	246	15
Carrots (r)	43	7.6	1.0	0.2	2.5	27	44	0.5	323	15
Cauliflower (c)	24	2.1	1.9	0.2	2.5	27	35	0.4	323	11
Celery (r)	16	2.1	0.7	0.1	1.5	36	26	0.5	284	12
Chicory (r)	15	3.2	1.0	0.1	–	–	21	0.5	182	13
Cucumber (r)	13	2.4	0.5	0.1	0.5	14	17	0.3	149	11
Garlick	149	31.6	6.4	0.5	1.5	181	153	1.7	401	25
Kale (c)	32	4.8	1.9	0.4	0.8	72	28	0.9	228	18
Leeks (r)	61	10.4	1.5	0.3	3.8	59	35	2.1	180	28
Lettuce	13	0.6	1.0	0.2	1.5	19	20	0.5	158	9
Mushrooms (r)	25	2.2	2.1	0.4	2.5	5	104	1.2	370	10
Okra (c)	32	4.0	1.9	0.2	3.2	63	56	0.5	322	57
Onions (r)	34	5.6	1.2	0.3	1.7	25	29	0.4	155	10
Onions, spring (r)	25	3.7	1.7	0.1	1.9	60	33	1.9	257	20
Parsley (r)	33	1.9	2.2	0.3	5.0	130	41	6.2	536	44
Parsnips (c)	81	16.2	1.3	0.3	3.3	37	69	0.6	367	29
Peas, fresh (c)	84	9.9	5.4	0.2	5.7	27	117	1.5	271	39
Peppers, green (r)	25	4.4	0.9	0.5	0.9	6	22	1.3	195	14
Peppers, red (r)	25	4.4	0.9	0.5	0.9	6	22	1.3	195	14
Potato, baked	109	22.7	2.3	0.1	2.5	10	57	1.4	418	27
Potato (c)	87	18.9	1.9	0.1	1.2	5	44	0.3	379	22
Pumpkin (summer) (c)	20	2.7	0.9	0.3	1.6	27	39	0.4	192	24
Pumpkin (winter) (c)	39	7.6	0.9	0.6	1.2	14	20	0.3	437	8
Radish (r)	17	2.8	0.6	0.5	0.8	21	18	0.3	232	9
Spinach (c)	23	1.1	3.0	0.3	2.7	136	56	3.6	466	87
Sweet potato (c)	105	22.0	1.7	0.3	2.3	21	27	0.6	184	10
Swiss chard (c)	20	3.2	1.9	0.1	0.9	58	33	2.3	549	86
Tomato (c)	25	4.5	1.1	0.3	1.1	8	29	0.6	260	14
Tomato (r)	19	2.8	0.9	0.2	1.5	7	23	0.5	207	11
Turnips (r)	27	2.8	0.9	0.1	3.4	30	27	0.3	191	11
Watercress (r)	11	0.0	2.3	0.1	1.8	120	60	0.2	330	21

r = raw, c = cooked.

Table 7.21 (Part 1). The composition of selected vegetables. The figures are for 100 g portions. (Adapted from ref. 37)

Vegetables	Zn (mg)	Vit.A (IU)	Vit.B1 (mg)	Vit.B2 (mg)	Vit.B3 (m)	Vit.B5 (mg)	Vit.B6 (mg)	Fol. (µg)	Vit.C (mg)	Vit.E (mg)
Alfalfa sprouts	0.92	155	0.08	0.13	0.5	0.56	0.034	36	8	–
Artichokes (c)	0.36	144	0.06	0.05	0.6	0.20	0.087	45	7	–
Asparagus (c)	0.48	829	0.10	0.12	1.1	0.16	0.141	98	27	2.50
Beans green (c)	0.36	666	0.07	0.10	0.6	0.07	0.056	33	10	0.23
Beetroot (c)	0.25	13	0.03	0.01	0.3	0.10	0.031	53	6	0.00
Brinjal (c)	0.15	64	0.08	0.02	0.6	0.08	0.086	14	1	–
Broccoli (c)	0.15	1409	0.08	0.21	0.8	0.29	0.198	68	63	1.10
Brussels sprouts (c)	0.33	719	0.11	0.08	0.6	0.25	0.178	60	62	1.34
Cabbage (c)	0.16	86	0.06	0.06	0.2	0.06	0.064	20	24	0.20
Cabbage (r)	0.18	126	0.05	0.03	0.3	0.14	0.095	57	47	0.13
Carrots (r)	0.20	28129	0.10	0.06	0.9	0.20	0.140	14	9	0.44
Cauliflower (c)	0.24	14	0.06	0.05	0.6	0.12	0.202	51	55	0.14
Celery (r)	0.17	127	0.03	0.03	0.3	0.17	0.030	9	6	0.36
Chicory (r)	0.26	0	0.07	0.14	0.5	–	0.045	67	10	–
Cucumber (r)	0.23	45	0.03	0.02	0.3	0.25	0.052	14	5	0.15
Garlick	–	0	0.20	0.11	0.7	–	–	3	31	0.01
Kale (c)	0.24	7400	0.05	0.07	0.5	0.05	0.138	13	41	–
Leeks (r)	0.12	95	0.06	0.03	0.4	0.15	0.304	64	12	0.92
Lettuce	0.22	330	0.05	0.03	0.2	0.05	0.040	56	4	0.40
Mushrooms (r)	0.73	0	0.10	0.45	4.1	2.20	0.097	21	4	0.00
Okra (c)	0.55	575	0.13	0.06	0.9	0.21	0.187	46	16	–
Onions (r)	0.18	0	0.06	0.01	0.1	0.13	0.157	20	8	0.31
Onions, spring (r)	0.44	5000	0.07	0.14	0.2	0.14	0.061	14	45	0.00
Parsley (r)	0.73	5200	0.08	0.11	0.7	0.30	0.164	183	90	1.74
Parsnips (c)	0.26	0	0.08	0.05	0.7	0.59	0.093	58	13	1.33
Peas, fresh (c)	1.19	597	0.26	0.15	2.0	0.15	0.216	63	14	0.00
Peppers, green (r)	0.18	530	0.09	0.05	0.6	0.04	0.164	17	128	0.68
Peppers, red (r)	0.18	5700	0.09	0.05	0.6	0.04	0.164	17	190	0.68
Potato, baked	0.32	0	0.11	0.03	1.6	0.56	0.347	11	13	0.10
Potato (c)	0.30	0	0.11	0.02	1.4	0.52	0.299	10	13	0.04
Pumpkin (summer) (c)	0.39	287	0.04	0.04	0.5	0.14	0.065	20	6	–
Pumpkin (winter) (c)	0.26	3557	0.09	0.02	0.7	0.35	0.072	28	10	0.12
Radish (r)	0.30	8	0.01	0.05	0.3	0.09	0.071	27	23	0.00
Spinach (c)	0.76	8190	0.10	0.24	0.5	0.15	0.242	146	10	1.18
Sweet potato (c)	0.27	17054	0.05	0.14	0.6	0.53	0.244	11	17	4.00
Swiss chard (c)	–	3139	0.03	0.09	0.4	0.16	–	–	18	–
Tomato (c)	0.13	1352	0.07	0.06	0.7	0.29	0.036	9	21	1.52
Tomato (r)	0.11	1133	0.06	0.06	0.6	0.25	0.048	9	18	0.34
Turnips (r)	–	0	0.04	0.03	0.4	0.20	0.090	15	21	0.00
Watercress (r)	–	4700	0.09	0.12	0.2	0.31	0.129	–	43	1.00

r = raw, c = cooked.

Table 7.21 (Part 2). The composition of selected vegetables. The figures are for 100 g portions. (Adapted from ref. 37)

minerals magnesium and manganese, and it also contains a fair amount of vitamin C. Beetroot can be grated and eaten raw in a salad or it can be cooked and served with a little lemon juice rather than vinegar. In Russia, beetroot forms the basis of the popular soup called **borsch**.

Another variety of *Beta vulgaris* produces Swiss chard, which is cultivated for its leaves and is easy to digest. Swiss chard is very nutritious and supplies good quantities of potassium, calcium, phosphorus and iron. It is one of the richest sources of magnesium. Moreover, this vegetable is very rich in vitamin A, supplying in excess of 3 000 IU per 100 g.

Spinach (*Spinacia oleracea*)

Spinach is native to Asia and was introduced into Europe in the late Middle Ages. Like Swiss chard, it is rich in magnesium, calcium, potassium, phosphorus, iron, copper and manganese. The vitamin A-content is exceptionally high (8 190 IU). Spinach is also a good source of vitamins B-6 and C. Spinach can be eaten cooked, and creamed with a little nut sauce it is particularly delicious. Raw spinach can be eaten in salads without fear of oxalic acid build-up, as the blend of nutrients in spinach will prevent oxalic acid accumulation, particularly in the vegetarian. People already suffering from gall and kidney stones, should, however, avoid all foods rich in oxalic acid.

Compositae (Sunflower family)

The family *compositae* is a huge family of plants, better known for the flowers and oilseeds which are derived from it. One important vegetable from this family is **chicory**, and what would our salad bars look like without the all important **lettuce**, which is also a member of this family.

Chicory (*Cichorium intybus*)

Chicory is native to Europe and Asia, but has only been used as a vegetable since the thirteenth century. Chicory is cultivated mainly for its large taproot which is used as a coffee substitute, but its leaves are also used as a vegetable. The leaves of chicory have a bitter taste and Pliny, in fact, mentions chicory as one of the bitter herbs used by the Jews during the Passover. Chicory is cultivated from harvested roots which are replanted in spring and covered with soil or sawdust. This blanches the leaves and reduces the bitter taste. Chicory is a good source of folic acid and it can be eaten like lettuce in a salad.

Lettuce (*Lactuca sativa*)

The leaves of lettuce can be cooked, but they are most commonly used for salads, and have been used in this way for thousands of years. Wild species have a bitter taste because they have higher concentrations of the **triterpenoid alcohols, sesquiterpene, lactone, lactucin** and **lactupicrin** than do cultivated varieties. These compounds occur in the white milky fluid, latex, and are also known to have sedative properties, and are frequently used as a remedy for coughs. Varieties of lettuce which are characterized by overlapping leaves are known as cabbage or **head lettuce**, and these are the most popular varieties. Lettuce with oblong leaves are known as **cos lettuce** and others do not form a head, but merely a loose rosette of leaves. Lettuce contains only 1% protein, very little complex carbohydrate and consists mainly of water, which is why it is compatible with fruits. Lettuce also contains reasonable quantities of minerals and vitamins, particularly silicon, vitamin A and folic acid.

Convolvulaceae (Morning glory family)

The family consists mainly of twining herbs that are often classed as weeds. Some members of this family are used medicinally or as hallucinogens but one species, the **sweet potato** is an important food source.

Sweet potato (*Ipomoea batatas*)

Sweet potatoes are not related to potatoes, and they are cultivated for their root tubers. The tubers of sweet potatoes contain free sugar as well as starch, and this gives them their sweet taste. The plant is native to tropical America and was introduced to Europe by Columbus. Sweet potatoes can be eaten boiled or baked, and they are a very nutritious food, very rich in vitamin A (17 054 IU per 100 g). Vitamin C is also well supplied.

Cucurbitaceae (Gourd family)

The gourd family includes plants that are utilized as a source of fruits such as the melons and watermelons, but also includes varieties such as **pumpkins, squashes, gherkins** and **cucumbers** that are regarded as vegetables. **Gourds**, on the other hand, are mainly ornamental.

Pumpkins and Squashes (*Cucurbita*)

Pumpkins and squashes are of American origin, and there are a number of species. In America, the terms winter and summer squash are used to differentiate between different varieties. The summer squash (*C. pepo*) is eaten in the immature stage whilst the other varieties of the same species, such as pumpkins and winter squash, are harvested when fully mature. These can be stored for use during winter, and are thus also known as winter squash. In Britain, summer squashes are called marrows and the term winter squash is not used.

Pumpkins and squashes are good sources of vitamin A, and the yellow varieties supply in excess of 3 500 IU of this vitamin per 100 g. Pumpkins are also a good source of the minerals calcium, potassium and silicon. Pumpkins can be eaten raw if grated into a salad, or they can be steamed or baked. Baked winter pumpkin is very nutritious and satisfying and supplies a high nutrient density.

Cucumber (*Cucumis sativa*)

Cucumbers have been used for thousands of years, and they were known to the ancient Egyptians. Today there are many different varieties that are cultivated for human consumption. They consist largely of water, minerals and vitamins, and are thus compatible with either fruits or vegetables, and can be used as a refreshing addition to salads or snacks. Cucumbers are mainly eaten raw, but they are also delicious when briefly cooked and prepared in a sweet and sour sauce. Some cultivars are pickled and preserved in vinegar, but it would be better to use brands that are preserved in brine, or to prepare one's own preserve substituting lemon juice for vinegar. Gherkins are also used for pickling, but they are derived from another species of *Cucumis*.

Cruciferae (Brassicaceae) (Mustard family)

This family includes some 350 genera and well over a thousand species, of which a number are utilized as vegetables. Cruciferous vegetables are rich in essential nutrients. They are known to reduce the risk of cancer,[81,82] and should therefore fill a prominent position in the diet. Because vegetables in general, and cruciferous vegetables in particular, contain substantial quantities of sulphur, the vitamin C-concentration does not decline as readily as it does in the case of fruits or vegetables with a lower sulphur content,[91] and this means that more of this vitamin is retained after storage and cooking.

Some of the common vegetables in this family are those which belong to genus *Brassica*, which includes **broccoli, brussels sprouts, cabbage, Chinese cabbage, cauliflower, kale, kohlrabi, rutabaga** and **turnips**. Some other important foods from this family include **cress, watercress,** and **radish**, which are eaten in salads, and **Japanese horseradish** and **mustard** which are used as condiments. The chemical components of the mustard family, to which its anti-cancer properties are attributed, are listed in table 7.18. One of these substances is mustard oil which also is responsible for the characteristic taste of the cabbage group, and the compounds attributed with anti-cancer activity are **isothiocyanytes, thiocyanates** and **dithiolthiones**.

Broccoli (*Brassica oleracea*)

Broccoli was developed in Italy and is well established as one of the major anti-cancer foods. It also stimulates the production of enzymes which rid the body of potentially harmful metabolites.[81] Broccoli contains some 3% of protein and is one of the richest vegetable sources of calcium, iron and magnesium. Moreover, broccoli is very rich in vitamins A and C, exceeding even oranges in the concentration of the latter. Broccoli can be eaten raw in salads or with dips, or it can be steamed and eaten as is, or served with a light nut, or similar sauce.

Brussels sprouts (*Brassica oleracea*)

Brussels sprouts was first developed in Belgium from where it also gets its name. Brussels sprouts is quite popular in Europe and its nutrient composition is similar to that of broccoli, except that the concentrations of vitamins and minerals tend to be lower. Use brussels sprouts as an alternative to provide variety, but try to use fresh or frozen sprouts as they lose their flavour and texture when canned.

Cabbage (*Brassica oleracea*)

Cabbage is yet another variety of the species *Brassica oleracea* which is rich in cleansing minerals such as sulphur. It is native to the Mediterranean region, England and France, but the cultivated form was introduced to Britain by the Romans. Cabbage can be eaten raw, pickled or cooked and is used in a great variety of ways. There are many varieties of cabbages but the **Savoy cabbage** is considered to be the best in terms of its nutrient content. Savoy cabbage contains some 157 mg of vitamin C per 100 g and is rich in sulphur, a cleansing mineral, which helps to retain this vitamin.

Cabbage can be fermented to produce **Sauerkraut**, a process whereby the bacterium *Lactobacillus* converts the sugars into lactic acid, which accounts for the sour taste of Sauerkraut. Lactic acid is a weak acid, and in spite of its presence, Sauerkraut still remains an extremely alkaline-forming food which supplies an abundance of vitamins and minerals. The body copes well with lactic acid, and Sauerkraut can be eaten without fear of acid build up. Red cabbage is another variety of cabbage which can also be eaten raw in salads, or it can be cooked with a little lemon juice, rather than vinegar, to give it a sour flavour. Another popular cabbage variety, that can be used to provide variety, is the **Chinese cabbage** which is good for making salads or cooked as a green vegetable.

Cauliflower (*Brassica oleracea*)

Cauliflower is probably native to Asia Minor but was known in Europe by the sixteenth century. Its nutrient composition does not compare with that of broccoli, but it is an excellent source of biotin, and other vitamins and minerals are in good supply. Cauliflower provides that necessary variety on the table and it can be eaten raw, cooked and served with a sauce or as a soup, and it lends itself to being crumbed.

Kale and collard (*Brassica oleracea*)

Kale is similar to cabbage, but the leaves, which are green, silver-green or purple, do not form a head. The varieties that are used for human consumption are usually those with the curled leaves, and in the USA there is a variety that also forms a rosette of leaves similar to cabbage, but not compact. This variety is known as collard. Kale is the oldest variety of *Brassica* and it is very rich in nutrients. Kale is rich in calcium, magnesium, vitamin B-6, and it contains over 7 400 IU of vitamin A per 100 g.

Kohlrabi (*Brassica oleracea*)

The name Kohlrabi is a German name which means 'cabbage turnip', and it is the swollen turnip-like stem which is used as a vegetable. The leaves are not usually eaten, but they are edible and do have considerable nutritive value. Kohlrabi is normally cooked and can be served with a white nut, or similar sauce, and it is excellent in soups.

Turnip (*Brassica rapa*)

The turnip has been used for thousands of years, and is native to temperate parts of Europe and Asia. The swollen base can be cooked and eaten sliced and the leaves can be used like spinach. Turnips are not used extensively except in poorer areas, and they do not excel in any particular nutritional component, although they do contain reasonable amounts of calcium and vitamin C.

Radish (*Raphanus sativus*)

Radishes were used by the ancient Egyptians and they are probably native to Asia. Their pungent taste is due to the mustard oil. Radishes are eaten raw, and when they are peeled, most of the enzyme responsible for the production of mustard oil is removed, and they have a milder taste. The leaves of the radish should not be thrown away, as they can be used in salads, but as they are slightly prickly, they are best used in soups to create a pleasant, spicy taste. Radish-leaf soup is pleasant as a starter to meals, and is prepared by cooking the leaves and creaming them in a blender. Radishes contain fair amounts of vitamin C, and the mineral silicon is also in good supply.

Cress (*Lepidium sativum*)

Both garden cress and watercress (*Nasturtium officinale*) are members of the cruciferous family and their taste is due to mustard oil. They are used raw in salads or in soups and stews, and have a fresh spicy taste. Watercress was originally used as a medicine, and in view of its superb composition, it should become a part of every household's menu. Watercress is an excellent source of calcium (120 mg per 100 g), magnesium and phosphorus, and it contains 4 700 IU of vitamin A per 100 g. The B-group vitamins are well supplied and the concentrations of vitamins C and E are also above average.

Leguminosae (Fabaceae) (Pea or Pulse family)

The family *Leguminosae* is a large family which also includes some varieties that are used as spices or that can be eaten fresh as sprouts. The legumes can all be sprouted and eaten raw or cooked, and **fenugreek** can in addition be used as a spice. Another important plant belonging to this family is **liquorice** (*Glycyrrhiza glabra*), of which the underground portions are used as a flavouring agent in confectionery. Liquorice is recognized as having anti-cancer properties subscribed to the flavonoids, coumarins, tri-terpenes and phenolic acids which the roots contain. Most of the pea and bean varieties are discussed in the section on legumes, and the only ones that will be discussed here are those varieties that are eaten fresh as vegetables, namely the green or **French beans** and the fresh **garden peas**.

French beans (*Phaseolus vulgaris*)

There are two varieties of French beans that are eaten in the immature stage, and a further one where the beans are eaten in the dry form. Only those that are eaten in the immature stages will be discussed here. Cultivars where the entire pod is consumed, are normally called **snap beans**, and there are stringed and stringless varieties. In the other group the pods are not eaten, but the seeds are eaten in the immature stage. This last group is not of great commercial significance. Green beans contain good quantities of calcium, iron, magnesium, and the levels of vitamins A and C are also high.

Peas (*Pisum sativum*)

Garden peas probably originate from Asia, and they reached significance in Europe during the Middle Ages. Unripe peas can be served as a vegetable, and in the case of sugar peas, the whole pod can be consumed. Sugar peas are particularly attractive and tasty in Chinese dishes. Peas contain good quantities of phosphorus, but the other minerals are also present in adequate amounts. The vitamins A and C are also well supplied. Fresh garden peas are always an attractive addition to the menu.

Liliaceae (Lily family)

The *Liliaceae* include a wide variety of edible, as well as medicinal and ornamental plants. From the genus *Allium* we obtain the **onion, garlic, leeks, shallots** and **chives**, and from the genus *Asparagus* we obtain, of course, **asparagus**. Besides their tremendous flavour-enhancing capabilities, these foods have been categorized as having exceptional anti-cancer properties,[82] and they also have cleansing and disinfectant qualities. The pungent smell of garlic, onions and the other members of the *Allium* genus is due to disulphide compounds known as **allicins**. The enzyme allinase starts to work on odourless compounds known as alliins when the plant is cut or damaged, and this produces the allicins. Allicins are powerful irritants, and that is why one tends to cry when one peals onions or other members of the *Allium* genus. Although garlic and chives are flavourants and are not strictly vegetables, they will be discussed here in view of their significance as disease preventers and flavour enhancers.

Chive (*Allium schoenoprasum*)

Chive is a herb native to Eurasia and is very popular in Europe, where it is finely chopped and eaten raw in salads, on boiled potatoes, as a garnish or as a flavourant for soups and stews. Chives have a fresh, mild onion flavour and are relatively easy to cultivate, even as a pot plant, so that no household need be without it.

Garlic (*Allium sativum*)

Garlic was already used by the ancient Egyptians and perhaps even contributed to the health of those individuals who helped to construct the pyramids. Garlic is rated as the number one anti-cancer food, and the **sulphides, phenolic acids**, and **mono-** and **triterpenes** present in garlic are attributed with this protective capacity. Moreover, garlic is much used as a medicine, as it also has bactericidal properties. Garlic can be added to many foods to enhance their flavour, and besides these virtues, garlic is one of the best sources of primary and secondary nutrients. Garlic contains over 6% high quality protein, is rich in carbohydrates and contains exceptional amounts of calcium, phosphorus, iron, magnesium, niacin and vitamin C. Prolonged slow cooking removes the pungency of garlic, but some nations find this quality of garlic endearing. To the novice, the taste of garlic may seem somewhat overwhelming, but once a palate for this flavourant has been developed, there will be no holding back, except perhaps in the romantic sphere.

Leeks (*Allium ampeloprasum*)

Leeks are native to the Mediterranean region and have been used as a vegetable since ancient times. Leeks can be eaten raw in salads, or they can be eaten cooked, and young leeks can substitute for asparagus. The green leaves at the top should not be discarded, as they contain most of the nutrients. If served with a nut sauce, tomato an olive oil dressing, or similar, it can provide a tasty variety to meals. Like all green vegetables, leeks are a good source of calcium, and the minerals iron and magnesium are also well supplied. Leeks are rich in folic acid and vitamin B-6, and also contain a fair amount of vitamin C.

Onions (*Allium cepa*)

Onions have been used since ancient times, and their use is recorded by the Egyptians. Strictly speaking, the onion is a condiment but it is used so extensively that it will here be treated as a vegetable. The edible bulb of the onion is really the thickened stem, and the fleshy leaves are the bases of normal leaves from the previous season. Onions are one of the plants listed by the NCI (National Cancer Institute) as having anti-cancer properties. Raw onions contain up to 2% protein, and useful amounts of calcium, vitamin B-6 and folic acid. Spring onions are even more nutritious than mature onions, and they should be incorporated into the diet whenever possible. Make them a part of crisp green salads and use them in Chinese dishes. Spring onions contain twice as much calcium as mature onions (up to 60 mg per 100 g) and they are rich in vitamin C and contain up to 5 000 IU of vitamin A, whereas mature onions contain virtually no vitamin A.

Onions can be used raw, cooked or fried, and the taste of virtually all vegetable meals can be improved by the addition of onions. Onions need not be fried in oil to obtain that rich fried onion taste, but they can be simmered over low heat in waterless cookware or in a little soy sauce or yeast extract together with a small quantity of water until they become golden brown. This enhances their taste and lends a rich flavour to stews and sauces.

Asparagus (*Asparagus officinalis*)

Asparagus is native to Eurasia and it was regarded as a delicacy by the Romans. The most renowned type of asparagus is the **Argenteuil asparagus** which is cultivated in France. The part used as a vegetable is the young shoot, and if white, blanched asparagus is required, then the earth must be mounded up around the young plant so that the stem is not exposed to the sunlight. The plant is harvested when the tip of the asparagus appears above the mound. Fresh asparagus can be peeled and cooked, and served together with a creamy mayonnaise-type sauce (see recipes), or it can be used on Pizzas. Asparagus contains useful amounts of calcium, magnesium and iodine and is an excellent source of folic acid. Moreover, vitamins A, C and E are also well supplied.

Malvaceae (Mallow family)

The mallow family furnishes many ornamental plants as well as fibre, medicinal and food plants, but the family is most important as the source of cotton. Two frequently used food plants are **okra** and **roselle**, the latter being mainly used as a condiment. The edible calyces of the Roselle fruits are used to make jellies or a drink known as **sorrel**, or they are used as a flavourant in sauces.

Okra (*Abelmoschus esculentus*)

Okra is the large, green erect pod of *Abelmoschus (Hibiscus)* also known as gumbo or lady's-fingers. The pods are used in the green state for stews, or they are dried for winter and they contribute substantially to human nutritional needs in some areas. The capsules can be sliced and fried, but because they are highly mucilaginous, they are also used to thicken and flavour soups. In the Southern United States, they are used to make the well known gumbo soup. Okra is rich in calcium and phosphorus, and is also an excellent source of magnesium. The vitamins A, B-6, C and folic acid are also well supplied.

Solanaceae (Nightshade family)

This family abounds in ornamentals, plants with medicinal properties and a number of important food plants such as the **potato, tomato, egg-plant** (aubergine or brinjal) and **red pepper** (*Capsicum*). The vegetables belonging to this family have also been recognized by the NCI as having anti-cancer properties.

Capsicum (*Capsicum annuum*)

Green and red peppers, also known by their Hungarian name **Paprika** or the Spanish name **Pimento**, are native to South America from where they were introduced to most countries of the world. There are different varieties of peppers, ranging from the mild sweet pepper (*C. annuum* variety *grossum*) to the somewhat hotter Hungarian Paprika which was introduced to Hungary by the Turks. In Turkey, the pepper is a very important component of the everyday diet, and some of the best recipes for its use hail from that country. The fruits of this genus are not only used as vegetables, but are also used as condiments. Paprika powder is obtained by grinding the large, dried European variety of *Capsicum*, and it is a tremendous flavour enhancer. The red pepper, known as **chilli**, is derived from another species (*Capsicum frutescens*) and the fruits of this species are more pungent than sweet peppers. The fruits of chillies can be ground after thorough drying, to produce **cayenne** or red pepper, and Tabasco sauce is obtained by pickling the pulp of chillies in vinegar or brine. The hot taste of these condiments is due to a compound known as **capsaicin**.

Red and green peppers are very nutritious and they are very rich in vitamin C. The composition of the unripe green pepper is very similar to that of the ripe red pepper, but the levels of vitamins A and C are far higher in the red than in the green pepper. Green peppers contain 530 IU of vitamin A per 100 g as opposed to 5 700 IU in red peppers and the levels of vitamin C in the red pepper exceeds that in the green pepper by more than 60 mg per 100 g. Peppers can be eaten raw, stuffed, or as garnish and flavourant in a host of dishes. They are also used as stuffing for green olives.

Egg plant (*Solanum melongena*)

The egg plant, also known as **aubergine** or **brinjal**, probably originated in tropical Asia and is extensively used in India and the Far East. The edible part is the egg-shaped fruit, which is a berry. Different cultivars have different colours ranging from white to yellow, dark purple and black. The most common variety, however, is purple. The fruit is eaten boiled, stuffed or baked, and it can be used in stews or sauces. In Turkey, brinjals are roasted directly on a hot stove plate until the outer skin is burnt black. The fruit is frequently turned during this process to prevent too much burning, and the inner flesh is then scooped out and added to dishes such as rice salads. It imparts a unique, smoked flavour to the dish. Brinjals do not excel in any particular nutrient, but they do add variety to the table, and contain compounds that act as cleansers and prevents disease such as cancer.

Potato (*Solanum tuberosum*)

The potato is native to tropical America and it was the staple food of the Incas. When potatoes were first introduced to Europe, they were only used as ornaments, but today they are one of the most important vegetables which are used in virtually all the countries of the world. The potato plant produces white, yellow or purple flowers, and the fruits, which are small berries, are very poisonous as they contain **solanine**, which is an alkaloidal sapotoxin. The edible part of the potato is the underground stem tuber which can have a whitish, yellow, brown or red skin, depending on the variety. Because the potato grows in the dark, it is not green, and it should be kept in the dark after harvesting to prevent it from going green. Green potatoes should never be eaten, as they also synthesize the toxin solanine.

Potatoes are rich in starch and contain some 2% protein. They contain fair amounts of potassium, B-group vitamins and vitamin C. Baked potatoes are more energy rich than boiled potatoes because of the lower water content. Potatoes can be prepared in so many different ways that one could fill a book just listing the recipes, but some dishes, such as French fries, have become international favourites. French fries are probably the unhealthiest way of consuming potatoes, as the impregnation with oil makes the potato very difficult to digest, and deep frying in oils, rich in polyunsaturated fats, has been linked to cancer. The use of free fats and oils should be avoided altogether, but if on occasion french fries are desired, then they can be prepared by giving the sliced potatoes a light coating of cold pressed olive oil (a monounsaturated oil) and baking them in the oven at 200 °C (400 °F) rather than deep frying them. The taste of this variety of fries is also superior to that of deep-fried French fries and will be less detrimental to health.

Tomatoes (*Lycopersicon esculentum*)

The tomato is also native to South America where it grows wild on the slopes of the Andes. Tomatoes were only brought to Europe in 1523 after the conquest of Mexico, and did not really become a part of the diet until the nineteenth century. The fruits of the tomato are used primarily as a vegetable, and they can be eaten raw or cooked. Like most vegetables, tomatoes contain a fair amount of sulphur compounds which act as cleansers, and the red colour of the tomato is due to the presence of the tetra-terpene **lycopene**.

Today, there are many varieties of tomatoes on the market and they are processed into pastes and sauces. Canned tomatoes and purees are also readily available. Tomatoes have become essential ingredients of salads, stews and sauces, and have a tremendous potential for enhancing the flavour of virtually any dish. Italians have become past masters in utilizing the tomato, and much can be learnt from their approach. Tomatoes contain about 1% protein and are a good source of vitamin A and C.

Umbelliferae (Apiaceae) (Parsley or Carrot family)

The *umbelliferae* are an important family, comprising some 250 genera and 2 800 species, the flowers of which look like small umbrellas or umbels. The plants often have a pungent odour and they are used as food source, flavourants, scent or for their medicinal value, but some of them are poisonous. Depending on the type of plant, the roots, leaves or seeds can be utilized as foods and flavourants. The plants of this family are recognized by the NCI as having cancer-preventive properties as they produce anti-cancer phytochemicals such as **flavonoids, carotenoids, coumarins, mono- and triterpens, phenolic acids, phthalides** and **polyacetylenes**. Many members of this family are used as herbs to improve the flavour of foods, and, in the interest of good health, this practice can only be encouraged.

Some of the more common herbs and foods belonging to this family are: **angelica, aniseed, caraway, carrots, celery, chervil, coriander, cumin, dill, fennel, lovage, parsley** and **parsnip**. Many of these are only used as flavourants, but carrots and parsnips are used as vegetables. As some of the flavourants, however, also enjoy extensive use, and in some cases are also consumed as vegetables, they will be briefly discussed here.

Angelica (*Angelica archangelica*)

Angelica is believed to be a good antidote for poison. Today it is used as a condiment and is often candied. In some areas it is, however, used as a vegetable.

Aniseed (*Pimpinella anisum*)

Aniseed is a fruit and is used as a spice in cakes and pastries.

Caraway (*Carum carvi*)

Caraway is not a seed, but a fruit, and is used as a spice in bread or to add flavour to vegetables such as potatoes and cabbage.

Carrots (*Daucus carota*)

Carrots are an important vegetable, and although they were known to the ancient Greeks and Romans, they were not introduced to Europe until the Middle Ages. The orange-coloured taproot of the carrot contains a high concentration of β-carotene, which is the precursor to vitamin A. Carrots can be eaten raw or cooked, but to obtain maximum benefit it is best to eat them raw. Carrots contain cleansing sulphur compounds and the main minerals and vitamins are well supplied. However, in its potential to supply vitamin A, the carrot is unbeatable, supplying in excess of 28 000 IU per 100 g portion of this important component. Different cultivars, as well as older and younger plants, vary in the amount of β-carotene which they contain, and the younger roots are also sweeter than the older ones.

Celery (*Apium graveolens*)

Celery is one of the most alkaline-forming foods as it is rich in alkaline minerals. Celery has remedial qualities, and extracts of celery are even used to combat arthritis. The variety of *Apium graveolens* known as **celeriac** is cultured mainly for its turnip-like swelling, which is fried or cooked as a vegetable and is very popular in Europe, where it is also used to liven up potato salads. Celery is, however, grown mainly for its stalks and leaves. Blanched celery is formed by earthing up the stems, and is more delicate in its flavour and also has a higher nutritional value in that it contains more vitamin A than the green stalks. Celery can be used raw as a salad or together with dips, but it also imparts a unique flavour to stews and soups.

Chervil (*Anthriscus cerefolium*)

Chervil is similar to parsley and is used as garnish or flavourant.

Coriander (*Coriandrum sativum*)

Coriander, which is a fruit, is used whole or ground in pickles and other foods as a flavourant.

Cumin (*Cuminum cyminum*)

Cumin also produces a fruit that is used as a spice and its use is similar to that of caraway.

Dill (*Anethum graveolens*)

In the case of dill, either the leaves or the fruits can be used as a flavourant in pickles, sauces and green salads to impart a pleasant, refreshing flavour.

Fennel (*Foeniculum vulgare*)

Fennel is used to flavour sweets, sauces and soups. In some areas it is used as a vegetable. However, as a vegetable, it has a somewhat overpowering taste for which one must develop a palate.

Lovage (*Levisticum officinale*)

Lovage is native to Southern Europe and is used as a spice to enhance the flavour of soups and stews. In Germany it is known as Maggi-Wurzel.

Parsley (*Petroselinum crispum*)

The ancient Greeks used parsley as medicine, but today it is extensively used as a condiment. Its distinctive flavour is due to **apiol**. Parsley should become a regular household commodity, as it is exceptionally rich in calcium (130 mg per 100 g), iron, potassium, magnesium and trace elements, although the other minerals are also present in useful amounts. Parsley is also an excellent source of vitamins, particularly vitamin A, vitamin B-2, folic acid and vitamin C. Parsley can be included in soups and stews, and finely chopped parsley on savoury sandwiches and in salads adds flavour and essential minerals.

Parsnip (*Pastinaca sativa*)

Parsnips are native to Eurasia, and the edible portion is the swollen taproot which is used as a vegetable or flavourant. Parsnips contain reasonable amounts of calcium, phosphorus, folic acid and vitamin C, and before the introduction of the potato to Europe it was quite an important vegetable.

There are many other varieties of vegetables that could be included here, but it is not the purpose of this book to supply an exhaustive list of edible vegetables. It is rather envisaged that the list supplied should encourage the readers to include a variety of foods in their diet and to point out why this variety is so essential to a healthy lifestyle.

References

1. Dwyer, J.T. 1986. Promoting good nutrition for today and the year 2000. *Pediatr. Clin. North Am.* 33: 799–822.

2. Bray, G.A. 1992. Pathophysiology of obesity. *Am.J.Clin.Nutr*. 55:488S-94S.

3. Dunn Clinical Nutrition Centre. 1995. Obesity damages your health. *Feedback Newsletter for Nutrition Research Volunteers*. (6) Autumn 1995.

4. Bray, G.A., York, B. and De Lany, J. 1992. A survey of the opinions of obesity experts on the causes and treatment of obesity. *Am.J.Clin.Nutr*. 55:151S–4S.

5. Blackburn, G.L., Wilson, G.T., Kanders, B.S., Stein, L.J., Lavin, P.T., Adler, J., Brownell, K.D. 1989. Weight cycling: the experience of human dieters. *Am.J.Clin.Nutr*. 49: 1105–1109.

6. Goodrick, G.K. and Foreyt, J.P. 1991. Why treatments for obesity don't last. *J.Am.Diet.Assoc*. 91 (10):1243–1247.

7. Pace, P.W., Bolton, M.P., Reeves, R.S. 1991. Ethics of obesity treatment: Implications for dieticians. *J.Am.Diet.Assoc*. 91 (10): 1258–1260.

8. Lustig, A. 1991. Weight loss programmes: Failing to meet ethical standards. *J.Am.Diet.Assoc*. 91 (10):1252–1254.

9. Wooley, S.C. and Garner, D.M. 1991. Obesity treatment: The high cost of false hope. *J.Am.Diet.Assoc*. 91 (10):1248–2251.

10. Ernsberger, P. and Haskew, P. 1987. Health implications of obesity: an alternative view. *Obes. Weight Reg*. 6: 58,137.

11. Begley, C.E. 1991. Government should strengthen regulations in the weight loss industry. *J.Am.Diet.Assoc*. 91(10):1255–1257.

12. Nutrition Today Newsbreaks. 1996. Concept of dysfunctional eating proposed. *Nutrition Today*. 31 (6) November/December 1996.

13. A.D.A. Report. 1980. Position paper on the vegetarian approach to eating. *J.Am.Diet.Assoc*. 77:61–69.

14. Butrum, R.R., Clifford, C.K. and Lanza, E. 1988. NCI dietary guidelines: rationale. *Am.J.Clin.Nutr*. 48:888–95.

15. Lancet July 13, 1991. Notice board: Eating for a healthier life. *Lancet*. 338:111.

16. Jacobs, C. and Dwyer, J.T. 1988. Vegetarian children. Appropriate and inappropriate diets. *Am.J.Clin.Nutr*. 48:811–818.

17. Olson, R.E. 1995. The folly of restricting fat in the diet of children. *Nutrition Today*. 30 (6) November/December 1995

18. Bushinsky, D.A., Krieger, N.S., Geisser, D.I.,Grossman, E.B., and Coe, F.L. 1983. Effect of pH on bone calcium and proton fluxes in vitro. *Am. J. Physiol*. 245:F204–F209.

19. Williams, S.R. 1989. Nutrition and diet therapy. 6th. ed. Times Mirror/Mosby College Publishing. St. Louis.

20. Mayo Clinic Diet Manual. 1961. 3rd. ed. Philadelphia, W.B.Saunders Company.

21. Coe, F.L., Moran, E. Kavalich, A. 1976. The contribution of dietary purine over-consumption to hyperuricosuria in calcium oxalate stone-formers. *J.Chron.Dis*. 29:793.

22. Robertson, W.G., Peacock, M., Heyburn, P.J., Hanes, F.A. 1980. Epidemiological risk factors in calcium stone disease. *Scand.J.Urol.Nephrol*. 53(Suppl.):15–30.

23. Bennion, L.J., Grundy, S.M. 1978. Risk factors for the development of cholelithiasis in man. *N.Engl.J.Med*. 299:1221–7.

24. Marsh, A.G., Sanches, T.V., Michelson, O., Chaffee, F.L. and Fagal, S.M. 1988. Vegetarian lifestyle and bone mineral density. *Am.J.Clin.Nutr*. 48:837–41.

25. Wachman, A. and Bernstein, D.S. 1968. Diet and osteoporosis. *Lancet*. 1:958–9.

26. Zemel, M.B. 1988. Calcium utilization: effect of varying levels and source of dietary protein. *Am.J.Clin.Nutr*. 48:880–3.

27. Dwyer, J.T. 1988. Health aspects of vegetarian diets. *Am.J.Clin.Nutr*. 48:712–38.

28. Finch, A.M., Kasidas, G.P., Rose, G.A. 1981. Urine composition in normal subjects after oral ingestion of oxalate rich foods. *Clin.Sci*. 60:411–8.

29. Breslau, N.A., Brinkley, L. Hill, K.D., and Pak, C.Y.S. 1988. Relationship of animal protein-rich diet to kidney stone formation and calcium metabolism. *J.Clin.Endocrinol.Metab*. 66:140–146.

30. Kok, D.J., Iestra, J.A., Doorenbos, C.J. and Papapoulos, S.E. 1990. The effects of dietary excesses in animal protein and in sodium on the composition and the crystallization kinetics of calcium oxalate monohydrate in urine of healthy men. *J.Clin.Endocrinol.Metab*. 71:861–867.

31. Register, U.D. and Sonnenberg, L.M. 1973. The vegetarian diet. Scientific and practical considerations. *J.Am.Diet.A*. 62:253.

32. Hardinge, M.G., Crooks,H., and Stare, F.J. 1966. Nutritional studies of vegetarians. 5. Proteins and essential amino acids. *J.Am.Diet.A*. 48:25.

33. Whitaker, J.R. and Feeney, R.E. 1973. Enzyme inhibitors in foods. In: Committee on Food protection, Food and Nutrition Board, National Research council. Toxicants occurring naturally in foods. 2nd. ed. Washington, DC: National Academy Press.

References

34. Acosta, P.B. 1988. Availability of essential amino acids and nitrogen in vegan diets. *Am.J.Clin.Nutr.* 48:868–74.

35. American diabetes association, Inc. The American dietetic association. 1988. Nutrition Guide for professionals. Ed. M.A.Powers.

36. Green, M.L. and Harry, J. 1987. Nutrition in contemporary nursing practice. 2nd. ed. John Wiley & Sons, New York.

37. NRIND. 1986. Food composition tables 2nd. ed. South African Medical Research Council.

38. Brouk, B. 1975. Plants consumed by man. Academic Press. London.

39. Jacobs, C. and Dwyer, J.T. 1988. Vegetarian children appropriate and inappropriate diets. *Am.J.Clin.Nutr.* 48:811–8.

40. Truesdell, D.D. 1985. Feeding the vegan infant and child. *J.Am.Diet.Assoc.* 85:837–40.

41. Wood, P.J., Braaten, J.T., Scott, F.W., Riedel, D., Poste, L.M. 1990. Comparisons of viscous properties of oat and guar gum and the effects of these and oat bran on glycemic index. *J.Agric. Food Chem.* 38:753–7.

42. Cara, L., Dubois, C., Bprel, P., Armand, M., Senft, M. et al. 1992. Effect of oat bran, wheat fiber, and wheat germ on postprandial lipemia in healthy adults. *Am.J.Clin.Nutr.* 55:81–8.

43. Grant, K.I. 1993. Oat bran – panacea or placebo? *S.Afr.Med.J.* In press.

44. Holm, J. and I. Björck, 1992. Bioavailability of starch in various wheat-based bread products: evaluation of metabolic responses in healthy subjects and rate and extent of in vitro starch digestion. *Am.J.Clin.Nutr.* 55:420–9.

45. Schäfer, W. 1980. Brot backen. Otto Maier Verlag, Ravensburg, Germany.

46. Meyer, L.H. 1964. Food chemistry. Reinhold organic chemistry and biochemistry textbook series. Reinhold Publishing corporation. New York.

47. Sanders, T.A.B. 1985. Growth and development of British vegan children. *Am.J.Clin.Nutr.* 48:822–5.

48. Whittaker, J.R., Feeney, R.E. 1973. Enzyme inhibitors in food. In.: Committee on food Protection. Food and Nutrition Board, National Research Council. Toxicants occurring naturally in foods. 2nd. ed. Washington, DC: National Academic Press.

49. Gargouri, Y., Julien, R., Pieroni, G., Verger, R., Sarda, L. 1984. Studies on the inhibition of pancreatic and microbial lipases by soybean proteins. *J.Lipid Res.* 25:1214–21.

50. Savage, G.P. 1990. Nutritional value of sprouted mung beans. *Nutrition Today.* May/June: 21–24.

51. Farhangi, M., Valadon, L.R.G. 1982. Effects of acidified processing and storage on the proteins and lipids in mung bean sprouts. *J.Food Sci.* 47:1158–63.

52. Geervani, P., Theophilus, F. 1980. Effect of home processing on the protein quality of selected legumes. *J.Food.Sci.* 45:707–10.

53. Bingham, S.A. 1984. Meat, starch and non starch polysaccharides and large bowel cancer. *Am.J.Clin.Nutr.* 48:762–7.

54. Kruh, J. 1982. Effects of sodium butyrate, a new pharmacological agent, on cell in culture. *Mol.Cell.Biochem.* 42:65–82.

55. Mc Burney, M.I., Horvath, P.J., Jeraci, J.L., Van Soest, P.J. 1985. Effect of in vivo fermentation using human faecal inoculum on the water holding capacity of dietary fibre. *Br. J. Nutr.* 53:17–24.

56. Bingham, S.A. 1996. Epidemiology and mechanisms relating diet to risk of colorectal cancer. *Nutrition Research Review* (1996), 9: 197-239.

57. Erdman, J.W. and Fordyce, E.J. 1989. Soy products and the human diet. *Am.J.Clin.Nutr.* 49:725–737.

58. Graf, E. and Eaton, J.W. 1990. Antioxidant function of phytic acid. *Free Radical Biol.Med.*8: 61–69.

59. Anderson, J.W., Story. L., Sieling, B., Chen, W-J.L., Petro, M.S., Story, G. 1984. Hypocholesterolemic effects of oat-bran or bean intake for hypercholesterolemic men. *Am.J.Clin.Nutr.* 40:1146–55.

60. Anderson, J.W. 1985. Cholesterol-lowering effect of canned beans for hypercholesterolemic men. *Clin.Res.* 33:871A (abstr)

61. Anderson, J.W., and Gustafson, N.J. 1988. Hypocholesterolemic effect of oat and bean products. *Am.J.Clin.Nutr.* 48:749 53.

62. Smith, M.V. 1988. Development of a quick reference guide to accommodate vegetarianism in diet therapy for multiple disease conditions. *Am.J.Clin.Nutr.* 48:906–9.

63. Akinyele, I.O. and Abudu. I.A. 1990. Acceptability and nutrient content of milk substitutes from four cultivars of cowpeas (Vignia unguiculata). *J. Food. Sci.* 55:701–702,707.

64. Messina, M. and Messina, V. 1991. Increasing use of soyfoods and their potential role in cancer prevention. *J.Am.Diet.Assoc.* 91(7):836–840.

65. Slavin, J. 1991. Nutritional benefit of soy

protein and soy fiber. *J.Am.Diet.Assoc*. 91:816–819

66. Messina, M. and Barnes, S. 1991. The role of soy products in reducing cancer risk. *J.Natl. Cancer.Inst*. 83:541–546.

67. Carroll, K.K. 1991. Review of clinical studies on cholesterol-lowering response to soy protein. *J.Am.Diet.Assoc*. 91:820-827.

68. Herbert, V. 1988. Vitamin B-12: plant sources, requirements and assay. *Am.J.Clin.Nutr*. 48:852–858.

69. Xie, Z.L. and Fretzdorff, B. 1992. Optimierung des Blanchierens von Sojabohnen bezüglich Lipoxygenase-Inaktivierung und Proteinlöslichkeit zur Herstellung von Sojamilch. *Z.Lebensm.-Unters. Forsch*. 194(1):43–46.

70. Omura, Y. and Takechi, H. 1990. Effect of hot water treatment on flavour of soymilk. *J.Jap. Soc.Sci.and Techn*. 37(4):278–280.

71. Fourie, P.C., Basson, D.S. 1990. Application of a rapid transestirification method for identification of individual fatty acids by gas chromatography on three different nuts. *J.Amer.Oil Chem. Soc*. 67(1):18–20.

72. Spiller, G. 1991. Recent nutrition research on almonds. *Europ. Food Drink Rev*. 46:48,50.

73. Ahn, C.Y., Hyun, K.H. Park, K.H. 1992. Investigation of antioxidant substances in black sesame seeds. *Korean J.Food Sci.and Technol*. 24(1):31–36.

74. Hirose, N., Inoue, T. Nishihara, K. et.al. 1991. Inhibition of cholesterol absorption and synthesis in rats by sesamin. *J.Lipid Res*. 32(4):629–638.

75. Young, C.K. and Cunningham, S. 1991. Exploring the partnership of almonds with cereal foods. *Cereal Foods World*. 36(5):412,414–415,417–418.

76. Duxbury, D.D. 1992. Pistachios – snack nuts now healthy ingredients. *Food processing. USA* 53:(2):92–93.

77. California Walnut Commission, USA, 1991. The California Walnut – the wonder nut. *Food Trade Rev*. 61(1):25–72.

78. Pisani, P. Berrino, F. Macaluso, M. et al. 1986. Carrots, green vegetables and lung cancer: a case study. *Int. J. Epidemol*. 15:463–8.

79. Kvale, G. Bjelke, E., Gart, J.J. 1979. Dietary habits and lung cancer. *Int. J. Cancer*. 62:1435-8.

80. Hemeda, H.M. and Klein, B.P. 1990. Effects of naturally occurring antioxidants on peroxidase activity of vegetable extracts. *J.Food Sci*. 55:184–185,192.

81. Zhang, Y.S., Talalay, P., Cho., C.G., Posner, G.H. 1992. A major inducer of anti-carcinogenic protective enzymes from broccoli: isolation and elucidation of structure. *Proc.Nat.Acad.Sci.USA*. 89(6):2399–2403.

82. Caragay, A.B. 1992. Cancer-preventive foods and ingredients. Food Tech. April 1992

83. Sestofft, L. 1983. *Fructose and health. Nutrition Update*, 1:39–54.

84. Swanson, J.E., Laine, D.C./ Thomas, W., Bantle, J.P. 1992. Metabolic effects of dietary fructose in healthy subjects. *Am.J.Clin.Nutr*. 55:851–856.

85. Scrimshaw, N.S. Nutrition and health from womb to tomb. *Nutrition Today*. 31 (2) March/April. 1996.

86. Spiller, G.A. 1991. Health effects of Mediterranean diets and monounsaturated fats. *Cereal Foods World*. 36(9):812–814.

87. Doll, R. and Peto, R. 1981. The causes of cancer: quantitative estimates of avoidable risks of cancer in the United States today. *JNCI*. 66:1191-308.

88. Fraser, G.E. 1981. The effect of various vegetable supplements on serum cholesterol. *Am.J. Clin.Nutr*. 34:1272–7.

89. Bakhsh, R., Khan, S. 1990. Influence of onions (Allium cepa) and chaunga (Caraluma tubercula) on serum cholesterol, triglycerides, total lipids in human subjects. *Sarhad J. of Agriculture*. 6(5):425–428.

90. Pither, R. Hall, M.N. 1990. Analytical survey of the nutritional composition of organically grown fruits and vegetables. *Technical memorandum, Campden Food & Drink Research Association*. 597:99 pp.

91. Albrecht, J.A., Schafer, H.W., Zottola, E.A. 1990. Relationship of total sulphur to initial and retained ascorbic acid in selected cruciferous and noncruciferous vegetables. *J.Food. Sci*. 55:181-183

Part 3

Applying the concept

Chapter 8
Guidelines and Recipes

Introduction

This section is not a recipe book as such, but merely a compilation of a few very basic ideas and recipes to help the reader get acquainted with a whole food lifestyle. Lifestyle changes should be well thought through and should be introduced gradually to enable the body to adapt. If animal products and free fats are to be replaced in the diet, then acceptable alternative foods, prepared in such a way that taste is not sacrificed, must be supplied. Moreover, the new diet must allow for flexibility, as the needs of different individuals vary. People tending towards obesity would have to limit the quantities of foods rich in fats, whereas the opposite is true for people with a low BMI. Free fats and oils and all animal products have been omitted from the recipes in this section, but taste is not sacrificed. Eating, after all is one of the pleasures of life, and healthy food should not be synonymous with drab food. The omission of free fats calls for ingenuity, but that fried taste can still be obtained by employing different techniques; e.g. onions browned in a little soy sauce also impart a rich flavour.

Some of the recipes described here are designed to meet the demands of a Western lifestyle without the associated pitfalls, and as such may require the use of some basic household equipment and the gourmet may even require some sophisticated appliances. Whole food cooking can however be very simple, requiring the minimum in terms of equipment. Not all people can afford the appliances, to process some of the foods described here, and some of the more expensive ingredients, such as nuts, can be replaced by cheaper alternatives such as seeds and certain legumes. Where recipes call for the use of a blender, it is possible to make the dishes discussed equally interesting and healthful by using legume and grain flours or cooked and mashed whole foods. This simple lifestyle makes even camping and hiking a lot easier – no more fuss about keeping perishables frozen, and what can be more pleasant, satisfying and nutritious than a freshly-baked pot bread baked in the camp-fire eaten together with a rich pot-casserole. It only requires a pan or even a flat iron sheet to bake flapjacks and other interesting foods over the coals.

Finally, the recipes described are, wherever possible, quick and easy to prepare, particularly once one is organized. Some of the criticisms against healthful cooking practices are that they are expensive and time-consuming. As far as the first of these criticisms is concerned, it must be remembered that some of the more expensive items such as the nuts are used to replace equally expensive animal products, but that there is no wastage. Moreover, the nutritive value on a weight-for-weight basis exceeds that of animal products, and one uses small quantities to achieve one's objectives. A small quantity of nuts will make a large quantity of nut milk or sauce, and the overall expense of cooking with whole foods will indeed be considerably less than that of conventional cooking. As regards the second criticism, it is indeed so that there is more to life than slaving over a hot stove.

Hopefully, the hints and recipes described will not only make cooking an enjoyable experience, but will also enable the "busy" people to adopt this lifestyle.

Useful equipment

1. A good blender
2. A heavy-base or non-stick frying pan
3. Waterless cookware
4. Optional: waffle iron
5. Optional: food processor (flat blade variety) to chop nuts and seeds till "butter" is formed
6. Optional: wheat mill.

Basic shopping list

Unfortunately, healthy foods are not always readily available in supermarkets and conventional stores and some health shops can be very expensive. Don't despair, do some detective work – if there are some Middle Eastern or Eastern communities in your country, they will have stores where whole foods can be bought in bulk at very reasonable prices. Moreover, many farming cooperatives and farm outlets supply many of the foods required, and it is also possible to purchase some foods directly from processing factories or factory outlets. Fortunately, the tide is turning, and more and more supermarkets are catering for whole food shoppers as public demand increases.

Shopping list

1. **Stone-ground wheat flour** (large quantity)

2. Other whole-ground flours, e. g. rye, millet, barley, corn, soy, garbanzo (chick pea), rice (small quantities)

3. **Whole grains:** barley, millet (dehusked!), brown rice, groats (dehusked whole oats) and also rolled oats, cracked wheat (bulgur) etc.

4. **Legumes:** soy beans, chick peas, mung beans (for stews and sprouts), lentils, other varieties of beans, split peas, peanuts

5. **Seeds:** sesame, sunflower, alfalfa (for sprouting), linseed, poppy seed

6. **Nuts:** cashew (pieces are cheaper), macadamia (for butter), almonds, pecan (find a wholesale supplier)

7. **Dried fruit:** raisins, sun-dried prunes, peaches, apricots, pears, apples, dates, etc. (for the lunch box, muesli, as stewed fruit or for fruit chutney or jam)

8. **Shredded coconut:** for cookies, muesli, etc.

9. **Carob powder:** for puddings, milk shakes, cookies

10. **Honey/ raw sugar/ molasses**

11. **Healthy peanut butter** (with no additives) and Tahini (sesame butter) and nut butters

12. **Agar-agar:** as a gelatine substitute

13. Concentrated fruit juice (if available): useful for puddings, ice-creams, etc.

14. **Natural vanilla essence** (from health shops)

15. **Active yeast:** for bread and cake

16. **Nutritional yeast** (food yeast): for flavouring savoury dishes. Available at health shops, and is not the same as Brewer's Yeast or Torilla Yeast.

17. **Soy Sauce** (without preservatives or other additives)

18. **Herbs**, fresh and dried

19. Some **spices**, such as coriander, cayenne pepper, paprika, cardamom, turmeric, cumin, aniseed

20. **Tinned tomato paste**/puree for sauces

21. **Olives** in brine, not vinegar

22. **Garlic** (powder and fresh)

23. **Onion powder**

24. **Gluten flour**

25. **Fresh fruits:** have a variety, but always have at hand avocados for butter, bananas for milk shakes and puddings and lemons for sauces

26. **Fresh vegetables**

27. **Tofu:** for salad dressings, omelets, quiches, etc.

List of abbreviations

c = cup
l = litre
min. = minutes
t = teaspoon
T = tablespoon
pkt = packet

Recipe table of contents

A. Bread 215

    Perfect whole wheat bread 216
    Pot bread 217
    Pita bread 218
    Easy no-knead bread 218
    Mealie (corn) bread 219
    Savoury sweet bagels 219
    Muffins 220

B. Spreads 221

    Millet spread 221
    Cheesy spread 222
    Breakfast butter 222
    Date spread 222
    Easy jam 223
    Savoury spread 223
    Mock Leberwurst 224

C. Sauces 225

    Nut mayonnaise 225
    Tofu mayonnaise 225
    Soy mayonnaise 226
    Garbanzo (chick pea) mayonnaise 226
    Tartare sauce 226
    Tomato and onion sauce 227
    Quick Tomato sauce 227
    Pink sauce 228
    "Thousand island dressing" 228
    Dried fruit chutney 228
    Pimento cream sauce 229
    Chick pea cream sauce 229
    Brown gravy 230
    Mushroom sauce 230

Simple sour cream	230
Substitute chocolate sauce	231
Easy fruit sauce	231
Substitute custard	231
Orange sauce	232

D. Milks and Creams 233

Soy concentrate	234
Soy milk	235
Nut milk	235
Coconut milk	236
Sesame milk	236
Milk shakes	236
Sweet soy cream	237
Sour soy cream	237
Sweet nut cream	237

E. Breakfast 239

Groats porridge	240
Muesli	240
Delicious creamy Muesli	241
Granola	242
Breakfast pudding	243
Putu	243
Soy waffles	244
Sunflower seed waffles	244
Savoury breakfast	245

F. Main meals 247

1. Casseroles and stews 247

Bean stroganoff	248
Garbanzo-A-La-King	249
Lentils Bolognaise	249
Moussaka	250

2. Patties and loaves 250

| Basic recipe | 251 |
| Potato balls | 252 |

3. Cheesy dishes ... 252

Lasagne ... 252
Sesamsan "cheese" ... 253
Pizza ... 253
Fondue ... 253
Cannelloni ... 254

4. Quiches, Pies and other Tofu dishes ... 255

Scrambled Tofu ... 255
Tofu cottage cheese ... 256
Baked Tofu ... 256
Tofu omelet ... 256
Soy omelet ... 257
Onion quiche ... 257

5. Miscellaneous ... 258

Bulgur Pilavi ... 258
Kisir ... 258
Baked potato dish ... 259
Vegetables ... 259
Fruits ... 260

G. *Desserts and cookies* ... 261

Fruit sponge ... 261
Carob sponge ... 262
No-bake tofu cheesecake ... 262
Basic pie crust ... 263
Easy apple crumble ... 264
Apple cake ... 264
Carob millet pudding ... 265
Milk tart ... 266
Ice-cream ... 266
Pancakes/flapjacks (crêpes) ... 267
Easy pancakes ... 267
Cookies ... 268
Coconut cookies ... 268
Carob oat cookies ... 269

Basic Recipes

A. Bread

Right through the ages bread has formed an important part of the human diet. With today's refining of flours and harmful chemical additions to most breads, bread has lost its original meaning and healthful qualities. With a little practice bread can be provided for the family which will be highly nutritious. Instead of a cooked meal with vegetables the table can be set with home-baked bread, nut butter, avocado, sprouts, home-made jam, honey, healthy peanut butter, a bean or lentil spread (for balanced protein) and a large bowl of fresh fruit, served with a delicious nut or other cream. And if the bread is baked with stone-ground flours, one can rest assured that the family is getting a meal that will supply natural fibres and nutrients in balanced proportions. By introducing such meals on a regular basis, one can save time, as the time will not be spent cooking elaborate meals.

When making bread, one must remember that all flours do not absorb the same amount of water – a fine flour will absorb more moisture than a coarse flour. If one decides to add some rye flour, rice, millet, soy flour etc., this may affect the moisture balance, and adjustments to the amounts of water may have to be made, depending on the quality of the flour. One should always add a little less water than the recipes requires and test first. Bread baked from stone-ground flour has better keeping qualities than one might expect, and can still be perfectly edible after three days. To save time, a number of loaves can be baked simultaneously and some of these stored in the refrigerator and freezer for later use.

Finally, there is a tendency in health food circles to bake bread that contains virtually everything that is required for a balanced meal. Loaves will thus contain numerous grains, legume flours, and other ingredients that will make them "health loaves". It should be remembered, that each addition to wheat flour will affect the quality of the loaf, and some "health loaves" can become so dense and heavy as to be a positive health hazard. If a varied diet is followed, there is no need to bake fully balanced meals into one bread, as the other nutrients will be supplied by the other foods consumed. A simple, light loaf of bread need therefore not be shunned.

Perfect whole-wheat bread

The following recipe is only a basic recipe. For a more balanced protein content, replace not more than 1/3 of the wheat flour with any other grain flour(s). Legume flours can also be added in very small amounts, about 1/2 c to every 1 kg grain flour.

Mix:

1 kg	stone-ground whole-wheat flour (approximately 10 c)
1 pkt	instant active yeast (10 g or 1 T)
1 1/2 T	salt

Blend:

900 ml	warm water
1	apple (optional)
1/2 c	raisins or 1T raw brown sugar/honey/molasses

Add the liquid to the dry ingredients and mix well with a wooden spoon. Turn out onto a floured surface and divide into two parts. If you have a mixer with a dough hook, this will make the kneading much easier, but if not, knead each half with a rolling action, adding more flour to the surface to prevent sticking. If the dough is getting too firm, dip hands into warm water when necessary and knead without flouring the surface. Keep on kneading until the dough can be pulled apart like chewing gum without breaking. This is probably the most important step, since the bread will not be a success if the gluten has not been developed during the kneading process. Place into large bowl, cover and let rise till double in size in a warm place, knead down, shape into 2 loaves and place in bread pans (greased lightly with cold-pressed olive oil or sprayed with a lecithin spray). Let rise till almost double (but not high above top rim, or you will not have a nicely rounded bread but one with a dip in the middle). Bake at 220 °C for 10 min., then at 200 °C for the next 10 min., then at 180 °C (350 °F) for the last 30 min. (or more if the bread pans are large).

Remember to pre-heat the oven to at least 240 °C to compensate for loss of heat when placing bread in the oven.

Variations:

This same recipe can be used to make **Pizza dough**, or **whole-wheat rolls** for hamburgers. The dough may also be sweetened with dates, raisins or bananas for a **banana bread**. For a German-style **rye bread**, use 1/3 fine rye flour and 2/3 stone-ground wheat flour and use less water (about 800 ml). Do not place dough in bread pans, but shape into round or oblong shapes, place on greased cookie sheet and cut 1 cm deep cross-wise cuts into top of bread before letting it rise for the last time.

Pot bread
(for the camp-fire)

Make the fire with hard wood that will yield good lasting coals. While waiting for the coals, make up a 1 kg batch of **Perfect Whole-wheat Bread**, using a large mixing bowl to do the kneading in. Let rise next to the fire (may rise more than once). Just before the fire is ready, place the dough in a well-sprayed or oiled flat-based cast iron camping pot, the top rim diameter being about 32 cm. If you have a smaller pot, make up less dough. Let rise by the fire with the lid on till double in size. Work carefully with the pot, since jolts could affect the rising of the bread. Place pot on a tripod about 15 cm above the coals and place one layer of coals on top of lid for heat from the top and the bottom (not too much heat from the bottom, or else the base of the bread will be burnt black). Bake bread for about 50 min., checking and replacing coals when too cold. The baking procedure will take some practice but your efforts will be rewarded, since this bread excels in flavour and texture.

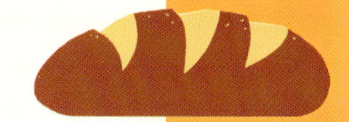

Pita bread
(for the camp-fire or at home in the oven)

Make up 1/2 kg of **Perfect Whole-wheat Bread**, divide into equal sections and roll little balls about the size of golf balls. Flatten, keeping hands well-floured. Place on kitchen towels – the bonnet of your car makes a good table – and let rise for 15 min. Bake on flat cast iron surface over the fire or over a gas cooker. Leave pitas for a few minutes on one side till they puff up, then turn and do the other side. When eating, cut a small slit in the side and stuff your favourite filling into the bread "pocket", e.g. patty, lettuce, sauce and tomato, or even peanut butter and honey. At home, bake pitas in a very hot oven (240 °C /460 °F) till they puff up.

Easy no-knead raisin bread

1) Mix and let stand:

1 c	warm water
2 pkts	yeast (2 T)

2) Cook till soft or blend the dates with hot water

4 c	water
1/2 c	dates

3) Mix:

7 c	whole-wheat flour
2 c	oatmeal
1/2 c	sesame seeds
1/2 c	walnuts (sunflower seeds or other nuts)
1 c	raisins
2 T	salt

Mix 2) and 3) lightly, then add 1). Makes a soft dough. Spoon into baking pans and let rise to top of pans. Bake at 200 °C for 10 min., then at 180 °C for 30–35 min.

Mealie (corn) bread

1) Blend:

1 c	warm water
1 pkt	yeast
1 T	honey
1 tin	sweetcorn (or 1 c frozen – warm first!)

2) Mix:

2 1/2 c	whole-wheat flour
1 1/2 c	cornflour
1 c	wheat-germ
2 t	salt

Mix 1 and 2 together and knead well. Let rise till double and bake at 190 °C (about 375 °F) for 35 min.

Savoury-sweet bagels

1) Beat:

2 T	yeast
3 c	whole-wheat flour
1 1/2 c	warm water (or 1 c water, 1/2 c tomato juice)
3 T	honey
1 T	salt

2) Add to above mixture:

1	chopped onion
1 T	chives or parsley

3) Bring to boil (in large pot):

4 l	water
1 T	honey

4) Extra flour, about 1 cup

Beat 1) and 2) for 3 min. at high speed. Add about 1 cup flour to make a fairly stiff dough. Knead again 3 min. Let rise 15 min., then cut into 12 portions and shape into smooth balls. Punch a hole into middle with finger and pull gently to enlarge hole. Cover, let rise 20 min. Drop bagels gently into simmering water, 4 at a time and cook for 7 min, turning once. Drain and place on cookie sheet. Bake at 190 °C (375 °F) for 30 to 40 min.

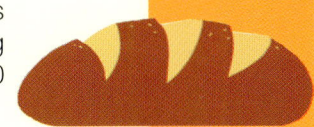

Variations:
This same recipe can be used to make **dumplings** or a form of pasta, called **Spätzle** in German. For dumplings, shape the dough into small balls, let rise for 20 min. and cook in same way in the boiling water. For Spätzle, cut the dough into small strips about the length of one's small finger, but thinner, let rise and cook in the water. Cooking time will be less than for bagels. No need to bake in oven, just drain and serve with your favourite sauce or gravy.

Muffins

2 c	whole-wheat flour
2 c	wheat-germ
1 T	soy flour
4 t	active yeast
6 T	honey
2 t	salt
2 1/2 c	warm water
1/3 c	raisins
1/3 c	chopped dates

Mix all ingredients gently with folding action. Fill muffin tins 2/3 full and let rise for 10 min. Bake at 165 °C (325 °F) for 10–15 min.

B. Spreads

If you have decided to eliminate butter and margarine from your diet, but you like the oily texture, a great substitute is nut or seed butter. Tahini (sesame seed butter), sunflower seed and almond butter can be bought at some health stores, but they are normally quite expensive. To make your own butters you will need a food processor which chops nuts and seeds at such a high speed, that the oil is pressed out and a rich smooth butter is formed. The macadamia nut has the highest oil content and is therefore excellent for butter-making. If, however, you do not have the equipment, substitute butter and spreads can be made with your blender.

Millet spread

Cook together till soft

1 c	millet (dehusked)
1/2 t	salt
1/4 t	turmeric
4 c	water

Blend till smooth

2 c	hot cooked millet
2/3 c	water

(optional: 2/3 c shredded coconut)

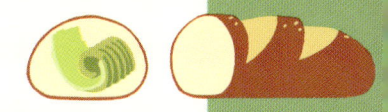

Cheesy spread

Prepare in the same way as for Pimento Cream Sauce (see section on sauces), except use only 2 cups of water instead of 3.

Breakfast butter

This butter can be made from any left-over grain porridge: corn meal, oats, millet, rice, etc.

1 c	cooked millet or other cooked grain
1 c	boiling water
1/4 c	cold water
2 t	agar-agar powder (2 T flakes)
1/4 c	cashews/sunflower seeds
1 T	lemon juice
1/4 t	turmeric (for yellow colour)

Measure agar and 1/4 c water into blender and soak for 1 min. Pour the boiling water into the blender and blend to dissolve. Add all remaining ingredients and blend till very smooth. Pour into rectangular plastic container, chill well. To serve, bend sides of container slightly and slide the block of "butter" onto a serving dish. Your guests will be surprised at this clever substitute.

Variations:

Add garlic and onion for garlic butter, herbs and food yeast for herb butter, or leave out lemon juice and add some honey, dates or raw sugar for a sweet spread or pie filling (see Milk Tart in the section on Desserts).

Date spread

Useful for sweetening breakfast cereals and as a sweet spread on bread.

1 c pitted dates
1 c hot water

Pour the hot water onto the dates in the blender, let soak a little and blend. Without blender, the dates can be cooked in the water till soft and then mashed.

Variations:

Add a quarter cup carob powder, 1/2 c peanut butter and a few drops of vanilla essence for a chocolate-flavoured spread.

Easy jam

Who says jams have to be cooked for hours! Make delicious jams by cooking the fruit gently till soft and adding enough dates to sweeten, then cook together for a few more minutes, mash fruit and dates with a potato masher or in food processor. Berries, especially mulberries, make an excellent jam.

Savoury spread

Can be made from any cooked legumes, e.g. beans, chick peas, lentils. This is where a food processor comes in handy. Also nice as a dip when blended with one of the mayonnaises in the section on sauces.

1 c	cooked, mashed (preferably in food processor) soy beans, chick peas or other legume
1/2 t	salt
1/2 t	sweet basil
1/2 t	oregano
1 T	tomato paste
1/8 t	garlic powder or small clove fresh garlic
1/2 c	finely chopped onion
2 T	finely chopped celery
1 t	food yeast

Mix all ingredients well. Use for sandwiches, on toast and in cooked savoury dishes.

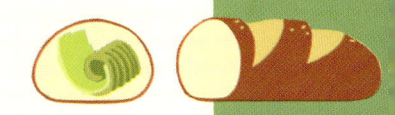

Mock "Leberwurst"
(substitute liver paté)

1 c	cooked lentils
3/4 c	stiff, cold, cooked oat porridge
1/2	finely chopped onion
2 t	marjoram
1	large clove garlic
	salt to taste

Chop lentils, garlic and marjoram till smooth in food processor. Add oats, onion and salt and blend briefly till mixed. (The oats and onion must not be smooth, since they give the "Leberwurst" its texture.) Use as spread on bread.

C. Sauces

In this section both fruit- and vegetable-compatible sauces are discussed. It is important to note that if whole fruits or vegetables are used in the recipes, then the sauce is only compatible with either the fruits or the vegetables. The juice of a lemon, herbs, garlic, onion salt can be used with both fruits or vegetables without ill effect.

Nut "Mayonnaise"

1/2 c	cashews (or sunflower seeds)
1 c	water
1/8 t	garlic powder (or fresh garlic)
1/4 t	onion powder
1/2 t	salt
	juice of 1/2 lemon
	(honey or raw sugar for sweet-sour taste)

Blend cashews in water till smooth and cook in sauce-pan till thick. Let cool a little, add lemon juice, (honey), salt, garlic and onion powder.

Tofu "Mayonnaise"

2 c	soft Tofu
1/4 c	water
1 t	onion salt
1/8 t	garlic powder
1/4 c	lemon juice
	(honey or raw sugar to taste)

Blend or beat all ingredients well together.

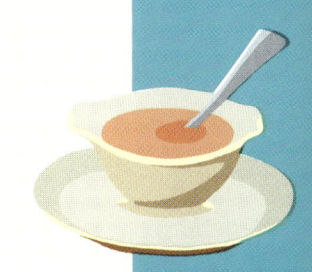

Soy "Mayonnaise"

3 c	water
3 T	corn flour
2 c	rich soy milk (see Creams and Milks)
2 c	cashews
3/4 c	lemon juice
1 T	salt
2 t	garlic powder
	(honey or raw sugar for sweet-sour taste)

Make a paste with corn flour and a little water. Add the rest of the 3 c of water or soy milk and cook till thick. Blend rest of ingredients in blender and add to the corn flour mixture. Mix well and chill.

Garbanzo (chick pea) "Mayonnaise"

1 c	soaked raw garbanzos
2 c	water
1	clove garlic
1 t	onion powder
1 t	salt
1/4 c	lemon juice
	herbs, e.g. dill
	(honey for sweet-sour taste)

Blend garbanzos, garlic, onion powder, salt and herbs with half of the water till smooth, add rest of the water and cook till thick. Let cool slightly, then add the lemon juice and honey and mix well. A dash of turmeric will give a soft yellow colour.

Tartare sauce

Add finely chopped raw onion or spring onion, green pepper, parsley, olives, and cucumber to any of the "Mayonnaises".

Tomato and onion sauce

Cooking procedure:

The onions are not fried in oil, but cooked in about 2 T of soy sauce (for 4 medium onions) and about 1 T of water, in a frying pan with the lid on, till all the fluid has been absorbed. Brown the onions uncovered a few minutes longer on high, stirring frequently, then add chopped tomatoes, pinch of oregano, thyme, basil, some crushed garlic and salt to taste. Cover with lid and simmer on low till cooked. Sweeten with brown sugar or honey for a tangy taste. Thicken with corn flour or other flour if necessary.

Quick tomato sauce
(for burgers, pizza, etc.)

1 can/tin	of tomato puree
10	pitted dates, softened in a little boiling water
1/2 t	onion powder
1 t	salt
	paprika
	pinch of basil, oregano

Blend all ingredients together till smooth.

The Quick Tomato Sauce should be used at a **fruit-based** meal, since the dates could cause gas-formation when eaten in large amounts together with vegetables. Use honey in the place of dates and thicken with some cooked corn flour and water (see **Soy "Mayonnaise"**) when needed for a vegetable patty (burger) or roast.

Example:

On a hamburger roll one may have the following fruit-compatible foods: avocado or nut/seed butter; a patty made without vegetables (small quantities of onion and garlic powder are not considered vegetables, but flavourants); Quick Tomato Sauce, any of the Mayonnaises, or Dried Fruit Chutney; lettuce; cucumber; sliced tomato; sliced pineapple. This hamburger may now be eaten together with a fruit salad or an apple pie and nut cream without any ill effects.

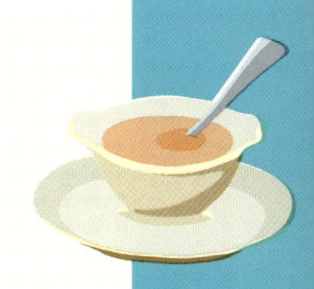

Pink sauce

1/2 c	Quick Tomato Sauce (for fruit meal)
or	Tomato and Onion Sauce (for vegetable meal)
1 c	nut/seed, chick pea or Soy Mayonnaise

Blend everything well together. Adjust the taste if necessary for salads or burgers, or blend tomato sauce with some cashew nuts till smooth if Mayonnaise is not available.

"Thousand island dressing"

Add chopped onion, garlic, green peppers, red bell peppers, olives, cucumber, and celery to **Pink Sauce**.

Dried fruit chutney

2 c	soaked mixed dried fruit (e.g. prunes, apricots, peaches)
5 c	cold water
1/2 t	salt
1/2 t	mixed herbs
good pinch of cayenne pepper (optional)	
good pinch of cumin	
2 T	lemon juice (omit if apricots are used)
1 T	soy sauce

Wash dried fruit well in a bowl. Most dried fruit has been treated with sulphur dioxide. If untreated fruit is unavailable, soak for an hour, wash well and discard the water. Now soak fruit in fresh water overnight, remove the pips from the prunes, bring to boil for a few minutes and blend 1 cup of the fruit with enough of the same water used for soaking (about 2/3 cup), or use fruit juice to blend easily. Add all ingredients, blend. Lastly add rest of fruit and blend very briefly for a chunky chutney. To preserve, bring to boiling point once again, pour into sterilized bottles and seal. Refrigerate after opening.

Pimento cream sauce
("cheese" sauce)

2 c	cashews or sunflower seeds
3 c	water or more
1/2	onion
1/8 t	garlic powder/fresh garlic
1 t	food yeast
1 T	chopped parsley/celery/ herbs (optional)
1/2-1	pimento (red bell pepper)
1/4 c	lemon juice
1 t	salt (or to taste)

Blend all ingredients together, except lemon juice and parsley. Cook till thick, then add lemon and parsley. For a white sauce on broccoli or cauliflower, omit the pimento and lemon juice.

Chick pea cream sauce

2 c	cooked chick peas
1 1/2 c	soy or nut milk
2 t	food yeast
1/2	onion
	salt to taste

or

1 c	raw soaked chick peas
2 t	food yeast
2 1/2 c	water/ milk
1/2	onion
1 t	salt

For the cooked chick peas, blend all ingredients together, warm in a saucepan and serve; for the raw chick peas, blend together, pour into saucepan and simmer for 5 min. Serve.

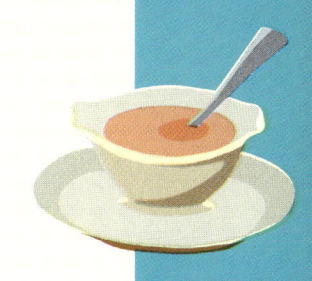

Brown gravy

2 c	water
1/3 c	whole-wheat or barley flour
1	onion
3 T	soy sauce
1 t	food yeast
	salt to taste

Brown flour gently in saucepan. Blend all ingredients together and cook over low heat for 5-10 min.

Simple sour cream

2 c	sunflower seeds
3 c	water
1-2	cloves garlic
	juice of 1 1/2 lemons
1 t	salt

Blend everything well together till the cream is white and smooth.

Mushroom sauce

Brown some onions and mushrooms in a little soy sauce. When cooked add soy concentrate and thicken with corn flour; or add thin cashew nut cream (about 1 c cashews blended with 2–3 c water). Flavour to taste.

Substitute chocolate sauce

Delicious over home-made soft serve ice-cream, Carob Millet Pudding or Rich Fruit Cake (see section on desserts).

3/4 c	tightly packed pitted dates
2 c	boiling water
1/4 c	honey or 3 T raw brown sugar
1/4 c	carob powder
	a few drops natural vanilla
1/4 t	salt
	(optional: 1 t grain coffee (a coffee substitute)

Soak the dates for a few minutes in the boiling water, then blend. Add remaining ingredients and blend till smooth.

Substitute custard

5 T	maize flour (heaped)
5 c	rich soy or nut milk
	dash of salt
1/4 t	turmeric
	honey or other sweetener to taste

Blend all ingredients in blender and pour into sauce-pan. Bring to boil, stirring constantly. Cool and serve.

Easy fruit sauce

Canned fruit
(e.g. peaches, apricots, berries, cherries)

Honey or concentrated juice
(e.g. pineapple, granadilla)

Blend fruit in their own juice and sweeten with honey or concentrated juice. May be heated gently before serving over desserts or ice-cream. Blending bananas with the fruit will make the sauce rich and thick.

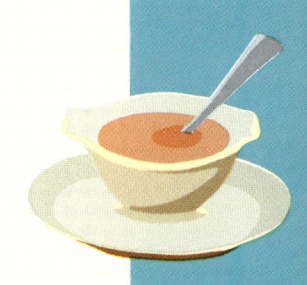

Orange sauce

2 T	corn flour
1 c	water
1 c	concentrated pineapple or orange juice
1 T	honey
	grated rind of 1 lemon or half an orange

Make a paste with the corn flour and a little of the water, add the rest of the water and cook till thick. Add remaining ingredients and heat gently.

Variations:

For a thick **apple sauce** use fresh, peeled apple pieces (2 apples) and simmer till cooked. Place in blender and blend with 1/2 cup pineapple concentrate and 1/2 cup water. Add together with only 1/2 t of lemon rind to the cooked corn flour and heat. For **strawberry** or **cherry sauce** use fresh or canned juice, add honey and cook in the same way as for Orange Sauce.

Guidelines and Recipes

D. Milks and Creams

The value of the soy bean in preparing a dairy milk substitute in the western world was discovered in the early 1930s, but soy milk has only recently been re-discovered and marketed in some countries. If you cannot obtain the milk in canned, frozen or powdered form, it can easily be made at home. The recipe for **Soy Concentrate** will form the basis for milk and cream.

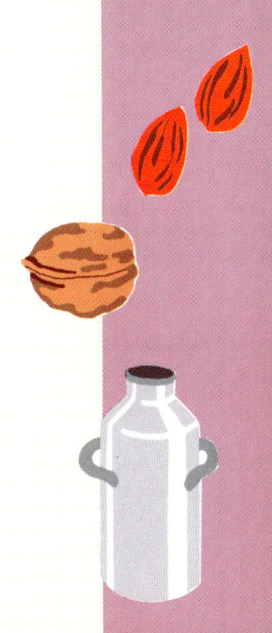

Soy concentrate

3 c	soaked raw soy beans (warm, not frozen)
4 c	boiling water

Blend beans in boiling water till very fine. (If your blender cannot handle boiling water, use hot water.) Pour into a fine-mesh cloth and let drain into a bowl. Meanwhile blend another batch and repeat procedure. Squeeze through cloth and turn pulp left in the cloth out into a separate bowl, add 2 cups cold water for every batch (= 2 c cold to 4 c boiling water used), mix well and return pulp to cloth and squeeze out as much fluid as possible. Discard the left-over dry pulp and boil the concentrated milk, stirring constantly for 10 min. (to prevent burning) or 5 min. in microwave. Watch carefully – it boils over easily! Some soy bean recipes in the literature leave out this final cooking procedure, but raw soy beans contain secondary compounds, which are destroyed during cooking. Some people react negatively (especially children) if the concentrate is not cooked. The Soy concentrate may be used in the concentrated form in various dishes, but has to be converted to soy milk for breakfast cereals etc.

1 c dried beans (150 g) = 2,5 c soaked = 850 ml soy concentrate = about 4 cups

Soy milk

350 ml	Soy Concentrate (about 1 part)
650 ml	water (about 2 parts)
1 T	honey
1/4 t	salt
	few drops natural vanilla or coconut flavouring

Blend all ingredients well together. Soy milk can be fortified with vitamin B-12 and vitamin D by dissolving one tablet in hot water and blending with the milk.

Nut milk

1 c	almonds or macadamias (or 2/3 c cashews)
2–3 c	water
1 T	honey/or a few dates
	pinch of salt
	natural vanilla

Blend nuts and water till smooth, then add enough water to make a total of 1 litre milk. For drinking purposes the milk can be strained through a fine-mesh cloth and returned to blender to blend in the rest of the ingredients. Use the left-over pulp in porridges, puddings, breads or even in savoury patties. For milk on breakfast cereals the straining may be omitted and when using cashew nuts the milk will be fine enough to drink without straining.

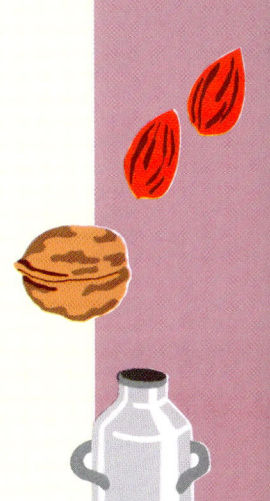

Coconut milk

1 c	shredded coconut
2 c	boiling water
2	dates (or 1T honey)
2	pinches salt

Blend all ingredients well for a few minutes. Add ice cubes and cold water to make 1 litre. Strain or use as is.

Sesame milk

1/2 c	sesame seeds
4 c	water
1/4 t	salt
	few drops of natural vanilla
	sweetener (honey, raw sugar or dates)

Blend all ingredients well for a few minutes and strain.

Milk shakes

Give yourself a treat! Blend soy, nut, sesame or coconut milk with ripe banana, strawberries, apricots or any other favourite fruit. For children this is a good way to get them to enjoy milks other than cow's milk.

Sweet soy cream

1 c	Soy Concentrate (chilled)
1 T	honey
	pinch of salt
	few drops of natural vanilla
	about 1/4 t of lemon juice

Blend first 4 ingredients well, then, blending slowly, add lemon juice to thicken. Stop blending immediately and chill. Use on puddings, fruit salad, especially good on warm apple pie.

Sour soy cream
(good on baked potatoes, even as salad dressing)

1 c	Soy Concentrate (chilled)
1/4 t	salt
1	small clove garlic
2 t	lemon juice
	chopped parsley

Blend first 3 ingredients very well. While still blending slowly, add lemon juice to thicken. Don't blend too long, since this will reverse the thickening process. Stir in chopped parsley or other fresh garden herbs.

Sweet nut cream

Use the ingredients as given for Nut Milk but use only enough water to cover the nuts in the blender and do not strain. Blend till very smooth and serve on desserts, such as Carob Millet Pudding, Rich Fruit Cake or apple pie. Cashew nuts or macadamia nuts make excellent nut creams.

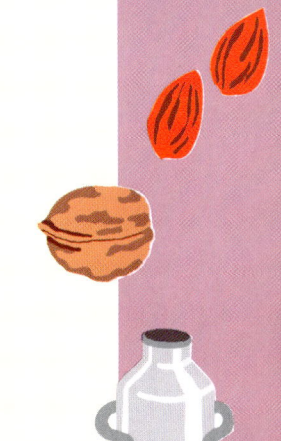

E. Breakfast

In planning your breakfast, the following list may provide you with ideas and variety:

Grains
groats (whole oats)
sorghum
mealiemeal
millet
whole-wheat kernels
ryekernels

Nuts and seeds
almonds
pecans
cashews
macadamias
sesame seeds
sunflower seeds

Fruit
fruits in season
bananas
raisins
dates
prunes

Additions to make the above complete and interesting:

soy milk
coconut
carob powder
honey
whole-wheat bread
peanut butter or nut butter

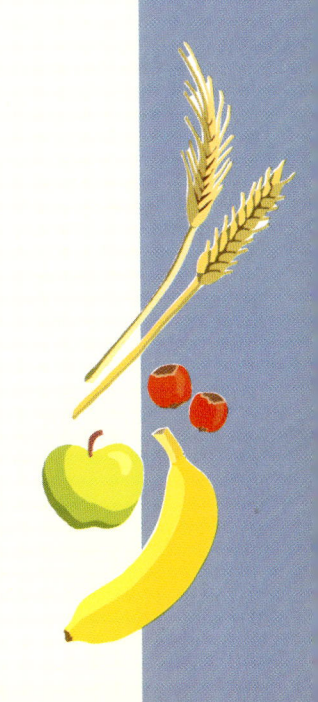

Groats porridge
(prepare the evening before)

1 c	groats (whole oat kernels)
6 c	water
	salt

Cook whole oat kernels as one would cook rice for approximately one hour, switch off, leave on stove with lid on. Next morning cook 1/2 hour till soft and fluffy. Alternatively, grind groats and cook to make a smooth porridge as one would cook commercial rolled oats.
Any of the other grains can be prepared in the same way, but it is better to cook millet just before eating it for about 40 min. (1 cup millet to 4 cups water.) Add to bowl of cooked porridge: nuts, bananas, raisins, coconut, dates/honey, carob (for chocolate flavour) and rich soy milk (home made-preferably) or nut milk.

Muesli

1 kg (14 c)	rolled oats
1 c	chopped nuts
1 c	seedless raisins
1/2 c	pumpkin seeds
1 c	chopped soft dried fruit (e.g. figs)
1 c	shredded coconut
1 c	sunflower seeds
1/2 c	sesame seeds

Toast the rolled oats under the grill, stirring frequently and watching closely. When lightly browned, spread the sunflower and sesame seeds and the coconut over the top of oats and toast lightly. Mix with all remaining ingredients. Very useful to take along on hikes and camps.

Delicious creamy muesli
(prepare the night before)

2 1/2	rolled oats
1/2 c	shredded coconut
3 c	rich soy milk or nut milk
	vanilla
1/2 t	salt
3/4 c	raisins
	juice of 1 small lemon, or to taste
3 T	honey/date spread/sugar
	diced fresh fruit
1/2 c	chopped pecans or walnuts

Prepare the oats and coconut as for **Muesli** in the oven. Blend the soy milk, vanilla, salt, lemon juice and mix well with oats, coconut and raisins and place in airtight container and refrigerate overnight. Next morning add honey or other sweetener, nuts and plenty of fresh diced fruit, e.g. bananas, peaches, papaya, melon, or any fruit in season (out of season use canned fruit) and serve cold.

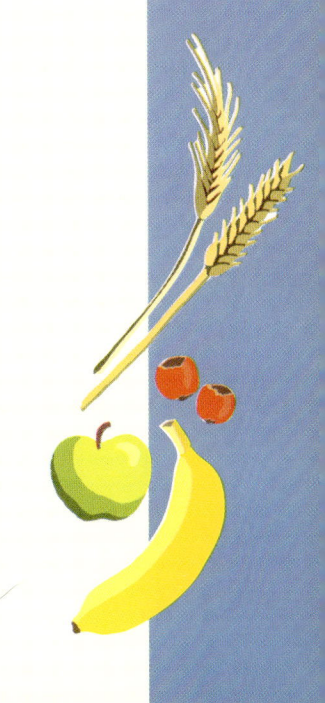

Granola

Mix well:

8 c	rolled oats
1 c	sunflower seeds
1 c	coconut
1 c	chopped nuts

Mix:

2	ripe bananas
1 1/2 c	chopped dates
1 1/2 t	salt
1/2 c	hot water
	natural vanilla

Stir the two mixtures together, spread onto cookie sheets and bake at 130 °C (250 °F) for 1 hour, stirring every half hour. Serve with soy milk, raisins, bananas etc. or with soy milkshake (see section on Milks and Creams). Also have a slice of whole-wheat toast and peanut butter, and a bowl of fruit for an energy-packed breakfast that will give you staying power.

Breakfast pudding

Blend:

1/2 c	nuts (cashews)
1 c	water/soy milk
2	bananas
2 T	honey
1 t	salt
	natural vanilla

Add above mixture to

3 1/4 c	quick oats
1/2 c	coconut
3/4 c	chopped dates
2	grated apples

Add 4 cups boiling water to above, mix thoroughly. Bake at approx. 200 °C (375–400 °F) for one hour. (Make before you go to bed and warm in oven next morning.) Serve with fruit cream (blended soy milk and bananas or other fruit) or soy cream, a nut cream (see section on Milks and Creams), or stewed fruit.

Putu

Putu is a stiff or crumbly maize meal porridge eaten by many African people.

1 3/4 c	maize meal
2 1/2 c	boiling water
3/4 t	salt

Boil water in saucepan and add salt. Place maize meal gently in a heap in the simmering water. Do not stir. Cook with lid on at low heat for 10–15 min. till skin forms. Stir to form crumbs, replace lid and cook for further 15–30 min. Stir well and serve with tomato and onion sauce or stew, or with soy/nut milk, honey and raisins for breakfast.

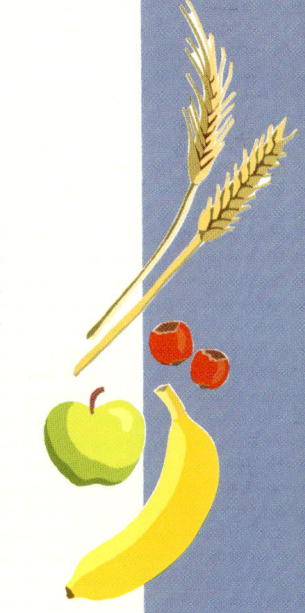

Waffles

Waffles can be made ahead of time and frozen. When needed, pop into toaster for a quick meal. Serve with Soy/Nut Cream, apple sauce with raisins, Carob Spread (see Spreads) or honey.

Soy waffles

Blend:
1 c	soaked soy beans
1 3/4 c	rolled oats
2 1/4 c	water (cold)
3/4 t	salt

Bake in hot waffle iron for approximately 8–10 min. or until waffle does not stick and is nicely browned.

Sunflower seed waffles

Blend:
2 1/2 c	water
2 1/4 c	rolled oats
1/4 c	sunflower seeds
1 t	ground sesame seeds (blend dry till fine in blender)
1 t	salt
5	chopped dates
	vanilla

Bake in hot waffle iron for approximately 8–10 min. or until waffle does not stick and is nicely browned.

Savoury breakfast

If you have one of those mornings when you do not feel like something sweet for breakfast, try the following "hay stack":

1. Brown plenty of onions in soy sauce. When cooked add mashed tofu and heat gently.
2. Make some **Chick Pea Cream Sauce** or **mushroom sauce** (see Sauces).
3. Chop tomato, lettuce, cucumber finely and avocado in larger pieces.
4. Make whole-wheat toast.

Now stack your hay stack:

First a slice of **toast**, then some of the **Chick Pea Cream Sauce**, then the **onion and tofu** mixture, followed by more **Chick Pea Sauce** and topped with the chopped **salad**. Sprinkle with **herbs, salt** and a few drops of **lemon juice**.

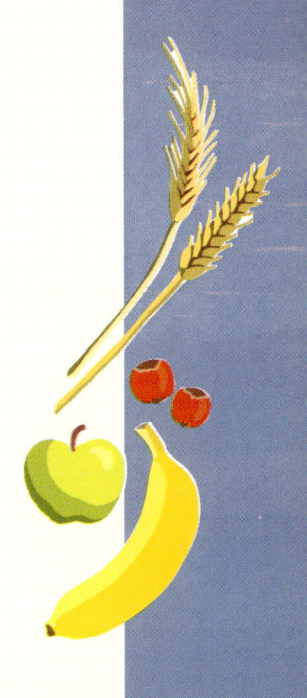

F. Main meal

Practical hint:

Soak large amounts of beans and chick peas and freeze them in plastic bags for future use. This will enable you to make quick nutritious meals within as little as half an hour.

This section is divided into 5 basic meal types:

1. Casseroles / stews / soups
2. Patties (burgers) / loaves
3. Cheesy dishes
4. Quiches, pies and other tofu dishes
5. Miscellaneous

1. Casseroles/stews

If you have a pressure cooker, most grains and legumes can be cooked in 20-25 min. For chick peas and most beans (except mung beans), it is wise to cook the legumes for half the time before adding the vegetables to keep vegetables from disintegrating.

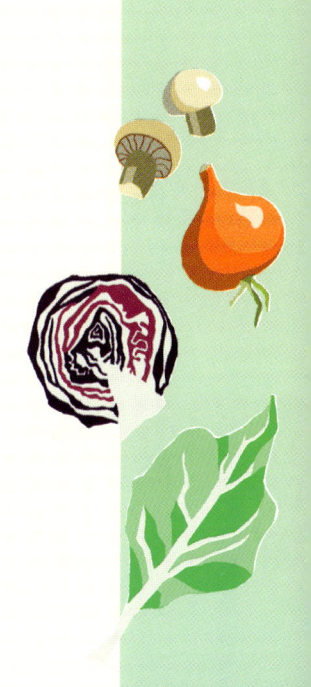

Bean stroganoff

3	onions
2 c	soaked beans (may be frozen)
	(optional: 1 c chick peas)
5	diced carrots
1 tin	tomato puree
1 small tin	tomato paste
(if preferred, use plenty of chopped fresh tomatoes)	
3 T	soy sauce
2 t	paprika
	herbs/parsley
	salt
2 t	food yeast
1/2 c	cashews or sunflower seeds
	water

Chop onions and brown in soy sauce, add beans, salt, paprika, stirring often. Cover with boiling water, bring pressure cooker to 2nd ring and cook for 10 min. Add vegetables and more salt, tomato paste and puree, herbs and more water to cover to about 3 cm above the ingredients. Pressure cook for a further 10-15 min. Cover cashew nuts (or sunflower seeds) with 1 cup water and blend till very smooth. Thicken stew with corn flour, if necessary, and add the blended cashew nuts to the stew together with the food yeast. Let simmer for 1 min. If sauce is too sour, it may be sweetened slightly with honey or brown sugar. Without a pressure cooker, the beans can be pre-cooked till almost done, then add all other ingredients and bake in a casserole dish for 1 hour. Serve with whole brown rice, barley rice, noodles or bulgur wheat (a very tasty, easy-to-cook Middle-Eastern dish – see recipes under Miscellaneous).

Variations:

Leave out the blended nuts and carrots, add some diced tomatoes for a rich tomato sauce on rice, spaghetti or whole-wheat toast. Unthickened, the stew can be served as a soup, served with home-baked whole-wheat bread and macadamia nut butter or a savoury spread.

Garbanzo-a-la-king

2 c	soaked chick peas (garbanzos)
3	large onions or plenty spring onions
2 T	soy sauce
2 c	cashews or sunflower seeds
3 c	water
1 T	food yeast
	pinch of thyme
1/4 t	oregano
1 can	asparagus salad cuts
	salt
	frozen green peas (optional)
	juice of 1/2 lemon

Cover chick peas with water, add salt and pressure cook for 20–25 min. Keep the juice. Brown the chopped onions in the soy sauce and add to the chick peas and their juice in the pot, plus the juice of the asparagus. Add the frozen green peas and cook gently. Meanwhile blend the cashews, food yeast, herbs and 3 c water till very smooth and add to the chick peas. Cook till thick, and lastly add asparagus pieces and lemon juice. If too thin, thicken before adding lemon juice, if too thick, merely add more water.

Lentils bolognaise

Use the recipe given for Bean Stroganoff, but substitute the beans and chick peas for one 500 g packet of washed, sorted and preferably soaked lentils. Cook all ingredients together in pressure cooker for 15 min. and leave out the blended cashew nuts.

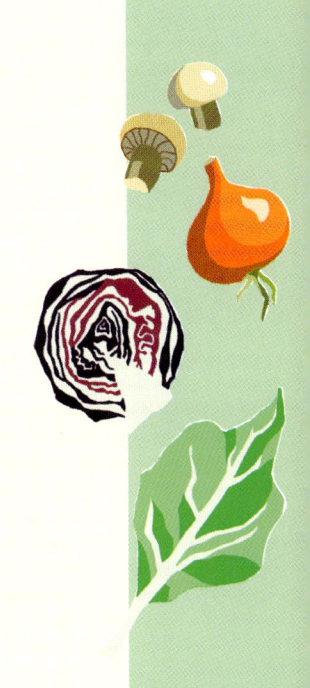

Moussaka

1	brinjal (egg plant)
1	large onion, diced
1	garlic clove, pressed
3	tomatoes, diced
1 T	tomato paste
1/2 t	coriander
4 T	red grape juice
1 c	cooked Adzuki, Lima or other beans
	salt
	herbs
about 2 c	simple sour cream

Slice brinjal thinly, rub with salt and let stand for 30 min. to draw out bitterness. Rinse and bake in oven at 180 °C (350 °F). Brown onions and garlic in saucepan, add tomatoes, tomato paste and grape juice. Let simmer for 5 min., then mix with cooked beans. Add salt and herbs to taste. Place half of the baked brinjal in a baking dish. Cover with half the bean mixture, followed by half of the simple sour cream. Repeat layers once more. Finally sprinkle herbs on top and dust with paprika. Bake at 180 °C (350 °F) for 45 min.

2. Patties and loaves

The following basic recipe applies both for patties (steamed in a frying pan) or loaves baked in the oven.

Basic recipe:

1 c	soaked soy beans or chick peas
1 c	water
2 t	food yeast (or Brewer's Yeast for brown colour)
1/2 t	salt
1/2	onion
1	clove garlic
1 c	rolled oats (or 1/8 c rice flour)
1 T	soy sauce
	Italian herbs

(Optional: for an extra rich flavour, add 2 T ground toasted pumpkin seeds – toast lightly under grill and blend dry in blender. Alternatively, 2 T of Sesamsan Cheese will also give a rich flavour)
Blend everything together, except the rolled oats or rice flour. Add mixture to the oats, mix well and let stand for about 5-10 min to allow the oats to absorb the moisture.

For **PATTIES** spray frying pan with lecithin spray or rub 1/2 t of olive oil over surface. Heat pan on high, then turn down to lowest setting. Drop spoonfuls of mixture into pan and flatten patty to about 1 cm thick. Cover with lid and let steam for 4-5 min. on one side, turn over and repeat on other side. Patties can also be shaped and baked in the oven at 190 °C (375 °F), but be careful that they do not dry out. Serve with **Pink Sauce**, **Quick Tomato Sauce** or any **mayonnaise**.

For **LOAF** spray a bread pan or baking dish, fill with mixture and bake in oven at 180 °C (350 °F) for 45 min. Let cool, loosen sides and slide up-side down onto serving plate. Cut into slices and garnish. Serve with hot **tomato and onion sauce, Brown Gravy** or white **nut or chick pea sauce**.

Variations
If you do not have a blender, substitute the soy beans/chick peas with 1 cup tofu and 1 cup finely ground nuts, or 1 cup tofu and 1/4 cup legume flour (e.g. soy, chick pea, lentil). A very easy patty can be made with left-over stew: mix 1/2 cup rolled oats or rice flour for every 1 cup thick stew and prepare as described above.

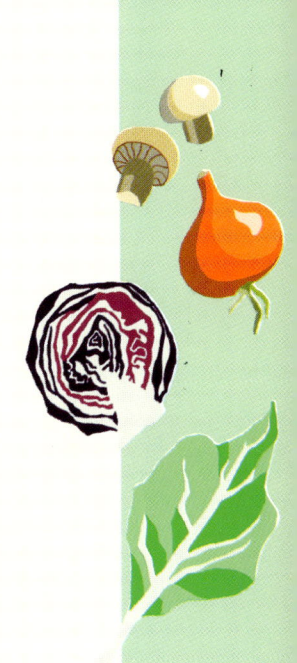

Potato balls
(very easy and tasty meat ball substitute - makes a good patty or loaf too)

1 c	grated potatoes
1 c	grated onion
2 t	soy flour
1/2 t	sage
1/2 t	marjoram
1 c	whole-wheat bread crumbs
1 c	ground walnuts
1/2 t	salt

Mix well and form into balls. Place in baking dish, cover with any gravy and bake at 180 °C (350 °F) for 30 min.

3. Cheesy Dishes

Lasagne

500 g	cooked spinach ribbon noodles (or other noodles)
4–5 c	tomato and onion sauce
1 c	cooked lentils (optional)
1 litre	thin, uncooked Pimento Cream Sauce
	Italian herbs
1 c	pitted olives, chopped (optional)

Spread 1 cup of tomato and onion sauce, 1/4 cup lentils and some of the olives and herbs over bottom of oven dish. Follow with a layer of noodles and pour 1/4 of the Pimento Cream Sauce over the noodles. Repeat the layers 3 more times, reserving some of the tomato-onion sauce for the top. Top off with the rest of the cream and sprinkle with paprika. Bake at 200 °C (400 °F) till cream has set and is golden brown (about 30 min.). Serve with salad and Sesamsan Cheese.

Sesamsan "cheese"

2 c	sesame seeds, lightly toasted in oven or frying pan
1 T	onion flakes
2 T	food yeast
1 t	salt
pinch	of garlic powder

Place all ingredients in blender and blend till fine, but not powdery. Use as substitute for Parmesan cheese.

Fondue

Something different and sociable for a special evening: Heat cooked Pimento Cream Sauce and pour into a heat-resistant pottery dish. Set the table attractively with candles, different kinds of green salads and dressings or even a big bowl of fruit salad and a basket with bread cubes. Place the dish over a heating candle to keep warm and dip the bread cubes into the cream sauce with your fondue fork.

Pizza

Dough:

Any regular bread dough may be used, but the **Perfect Whole-wheat Bread** dough makes an excellent base. When using the whole-wheat bread dough, the topping should be added gently after the dough has risen for the second time, and then baked together at 200 °C (400 °F) for about 25 min.

For a change try the following tender crust as a base.

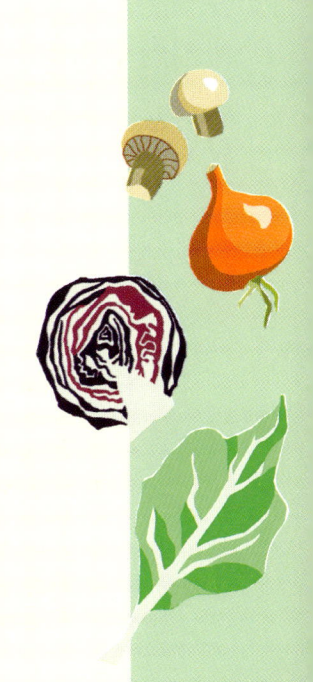

Yellow corn meal dough:

2 c	finely ground yellow corn flour
1 c	whole-wheat flour
2 T	gluten flour (because of lack of gluten in corn flour)
1 t	salt
2 T	food yeast (optional)
1 T	active yeast
1 T	honey
1/2 c	nut or seed butter (e.g. tahini)
1 1/3 c	warm water

Work butter into well-mixed dry ingredients. (If you do not have the butter, the nuts or seeds may be blended with water in the blender to cream and then worked into the flour mixture, in which case you will need about 1 cup of thick cream.) Blend water, honey, active yeast and gluten flour. Add yeast mixture to flour and knead well. Let rise for about 40 min. Make two equal balls, roll into flat circles and place on sprayed pizza plates. Let rise for 20 min. and bake at 200 °C (400 °F) for 8 min. Remove from oven, cover with topping and bake till pimento cream has set.

Topping:

Spread on baked crust: Tomato and Onion Sauce, or: Quick Tomato Sauce, or: Canned tomato puree/paste

Sprinkle with the following, finely chopped: celery, parsley, olives, tomatoes, onion/spring onion, green pepper, etc.

Top with:

Pimento Cream Sauce or **thick cashew nut cream** (see section on Sauces) and bake till golden brown.

Cannelloni

Easy Pancakes (see section on Desserts and Cookies)

Filling:

5	big onions
1 can	tomato paste (115 g)
5 c	cooked brown lentils

"Cheese" sauce:

Use **pimento Cream Sauce** (see section on sauces), but omit the pimento.

Chop onions finely, add salt and brown very well in a frying pan sprayed with a lecithin spray or a few tablespoons soy sauce. Add tomato paste and cooked lentils. Flavour to taste with herbs and salt.
Place about 3 T of the filling in centre of pancake, fold two sides one over the other, then fold the remaining two sides under the pancake. Place pancakes side by side in shallow casserole dish and cover with "cheese" sauce. Bake in oven at 180 °C for about 45 min.

4. Quiches, pies and other tofu dishes

Tofu is a very versatile food. Tofu blocks can be bought from health shops or some supermarkets and are a good stand-by for quick meals. It is made from soy bean milk and is very nutritious, but one must bear in mind that it is a partly refined product and should not be eaten too often.

Scrambled tofu

Brown chopped onions in soy sauce in a frying pan. Mash a few tofu blocks with a fork, add salt, a little lemon juice and heat together with onions in pan, stirring constantly. Herbs, garlic, etc. may be added to taste. Serve on hot toast.

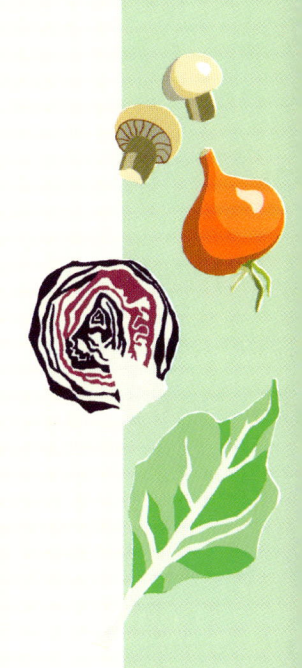

Tofu cottage cheese

Mashed cold tofu may be seasoned with salt, herbs, chives, garlic and lemon juice and eaten on bread as a very tasty substitute for cottage cheese.

Baked tofu

tofu blocks, cut into strips of about 1/2 cm thick
soy sauce
seasoned crumbs

Soak tofu in soy sauce for several hours, turning regularly. Roll blocks in bread crumbs and bake at 180 °C (350 °F) on a baking sheet till crumbs are light brown. Eat as is together with vegetables, or use as a filling in pita bread or on bread rolls.

Tofu omelet
(makes one omelet)

1/2 c	tofu
1/4 c	rice flour
1/2 c	cashews (or: increase rice flour to 1/8 cup)
1/2 c	water
1 t	salt
1 t	onion powder
1	large clove garlic
1/8 t	turmeric or
1/4	medium carrot (for yellow colour)

Blend all ingredients until smooth. Spray non-stick or heavy-base frying pan or spread 1/2 t olive oil over interior. Preheat pan, pour in omelet mixture, cover and cook on low heat for about 5 min till soft brown on bottom. Loosen around edges, flip over carefully and cook 5 min. on the other side. Serve with your favourite savoury sauce.

Soy omelet

See recipe for **soy waffles** and use the method as described above.

Onion quiche

Pie crust:
Basic Pie Crust or Yellow Corn Meal Pizza Crust

Filling:

1/2 c	cashews
1 c	water
500 g	tofu (about 2 cups)
2	onions, sliced and browned in soy sauce
2 t	onion powder/ 2 T onion flakes
1 T	lemon juice
2 t	salt
1/4 t	oregano
1 t	sweet basil
1/2	clove garlic
2 T	corn flour

Blend nuts and water till smooth. Add all ingredients, except browned onions. Blend, then stir in the onions, pour into pie dish lined with pie crust. Bake for 1 hour at 180 °C (350 °F). Sprinkle top with paprika and parsley. Also delicious eaten the following day, or even cold. The filling can be varied. Experiment with adding grated vegetables or diced tomato. Cover the rim with tin foil if it seems to be burning before cooked.

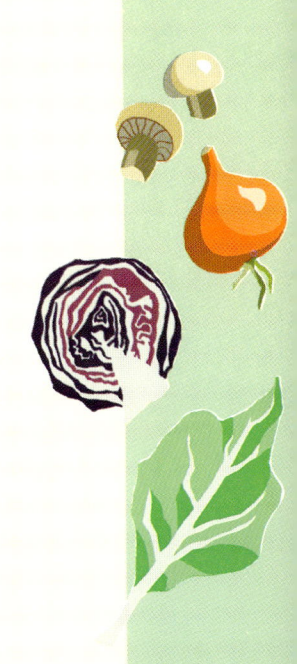

5. Miscellaneous
(This section will give you a few ideas on side dishes)

Bulgur pilavi

3 c	bulgur (cracked wheat)
5 c	boiling water
2	big onions
1	green pepper
2 T	soy sauce
1 t	tomato puree or 2 chopped tomatoes
	salt to taste

Chop onions, tomatoes and green pepper finely and stir-fry in soy sauce or a little water till fluid is absorbed. Add 5 cups boiling water and salt to taste. Add bulgur, stir, cover with lid and lower heat to lowest setting. When the water has been absorbed, the bulgur is cooked (about 10 min.)

Kisir
(bulgur salad)

Cook bulgur as for **Bulgur Pilavi** and add the following ingredients when cold:

1	tomato
1	green pepper
2	spring onions
	parsley, finely chopped
1 T	dried peppermint
1 t	paprika
pinch	cumin
	juice of 1/2 lemon

Chop tomato, pepper and onions finely and add together with rest of ingredients to cooked bulgur. Makes a very popular salad.

Baked potato dish

5	raw potatoes, peeled and sliced thinly
2	thinly sliced onions
4 c	of either one of the following:
	– Soy Sour Cream
	– Simple Sour Cream
	– thin Chick Pea Cream Sauce (raw or cooked)
	– thin Pimento Cream Sauce
	– a thin nut cream, lemon juice added
	salt
	paprika
	crushed garlic (optional)
	dill (optional)

Mix the potatoes, onions, salt, garlic and cream sauce well together and place into a sprayed casserole dish. The sauce must cover the potatoes – if not, add some nut or soy milk or more sauce to raise level. Sprinkle with paprika, cover with lid and bake at 200 °C (400 °F) till potatoes are soft right through.

Vegetables

Growing your own vegetables is of course ideal, but if you have to buy from the greengrocer, make sure you wash all vegetables well before placing in plastic bags in the refrigerator. This will wash away surface residues of pesticides and will keep vegetables fresher. Do not overcook, and try to eat more raw vegetables. Make cooked vegetable dishes palatable with nut or seed sauces and use sour soy or similar creams as basis for dips for raw vegetables.

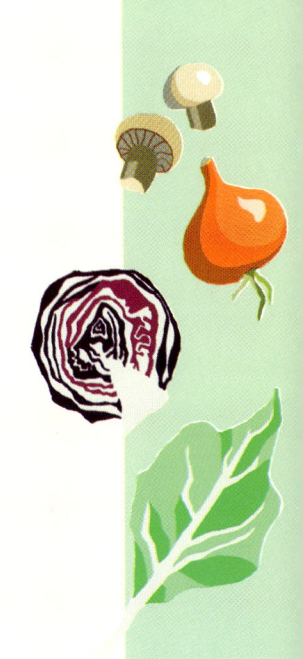

Fruits

Fruits should become a regular part of the diet and not just an afterthought or dessert, which in most cases, would be incompatible with the main meal. Design meals around a good wholesome bread and plenty of fruit. Remember to supply energy food such as a legume-based spread or fruit-compatible patty to ensure sufficient calories for young children. Fruit eaten together with "haystacks", such as a slice of whole-wheat bread or rice, followed by a legume patty (or spread), avocado, fruit chutneys, tomato, shredded lettuce, cucumber and a creamy topping is quick to prepare and will provide a welcome tangy change. Read the section on fruits in chapter 7 for more details.

G. Desserts and Cookies

Fruit sponge

2 t	agar-agar powder
1/2 c	water
1 1/2 c	rich soy/nut milk
1/2 c	fruit juice concentrate
	(e.g. granadilla, apple, pineapple)
	pinch of salt

Soak agar in the 1/2 cup of water for 1 min., then boil for a min. In blender blend the milk, juice and salt. Add the hot agar while blending slowly. Pour quickly into dish and chill. (Agar-agar sets very quickly.)

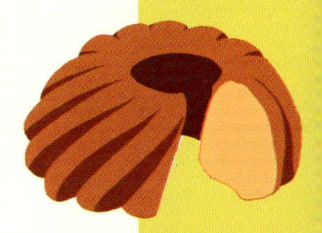

Carob sponge

4 t	agar-agar powder
1 c	water
3 c	rich soy milk
25	pitted dates (= 1 1/4 cup)
1 1/4 c	boiling water
3/4 c	carob powder
1/4 c	cashews
few drops	natural vanilla

Soak and boil agar as for Fruit Sponge. Soak dates for a few min. in the boiling water in the blender, then blend till fine. Add all remaining ingredients and the agar and blend till smooth. Pour into dish and chill.

No-bake tofu cheesecake

1 1/4 t	agar-agar powder (3 T flakes)
1 c	water
500 g	tofu
1/2 c	concentrated pineapple juice (or canned crushed pineapple)
1/3 c	honey
1 t	salt
	grated rind of 1 lemon
	shredded coconut, toasted lightly

Soak agar in water. Bring to boil and simmer 1 min. Add tofu and heat gently (to prevent rapid setting of mixture). Blend all ingredients till smooth and pour into pie dish, which has been sprinkled with toasted coconut or muesli. Refrigerate and decorate when set.

Basic pie crust
(makes 2 pie bases, or 1 base and crumble for the top)

1/2 c	macadamia butter (or other nut or seed butter)
2 c	whole-wheat flour
	(small quantities [± 1/2 c] of rice, millet, barley or oat flour may be substituted)
1 t	salt
1/2 c	water (approx.)
1 T	honey/brown sugar (for sweet pies)

(optional: one may add chopped nuts, coconut, lemon rind, etc.)

Mix dry ingredients well, then rub nut butter into flour mixture. Dissolve honey in the water and add to flour mixture. Knead and form 2 balls. For Apple Crumble roll out one ball for the base and grate the other for the crumble topping. (You might worry about the cost of so much nut butter, but firstly, consider the nutritional value compared to dairy butter, margarine or oil, and secondly, as mentioned before, do some detective work and find a cheap source of nuts and seeds and buy in bulk – then your butters will not be much more expensive than the conventional fats.) If you only have a blender, and cannot make nut butter, 1 c thick nut or seed cream (i.e. blending nuts/seeds with water till smooth) can be used instead of 1/2 c nut butter, which is then worked into the flour. Reduce the amount of water added.

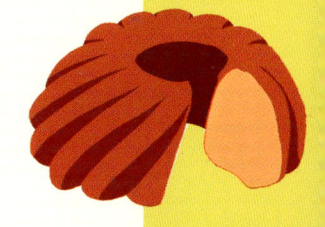

Easy apple crumble

Crust:
Basic Pie Crust

Filling:

5 c	peeled and sliced apples
1/2 c	grated pineapple (or crushed canned pineapple)
1/4 t	ground cardamom
1/8 t	salt
1/4 c	honey, brown sugar or
1/2 c	fruit sugar

Mix ingredients for filling well together, spread onto unbaked Basic Pie Crust and top liberally with grated pie crust. Bake at 190 °C (375 °F) for 35 min., or till apples are soft. Serve slightly warm with a nut or soy cream (see section on **Milks and Creams**)

Apple cake
(or any other fruit)

Crust:

Yellow Corn Meal Dough, but add 1/2 cup honey, raw brown sugar, dates or fruit sugar in the place of the 1 T honey (rice flour may be used instead of corn flour for an even lighter crust).

Topping:

Same as for **Easy apple crumble**, or vary with other fruit. Canned peaches or apricots make a pleasant change.

Make the dough as described in the section on main meals. After dough has risen once, roll out to thickness of about 1 cm and place in a sprayed shallow square dish. Do not line the sides as for a pie. Arrange the apples or other fruit neatly and close together on top of dough and sprinkle with sugar and cardamom, or drip with the honey. Let rise till double in size and bake at 190 °C (375 °F) for 35 min. or till fruit is cooked. Serve with Custard (see Sauces) or nut/soy cream.

Carob millet pudding

Cook together till soft

1 c	millet, dehusked
4 c	water
1/2 t	salt

Blend (one cup at a time):

1 c	hot cooked millet
2 T	peanut butter
2 T	carob powder
15–20	dates, softened in boiling water
	natural vanilla
	a little water (if necessary) to aid blending

(optional: a few drops peppermint oil/essence)

Blend till all the millet is used. The millet must be very smooth. Place a layer of sliced bananas in bottom of glass dessert bowl, followed by a layer of the carob-millet mixture. Repeat, ending with a layer of millet pudding. Sprinkle with shredded coconut. For special occasions, make a generous amount of nut or other sweet cream and repeat layers of banana, millet pudding, then cream, reserving some cream for the top. Sprinkle carob powder over cream and chill. This pudding is a definite hit with everyone.

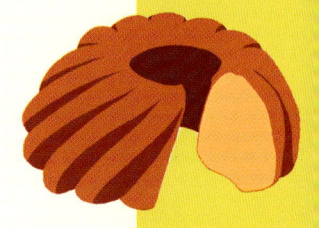

Milk tart

Crust:

Basic Pie Crust, or sprinkle base of pie dish with muesli or crumbled cookies

Filling:

Use **Breakfast Butter** (see Spreads) as base, but omit the turmeric and lemon juice and sweeten with honey. Pour into baked pie shell and leave to set.

or

If you wish to bake the pie, use the following ingredients:

1 c	cooked millet
1 c	cold water
1/4 c	cashews
1/4 c	honey
1 T	cornflour
1/4 t	salt (unless millet was cooked in salt water)

Blend all ingredients well together and pour into unbaked pie shell. Sprinkle with coriander or cardamom and bake at 190 °C (350 °F) for 30 min.

Ice-cream

Making ice-cream is much easier than you thought! Just peel and slice ripe bananas and freeze in plastic bags. When frozen, pour ice cold soy milk or nut milk (strained if desired) into blender and add frozen sliced bananas little by little while blender is blending. Add honey and vanilla if needed and continue blending until mixture is very thick. Can be eaten immediately or frozen slightly for later, but do not let the mixture freeze hard. For variety add a few drops of peppermint oil or add carob powder for chocolate flavour. Any other fruit (particularly apricots and strawberries) can be frozen (no need to cook) for other fruit flavours. Delicious served with hot Substitute Chocolate Sauce (see Sauces) and toasted sprinkle nuts.

Pancakes/flapjacks (crêpes)

As mentioned in the introduction many recipes are of such a nature that they can easily be adapted for a variety of dishes. The recipe given for Tofu Omelet (in the section under Quiches, Pies and other Tofu Dishes) can be adapted to make tender **pancakes** by adding a little water for a more fluid consistency, omitting the onion powder, garlic and half the salt and adding some sweetener. Pour a thin layer of the pancake mixture into the sprayed pan and flip over when light brown underneath. For **flapjacks** retain the thicker consistency and drop spoonfuls into the pan. Serve with **Orange Sauce** or honey and nut/soy cream.

Easy pancakes

1/2 c	cashews (or sunflower seeds)
3/4 c	white bread flour
1/4 c	soy flour
1/2 t	salt
2 c	water (1 1/2 c if using sunflower seeds)

Alternative recipe:

2 c	water
3/4 c	cashews or sunflower seeds
1 c	rice or millet flour
1 T	honey
	pinch of salt

Blend all ingredients together till very smooth. Use to make pancakes or flapjacks. Remember to whiz batter between each batch.

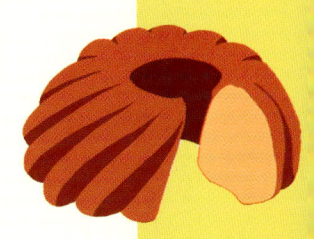

Cookies

The ingredient which makes cookies crispy, is the fat or oil. For a crispy cookie, try the Basic Pie Crust, where the nut butter takes the place of dairy butter and free oils.

Coconut cookies

2 3/4 c	dates
1 1/2 c	boiling water
1 t	salt
1 c	rice flour
2/3 c	nut or seed butter
3 c	shredded coconut

Measure flour into mixing bowl and rub butter into flour. Place dates in the boiling water in blender and soak to soften. Add salt and blend. Add dates and coconut to flour and mix well. Drop spoonfuls onto sprayed cookie sheet and press one almond into each cookie. Bake at 180 °C (350 °F) for 15 min., or until light brown.

Carob-oat cookies

1 1/2 c	rolled oats
3	ripe bananas
2 T	carob powder
	natural vanilla
1/2 c	date butter
1/2 t	salt

Blend rolled oats dry in blender or coffee grinder to make oat flour. Mash the bananas and combine all ingredients. Make heaps of the mixture on sprayed cookie sheet and bake at 180 °C (350 °F). Bake for about 15 min.

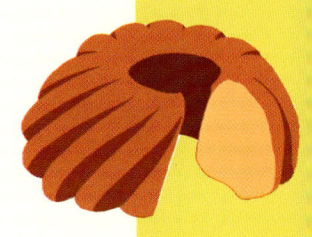

The ideas and recipes outlined above are by no means complete, but they should be comprehensive enough to provide an introduction to an alternative whole food lifestyle. Once the basic principles are understood and incorporated, then it is possible to glean ideas from many conventional and health orientated recipes and convert them to meet the desired criteria.

Register

A

abdominal cramps 84
Abelmoschus esculentus 198
Acanthos nigricans 139
acceptable daily intake 124
acesulfam-K 129
acetaldehyde 133
acid ashfood groups 145
– forming foods 142, 144
– urine 146
acidosis 142
Actinidia deliciosa 186
ADI see acceptable daily intake
adzuki bean 164
aflotoxins 91
agar 127
albedo 184
alcohol 130, 133
alitame 129
alkaline ash food groups 145
– forming foods 142, 144
alkaloid 130
alkalosis 142
Allium ampeloprasum 197
– cepa 197
– sativum 197
– schoenoprasum 197
almonds 170
Alzheimer's disease 90
amaranth 126
American Dietetic Association 129
American Society for Clinical Nutrition 129
amino acid composition of nuts 172
– – – of seeds 172
– – requirement 23
amino acids 17
– –, aromatic 20
– –, essential 18, 20, 25
– –, non-essential 18
– –, sulphur-containing 20, 25
ammonia 20, 66f.
– caramel 126
amylase 33
– inhibitors 160
Anacardium occidentale 172
Ananas comosus 188

Anethum graveolens 201
angelica 200
Angelica archangelica 200
angina 52
animal husbandry 84
– products 63f., 146
– proteins 20
aniseed 200
Anthriscus cerefolium 201
antibiotics 84ff.
–, resistance 87f.
anticancer 149
antimicrobial resistance 84
antioxidants 37, 58f., 122, 126
anti-promoters 51
Apiaceae 200
Apium graveolens 201
appendicitis 37, 39
apple 182
apple cake 264
– crumble, easy 264
– shaped 108
apricots 181
arachidonic acid 45
arginine 20
aromatic amino acids 20
arteriosclerosis 20, 52, 59, 73
–, ratio of lysine to arginine 21
arthritis 107
–, rheumatoid 113
asbestos 50
asparagus 198
Asparagus officinalis 198
aspartame 129
asthma 77, 126
athletes 29f.
atopic dermatitis 77
Avena sativa 152
avocados 102, 184
avoparcin 85
azorbin 126

B

bacillus bifidus 72
bacon 70
bacteria, drug-resistant 84
bagels, sweet 219

baked potato dish 259
– tofu 256
banana 185
– bread 217
barley 150
basal metabolic rate 104f.
– – –, multiple of 105
basic-four nutritional guide 98
– pie crust 263
– shopping list 208
bean stroganoff 248
beer 70
beetroot 190
benzo(a)pyrene 69
benzoic acid 128
berry fruit 183
Bertholletia excelsa 170
Beta vulgaris 190
BHA 126
BHT 126f.
bile acids 38
– –, secondary 108
– salts 47
biological magnification 70
– value 26
blackberries 183
black currants 183
– hebrews 101
bladder stones 25
blood pressure 111
blueberries 183
blurred vision 126
BMD see bone mineral density
BMI sie body mass index
BMR see basal metabolic rate
body mass index 106, 109f.
bone mineral density 112
boric acid 128
borsch 193
botulism 81
Bovine Spongiform Encephalitis 90f.
Bowman-Birk trypsin 167
boysenberries 183
brambles 183
bran 37
Brassicaceae 194
Brassica oleracea 195
– rapa 196

Register

brazil nuts 170
bread 156, 215ff.
–, perfect whole-wheat 216
breakfast 239, 245
– butter 222
– pudding 243
breast 51
– cancer 38
– feeding 101
– milk 75
brilliant black 126
broccoli 195
bronchitis, chronic 77
brown gravy 230
brussels sprouts 195
BSE see Bovine Spongiform Encephalitis
bulgur pilavi 258
– wheat 155
bulk sweeteners 129
butter beans 164
butylated hydroxyanisole 126
– hydroxytoluene 126
butyrate 39

C

cabbage 195
caffeine 35, 130ff.
– consumption 132
calcium 72, 74, 98, 111, 113, 117, 121, 132
– disodium EDTA 126
– efflux 144
– in dairy products 74f.
– levels in selected foods 74
– oxalate crystals 25
– supplementation 75
– utilization 74
calciuresis 112
calico beans 164
California 170
Campylobacter 82f.
cancer 21f., 37f., 43, 51f., 63ff., 68, 77, 98, 107, 139, 176
– and fats 50
–, colorectal, and meat consumption 68
–, initiation and promotion of 50
–, ovarian 52, 64ff.
–, preventive foods 177
–, prostate 52, 64, 66
–, rectal 133
cannelloni 254
canthaxanthin 126
capsicum 198
– annuum 198
caramels 126
caraway 200
carbohydrate 29, 107
– digestion 31
– foods 149
carboloading 29
carcass meal 89

carcinogenesis 59
cardiomyopathy 139
cardiovascular disease 22, 43, 53, 98, 110
– – and fats 52
Carica papaya 188
carmel 170
carmousine 126
carob 163
– millet pudding 265
– oat cookies 269
– powder 163
– sponge 262
carotene 184
β-carotene 118
carotenoids 149, 176, 200
carrots 200
Carum carvi 200
Carya illinoensis 173
casein 73f., 77, 113
cashew nuts 172
casseroles 247
Castanea sativa 173
cauliflower 195
celery 201
cellulase 33
cellulose 31f., 38
Ceratonia siliqua 163
cereals 98, 102
Chaij-Rhys 100
– – diet plan 99
cheesy dishes 252
– spread 222
chenopodiaceae 190
cholecystokinin-pancreozymin 49
cherries 182
chervil 201
chestnuts 173
chick pea 163
– – cream sauce 229
chicory 193
chills 84
chinese restaurant syndrome 129
chive 197
chocolate sauce, simple 231
– –, substitute 231
cholesterol 21, 36f., 39, 46, 48, 52, 57, 74, 107
chronic bronchitis 77
chymotrypsin inhibitor 167
Cicer arietinum 163
Cichorium intybus 193
citrus fruits 184
– limon 184
– sinensis 184
CJD see Creutzfeldt-Jacob disease
clenbuterol 89
Clostridium botulinum 81
– perfringens 84
cobalamin 119
cob nuts 173
cocoa 130
coconut 173

– cookies 268
– milk 236
Cocos nucifera 173
coefficient of digestibility 26
coffee 130f.
cold drink 36
– pressed oil 59
colds 47, 77
colic 77
colitis 37
collard 195
colon cancer 37, 51f., 64ff.
colorants 122, 125
colorectal cancer and meat consumption 68
colostrum 76
combining fruits 146
– grains 147
compatible combinations of plant foods 148
complete proteins 20
compositae 193
composition of dried fruits 180
– of fruits 178f.
– of legumes 161f.
– of nuts 171
– of rice 154
– of rye 155
– of seeds 171
– of sorghum 156
– of soyfoods 167f.
– of vegetables 191f.
– of wheat products 157
confusion 84
constipation 37f., 77
consumption of caffeine 132
– – dairy products and diseases 67
– – egg and diseases 66
– – meat and diseases 65, 68
convolvulaceae 193
cookies 261, 268
cooking 160
copper 40
coriander 201
Coriandrum sativum 201
corn 151
coronary heart disease 63
Corylus avellana 173
coumarins 200
cow pea 165
cow's milk 76, 78
cramps, abdominal 84
cranberries 183
creams 233
creamy muesli, delicious 241
crêpes 267
cresol 20, 68
cress 196
Creutzfeldt-Jacob disease 90f.
cruciferae 194
cruciferous vegetables 176
cryptoxanthin 149
cucumber 194

Register

Cucumis sativa 194
cucurbita 194
Cucurbitaceae 194
cumin 201
Cuminum cyminum 201
currants, black 183
–, red 183
–, white 183
curry beans 164
custard, substitute 231
cyclamate 129
Cydonia oblonga 183
cysteine 20

D

dairy products 65, 72, 98
– – and infertility 78
– – and the immune system 76
–, –, calcium content of 74f.
– –, consumption and disease 67
dates 186
date spread 222
Daucus carota 200
DDT 70f.
deficiency diseases 117
degenerative diseases 63
– – and fats 49
– –, vegetarians 105
dehidroacetic acid 128
delicious creamy muesli 241
depression 107
dermatitis, atopic 77
DES see diethylstilboestrol
desserts 261
Dhal 165
diabetes 22, 64, 107
–, insulin depended 109
– mellitus 34, 109, 139
–, non-insulin depended 109
diarrhoea 73, 77, 84
dienoestrol 88
dietary fatty acids 56
– patterns for infants 100
– – for lactating mothers 100
– – for pregnant women 100
– – for young children 100
diethylstilboestrol 88
diet plan for young vegan children 103
digestibility, coefficient 26
digestion of carbohydrates 31
– of fats 47
– of proteins 18
dill 201
Diospyros khaki 188
disodium guanylate 128
– inosinate 128
dithiolthiones 176
diverticulosis 37, 39
Dosa 165
dressing, thousand island 228
dried fruit 102

– – chutney 228
– – composition 180
drug-resistant bacteria 84
dysfunction, gonadal 139
–, pituitary 139
dysfunctional eating 140

E

ear infections 77
easy apple crumble 264
– fruit sauce 231
– jam 223
– no-knead raisin bread 218
– pancakes 267
EDTA, calcium disodium 126
egg consumption and diseases 66
– plant 199
eggs 65
eicosanoids 55
eicosopentanoic acid 45
embolus 52
emulsifiers 49, 122, 127
encephalopathy, transmissible mink 90
endopeptidases 18
energy intake, minimum 30
– requirements 104
enzyme suppressants 166
equipment 208
Eriobotrya japonica 187
erythrosine 126
Escherichia 82
– coli 83
essential amino acids 18, 20, 25
– fatty acids 45
17α-ethynyloestradiol 88
exopeptidases 18

F

Fabaceae 196
fats 43, 107
– and cancer 50
– and cardiovascular disease 52
– and degenerative disease 49
– and immune system 54
–, digestion 47
–, hydrogenated vegetable 53
–, monounsaturated 58
–, polyunsaturated 51, 58
–, processed 55
–, replacements 43
–, saturated 53, 58
fatigue 47
fatty acids
– –, cis 55
– –, cis-trans conversion 55
– –, dietary 56
– –, distribution in vegetable oils 46
– –, essential 45
– –, polyunsaturated 44, 53
– –, saturated 44, 51

– –, trans 53, 55, 57
– –, unsaturated 44
fennel 201
fenugreek 196
fermentation 19, 160
fever 84
fibres 35, 37ff., 43, 52, 66
–, soluble 40
–, water-insoluble 38
–, water-soluble 39
figs 186
filberts 173
finegold 125
fish 64, 70f.
– meal 89
flapjacks 267
flatulence 146, 159
flavones 176
flavonoids 200
flavour enhancers 128
flu 47
Foeniculum vulgare 201
fondue 253
food additives 122, 124
– allergy 125
– combinations 142
– pyramid 99
foodborne illness 81f.
free radicals 37, 59
french beans 163, 196
fructose 31f., 36, 180
fruit sauce, easy 231
– sponge 261
fruits 43, 64, 98, 176, 260
– composition 178f.
frying 49
– of food in oil 58

G

galactokinase 73
galactose 31f.
gallstone 107, 146
garbanzo 163
– a-la-king 249
– (chick pea) „Mayonnaise" 226
garden peas 196
garlic 197
gastric inhibitory peptide 49
gastrointestinal disease 84
– infection 82
genetic engineering 91
germination 160
Gerstman-Straussler syndrome 90
GIP see gastric inhibitory peptide
gliadin 158
globulins, immune- 76
glucagon 34
glucose 31
– level 34, 41
– surge 40
glutamate 129
glutamic acid 129

glutelins 158
gluten 158
glutenin 158
glycine 20
– max 165
glycogen 29f., 35
glycosidases 33
gonadal dysfunction 139
gooseberries 183
goosefoot family 190
gourd family 194
gourds 194
gout 107
grains 64, 149
granadilla 188
granola 242
granulocytes 54
grapes 183
green S 126
grilling 49
groats porridge 240
growth promoters 88
– retardation 77
guava 186
gums 39

H

haeme iron 121
haemolytic uraemic syndrome 83
haemorrhagic colitis 83
halitosis 146
halva 175
haricot beans 164
hay fever 77, 126
Hayward 186
hazel nuts 173
HDL see high-density lipoprotein
headaches 47
heartburn 19
heart disease 64
– –, coronary 63
heat damage sustained by oil 58
heavy metals 70
hebrews, black 101
Helianthus annuus 175
hemicelluloses 38f.
herbicides 70
hernias 39
heterocyclic amines 66, 69f.
hexaestrol 88
n-hexanal 169
hiatus hernia 37
high-density lipoprotein 47
honey 36
hospital epidemics 84
human milk 72, 76
hydrogenated oils 57
– vegetable fats 53
hydroxyanisole, butylated 126
4-hydroxybenzoates 128
hydroxytoluene, butylated 126
hyperactivity 126

hyperglycaemia 77
hypertension 107
hypertriglyceridaemia 107
hypoglycaemia 34ff., 39
–, symptoms of 34

I

ice-cream 266
IDD see insulin-dependent
    diabetes
Idli 165
immune function 53
– globulins 76
– system 133
– – and dairy products 76
– – and fats 54
immunosuppression 71
improving agents 122
incomplete proteins 20
indica 153
indigo carmine 126
indoles 176
infarct 52
infertility 78f., 107
– and dairy products 78
–, male 79
inflammation 59
inhibitors 166f.
initiation of cancer 50
inositol hexaphosphate 149
insulin 34
– dependent diabetes 77, 109
– level 41
– resistance 107
– surge 40
intelligence quotients 21, 78
intense sweeteners 129
interferon 54
interleukon 1 54
Ipomoea batatas 193
IQ see intelligence quotients
iron 40, 98, 100, 117, 120f.
ischaemia 52
isoflavins 166
isomalt 129
isothiocyanates 176

J

jam, easy 223
japanese and fat intake 49
japonica 153
Juglans regia 174

K

kale 195
ketosis 77
ketosteroids 88
kidney beans 163
– stones 25, 146
killer cells, natural 54, 133

kisir 258
kiwifruit 186
kohlrabi 195
kunitz trypsin inhibitor 167
kuru 90

L

lactase 72
lactitol 129
Lactobacillus 195
β-lactoglobulin 73
lactone 193
lacto-ovo-vegetarians 97
lactose 31, 33, 73
– intolerance 72
lacto vegetarians 97, 99
Lactuca sativa 193
lactucin 193
lactupicrin 193
lasagne 252
LDL see low-density lipoprotein
leberwurst 224
lecithin 47, 49
leeks 197
legumes 102, 147, 159
– composition 161f.
Leguminosae 196
lemons 184
Lens esculenta 164
lentils 164
– bolognaise 249
Lepidium sativum 196
lettuce 193
leucotrienes 55f.
Levisticum officinale 201
lignin 38
Liliaceae 197
lily family 197
lima beans 164
linoleic acid 45f., 53, 57, 169
linolenic acid 45f.
lipase inhibitors 160
lipases 47, 49
lipoproteins, high-density 47
–, low-density 47
lipoxygenase 168
liquorice 196
Listeria 81ff.
litchi 186
loaves 250
–, basic recipe 250
loquats 187
lovage 201
low-density lipoprotein 47
lycopene 200
Lycopersicon esculentum 200
lymphatic system 47
lymphocytes 54
T-lymphocytes 54, 77
lymphokines 54
lysine 24

Register

M

macadamia nuts 173
Macadamia ternifolia 173
macrophages 54
mad cow's disease 90
magnesium 40
main meal 247
maize 151
male infertility 79
mallow family 198
maltase 34
maltose 33
Malus domestica 182
Malvaceae 198
mandarins 184
manganese 40
Mangifera indica 187
mangoes 187
mannitol 129
margarine 57
marine pollution 71
mayonnaise 226
mealie 151
– (corn) bread 219
meat 49, 64, 66
– consumption and colorectal cancer 68
– – and diseases 65
mediterranean diets 53
– cultures 149
melons 187
methionine 20
methyl violet 126
mexican black beans 164
micelles 47
milk 66, 72, 233
–, mother's 72, 101
–, nut 235
– protein 73
– – intolerance 73
– shakes 236
– tart 266
millet 151f.
– spread 221
minerals in vegan diets 117
minimum energy intake 30
mink encephalopathy, transmissible 90
miso 166
mission 170
mock "leberwurst" 224
monocytes 54
monosaccharides 31
monosodium glutamate 128f.
monoterpens 200
monounsaturated fats 58
morning glory family 193
mother's milk 72, 101
moussaka 250
MSG see monosodium glutamate
mucus 77
muesli 240

mulberries 183
mung beans 165
musa 185
mushroom sauce 230
mustard family 194
mycotoxins 91

N

natural killer cells 54, 133
nausea 84
navy beans 164
NCI (National Cancer Institute of the US) 37
nectarines 182
net protein utilization 26
neutrophils 54
niacin 149
nightshade family 198
nitrates 128
nitrites 128
nitrosoamines 128
NK see natural killer cells
N-nitroso compounds 66, 70
no-bake tofu cheesecake 262
non-azo colours 126
– essential amino acids 18
– insulin dependent diabetes 109
nonhaeme iron 121
nonpareil 170
non starch polysaccharides 29, 38
NPU see net protein utilization
NSP see non starch polysaccharides
nut butters 102
– cream, sweet 237
– milk 235
nutritional guide, basic-four 98
nuts 169
–, amino acid composition 172
– composition 171

O

oat bran 40
oats 152
obesity 22, 106, 108, 113, 139
–, Acanthos nigricans 139
–, arthritis 107
–, cancer 107f., 139
–, cardiomyopathy 139
–, depression 107
–, diabetes 107
–, diabetes mellitus 139
–, gallstones 107
–, gonadal dysfunction 139
–, gout 107
–, hypertension 107
–, hypertriglyceridaemia 107
–, infertility 107
–, insulin resistance 107
–, osteoarthritis 139
–, pickwickian syndrome 139
–, pituitary dysfunction 139

–, renal failure 107
oestradiol 88
oestrogen 38, 79, 108
oil, hydrogenated 57
oil refining 55
oilseeds 169
okra 198
Olea europaea 187
oleic acid 45, 169
olives 187
onceau 4R 126
onion 197
– quiche 257
– sauce 227
Opuntia 189
oranges 184
orange sauce 232
Oryza sativa 153
osteoarthritis 139
osteoporosis 20, 25, 74ff., 111
ovarian cancer 52, 64ff.
ovo-lacto-vegetarians 97, 99, 110
oxalic acid 146, 159

P

PAH see polycyclic aromatic hydrocarbons
palmitic acid 44, 169
pancakes 267
–, easy 267
Panicum miliaceum 151
papayas 188
parachlorobenzoic acid 128
parsley 201
– or carrot family 200
parsnip 201
Passiflora 188
passionsfruit 188
Pastinaca sativa 201
patties 250
–, basic recipe 250
peaches 182
pea or pulse family 196
pears 183
pearshaped 108
peas 196
pecan nuts 173
pectin 39, 180
penicillin 87
pepsin 18f.
pepsinogen 18
peptide, gastric inhibitory 49
peptones 19
Persia americana 184
persimmons 188
pesticides 70
Petroselinum crispum 201
Phaseolus lunatus 164
– vulgaris 163, 196
phenol 20, 66, 68, 176
phenolic acid 166, 200
phenylalanine 20

Register

Phoenix dactylifera 186
phthalides 200
phytic acid 160f., 166
phytochemicals 21, 51, 176
phytoestrogen 166
phytosterols 166
pickled foods 43
pickwickian syndrome 139
pies 255
pimento cream sauce 229
Pimpinella anisum 200
pineapples 188
pink sauce 228
pinto beans 164
pip fruits 182
pistachio nuts 174
Pistacia vera 174
Pisum sativum 196
pita bread 218
pituitary dysfunction 139
pizza 217, 253
plant food, compatible combinations 148
– gums 127
– proteins 20
plums 182
pole beans 164
pollution, marine 71
polyacetylenes 200
polycyclic aromatic hydrocarbons 66, 69
polyphenols 130, 176
polysaccharidases 33
polysaccharides 31
–, non starch 29, 38
–, storage 39
polyunsaturated fats 51, 58
– fatty acids 44, 53
pomegranates 188
porridges 102, 240
potato 199
– balls 252
– dish, baked 259
–, sweet 193
pot bread 217
poultry 64
preservatives in foods 122, 128
prickly pears 189
primary foods 143
– proteins 20
prion diseases 89
prions 89
processed fats 55
progesterone 88
– acetate 88
prolamines 158
promoters for growth 88
promotion of cancer 50
pro-oxidants 58
propionic acid 128
prostaglandins 45, 54ff.
prostate cancer 51f., 64, 66
protease 166

– inhibitors 166
proteins 17, 98
–, complete 20
–, composition of selected protein food 27
–, digestion 18
–, incomplete 20
–, milk 73
–, net utilization of 26
–, of animals 20
–, of plants 20
–, primary 20
–, recommended daily allowance 22
–, requirement 21
–, secondary 20
proteoses 19
prunes 182
Prunus amygdalus 170
– armeniaca 181
– avium 182
– persica 182
Psidium guajava 186
PST 89
psychological disturbances 77
ptyalin 33
pulse family 196
pumpkins 194
pumpkin seeds 174
Punica granatum 188
purpura, thrombotic thrombocytopenic 83
putu 151, 243
pyrus communis 183

Q

quiches 255
quinces 183
quinoline yellow 126

R

radicals, free 37, 59
radish 196
raffinose 160
raisin bread, no-knead 218
raisins 183
Raphanus sativus 196
rashes 126
raspberries 183
rastafarians 101
RDA see recommended dietary allowance
recipes 207
recommended daily allowance for protein 22
recommended dietary allowance 117
rectal cancer 133
red currants 183
reduced-fat products 43
refined food 35, 38
refining of foods 141
renal failure 107

rennin 73
resistant starch 34, 39
retinol 118
rheumatoid arthritis 113
riboflavin 98, 149
rice 153
– composition 154
rickets 120
rolls 217
rye 154
– bread 217
– composition 155

S

saccharin 129
salicylic acid 128
Salmonella 82, 85
salted foods 43
saponins 166
satiety 19
saturated fats 53, 58
– fatty acids 44, 51
sauces 225ff.
sauerkraut 195
Secale cereale 154
secondary bile acids 108
– proteins 20
seeds 174
–, amino acid composition 172
– composition 171
selenium 52
semen quality 78
sesame milk 236
– seeds 175
sesamin 170, 175
sesamsan „cheese" 253
Sesanum indicum 175
sesquiterpene 193
Seventh-day-Adventists 106
sewage 71, 89
shell-fish 71
side dishes, miscellaneous 258
sieva beans 164
sinusitis 77
β-sitosterol 176
sleep apnea syndrome 139
smoked foods 43
snap beans 164
soaking 160
sodium 25
– diacetate 128
soft drinks 35, 131
Solanaceae 198
Solanum melongena 199
– tuberosum 199
soluble fibres 40
solvents 122, 127f.
sorbic acid 128
sorbitol 129
sorghum 154
– composition 156
– vulgare 154

sour cream 230
– –, simple 230
– soy cream 237
soy 25
– concentrate 234
– cream, sour 237
– –, sweet 237
– „mayonnaise" 226
– milk 166ff., 235
– omelet 257
– waffles 244
soya 21
– beans 74, 165
soyfoods composition 167f.
sperm concentrations 81
– count 78
– quality 80
spinach 193
Spinacia oleracea 193
spreads 221
sprouting 165
squashes 194
stabilizers 122, 127
stachyose 160
staggers 71
Staphylococcus 82
– aureus 84f., 87
starch 31f.
–, resistant 34, 39
stearic acid 44
stevioside 129
stews 247ff.
stilbene diethylstilboestrol 88
stomach 49
stone fruits 181
stool 37ff.
storage polysaccharides 39
strawberries 183
streptomycin 87
substitute chocolate sauce 231
– custard 231
subtropical fruits 184
sucralose 129
sucrose 31, 33, 36
sulphur-containing amino acids 20, 25
– dioxide 128
sultanas 183
sunflower family 193
– seeds 175
– seed waffles 244
sunset yellow 126
sweeteners 122, 129
sweet nut cream 237
– potato 193
– soy cream 237
swiss chard 190

T

Tahini 175
tannin 160
tartare sauce 226
tartrazine 126
TBT see tributyl tin
tea 130f.
teicoplanin 85
tempeh 166
testosterone 88
tetracycline 85, 87
thaumatin 129
theobromine 35
thiamin 149
thiocyanates 176
thousand island dressing 228
thrombosis 53
thrombotic thrombocytopenic purpura 83
thromboxanes 55f.
thrombus 52
thyroid function 73
tobacco smoke 50
tocopherols 149
tofu 25, 166
–, baked 256
– cheesecake, no-bake 262
– cottage cheese 256
– dishes 255
– omelet 256
–, scrambled 255
tomatoes 200
tomato sauce 227
transgenic animals 92
transmissible mink encephalopathy 90
trenbolone acetate 88
tributyl tin 71
triglyceride 44, 52
triterpenoid alcohols 193
triterpens 200
triticale 154
Triticum 155
tropical fruits 184
trypsin 18f.
tummy upsets 126
turnip 196
tyrosine 20

U

ulcer 19, 77
Umbelliferae 200
undernutrition 108
unsaturated fatty acids 44
urea 20
uric acid 133

V

vancomycin 85, 87
variation 147
varicose veins 39
varieties 170
variety of foods 140
vegan 98, 110, 113
– children, diet plan for 103
– diets, minerals 117
– –, vitamins 117
– vegetarian lifestyle 97
– vegetarians 53
vegetables 43, 64, 98, 146, 176, 189, 259
– composition 191f.
vegetarian dietary patterns for adults 98
vegetarians 52, 64, 97f.
–, degenerative diseases 105
–, lacto 97, 99
–, lacto-ovo- 97, 99, 110
–, vegan 53, 97
Vibrio vulnificus 84
Vignia aureus 165
viruses 50
vision, blurred 126
vitamin A 52, 117f., 149, 176
– B-6 117f., 149
– B-12 98, 100f., 117, 119f.
– C 52, 100, 149, 176
– D 100f., 117, 120, 149
– E 37, 52, 126, 176
vitamins in vegan diets 117
vomiting 77, 84

W

waffles 244
walnuts 174
water 19
– insoluble fibres 38
– soluble fibres 39
watermelons 187
wheat 155
– composition 157
wheatgerm 37
white currants 183
whole-food 30, 32, 139f.
– grains 37
– wheat bread 216

X

xanthophyll 184
xylitol 129

Y

Yersinia 82f.
youngberries 183

Z

zea mays 151
zen macrobiotics 101
– – diet 97
zeranol 88
zinc 117, 122f.